# Providing Expert Care for the Acutely Ill

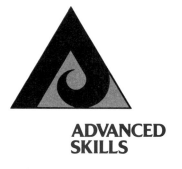

**ADVANCED
SKILLS**

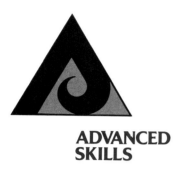

**ADVANCED
SKILLS**

# Providing Expert Care for the Acutely Ill

Springhouse Corporation
Springhouse, Pennsylvania

# Staff

**Executive Director, Editorial**
Stanley Loeb

**Senior Publisher**
Matthew Cahill

**Art Director**
John Hubbard

**Senior Editor**
Stephen Daly

**Clinical Project Director**
Patricia Dwyer Schull, RN, MSN

**Editors**
Neal Fandek, Kathy Goldberg, Elizabeth Mauro,
Jean Wallace

**Clinical Editors**
Sherri Inez Becker, RN, CCRN; Tina R. Dietrich,
RN, BSN, CCRN; Mary Jane McDevitt, RN, BS;
Linda Roy, RN, MSN

**Copy Editors**
Cynthia C. Breuninger *(supervisor)*, Priscilla
DeWitt, Traci A. Ginnona, Jennifer Mintzer,
Dorothy Oren, Nancy Papsin, Doris Weinstock

**Designers**
Stephanie Peters *(associate art director)*, Matie
Patterson *(senior designer)*, Linda Franklin, Joseph
Laufer

**Illustrators**
Jacalyn Facciolo, Jean Gardner, Linda Gist, Tom
Herbert, Bob Jackson, Robert Neumann

**Art Production**
Anet Oakes, Ann Raphun, Robert Wieder

**Typography**
David Kosten *(director)*, Diane Paluba *(manager)*,
Elizabeth Bergman, Joyce Rossi Biletz, Phyllis
Marron, Robin Mayer, Valerie Rosenberger

**Manufacturing**
Deborah Meiris *(director)*, T.A. Landis *(manager)*

**Production Coordination**
Patricia W. McCloskey

**Editorial Assistants**
Maree DeRosa, Beverly Lane, Mary Madden

Ⓡ A member of the Reed Elsevier plc group

**Library of Congress Cataloging-in-Publication Data**
Providing expert care for the acutely ill.
  p. cm. — (Advanced Skills)
  Includes bibliographical references and index.
  1. Catastrophic illness — Nursing.
  I. Springhouse Corporation.    II. Series.
  [DNLM: 1. Acute Disease — Nursing.
  2. Critical Illness — Nursing.
  WY 154 P969 1993]
RT42.P77  1993
616.028 — dc20
DNLM/DLC                 93-28363
ISBN 0-87434-556-1            CIP

# Contents

# Advisory board

**At the time of publication, the advisors held the following positions.**

### Cecelia Gatson Grindel, RN, PhD
Nurse Researcher
Lehigh Valley Hospital
Allentown, Pa.
President, Academy of Medical-Surgical Nurses

### Judith Ski Lower, RN, MSN, CCRN, CNRN
Nurse Manager, Neurology Critical Care Unit
Johns Hopkins Hospital
Baltimore

### Kathleen M. Malloch, RN, BSN, MBA, CNA
Vice President, Patient Care Services
Del Webb Memorial Hospital
Sun City West, Ariz.

### Marguerite K. Schlag, RN, MSN, EdD
Director, Nursing Education and Development
Robert Wood Johnson University Hospital
New Brunswick, N.J.

### Karen L. Then, RN, MN
Assistant Professor, Faculty of Nursing
University of Calgary, Alberta

# Contributors

At the time of publication, the contributors held the following positions.

**Barbara K. Blue, RN, MSN**
Pediatric Pulmonary Clinical Nurse Specialist
Phoenix Children's Hospital

**Vicki L. Buchda, RN, BSN, MS**
Director, Special Care Unit
Maryvale Samaritan Medical Center
Phoenix

**Cas Cahill-Wright, MS, ARNP, CNS**
Pain Management Consultant
Tampa, Fla.

**Marlene Ciranowicz, RN, MSN, CDE**
Nurse Consultant
Dresher, Pa.

**Mary Collins Derivan, RN, MSN, OCN**
Clinical Nurse Educator
Mercy Catholic Medical Center
Fitzgerald Mercy Division
Darby, Pa.

**Christine Ferrante, RN, BSN**
Nurse Manager
Mercy Catholic Medical Center
Fitzgerald Mercy Division
Darby, Pa.

**Betty Ferrell, PhD, FAAN**
Associate Research Scientist
City of Hope National Medical Center
Duarte, Calif.

**Ellie Z. Franges, RN, MSN, CCRN, CNRN**
Director, Patient Care Services, CNS Unit
Lehigh Valley Hospital
Allentown, Pa.

**Suzanne W. Gregonis, RN, MSN, CRNP**
Nurse Practitioner, Immunology Section
St. Christopher's Hospital for Children
Philadelphia

**Patti Hanisch, RN, MS, CCRN**
Nursing Instructor
Cardiac Rehabilitation Coordinator
Royal C. Johnson Veterans Administration Medical Center
Sioux Falls, S.D.

**Judith Anne Harris, RN, BSN**
Pulmonary Nurse Clinician
Phoenix Children's Hospital

**Margaret Lawler, RN, BSN, CPAN**
Staff Nurse, Post-Anesthesia Care Unit
Jeanes Hospital
Philadelphia

**Linda Leckrone, RN**
Head Nurse, Post-Anesthesia Care Unit
Providence Hospital
Sandusky, Ohio

**Margaret Massoni, RN, MSN, CS**
Assistant Professor
CUNY – The College of Staten Island (N.Y.)

**Claranne P. Mathiesen, RN, MSN**
Staff Nurse, Neurosurgical Intensive Care Unit
Lehigh Valley Hospital
Allentown, Pa.

**Margo McCaffery, RN, MS, FAAN**
Pain Management Consultant
Los Angeles

**Edwina A. McConnell, RN, PhD**
Nurse Consultant
Madison, Wis.

**Denise McNitt, RN, BSN, MS, OCN**
Oncology Clinician, Cancer Center
Good Samaritan Medical Center
Phoenix

**Judith E. Meissner, RN, MSN**
Senior Associate Professor
Bucks County Community College
Newtown, Pa.

**Deirdre P. Mountjoy, RN, BSN, MS, ANP,C**
Nurse Practitioner
CIGNA
Phoenix

**Catherine Paradiso, RN, MS, CCRN, CS**
Clinical Nurse Specialist, Critical Care
St. Vincent's Medical Center
Staten Island, N.Y.

**Carol F. Robinson, RN, MSN, RRT**
Pulmonary Nurse Specialist
Phoenix Children's Hospital

**Tammie S. Rottmann, RN, BSN, CCRN**
Staff Nurse, Intensive Care Unit
Maryvale Samaritan Medical Center
Phoenix

**Annette M. Szpiszar, RN, BSN, CNA, OCN**
Pediatric Pulmonary Clinical Nurse Specialist
Phoenix Children's Hospital

**Robyn Tyler, RN,C, MSN**
Clinical Nurse Specialist
Royal C. Johnson Veterans Administration
Medical Center
Sioux Falls, S.D.

**Richard E. Waltman, MD**
Family Physician, Geriatrician
Tacoma, Wash.

**Marla J. Weston, RN, MSN, CCRN**
Director, Nursing Systems & Education
Desert Samaritan Medical Center
Mesa, Ariz.

# FOREWORD

No matter what type of health care facility you work in, you're probably seeing more acutely ill patients than ever before. The aging of our population has contributed significantly to this trend, with the chronic illnesses of older adults often flaring up, causing acute episodes that require expert care. What's more, a great many of these patients are being shifted from critical and intensive care units to medical-surgical units, extended care facilities, ambulatory care centers, even their own homes.

Providing high-quality care for the acutely ill poses several challenges, and your ability to meet these new demands depends on a high degree of technical proficiency based on current knowledge. Not only must you constantly be sharpening your clinical skills, but you must also acquire new ones. In addition, you need to keep abreast of the newest insights into the causes and pathophysiology of illnesses, as well as the latest technological advances that might improve your patient's prognosis.

Where can you turn to for help? *Providing Expert Care for the Acutely Ill* is the perfect source with which to update your clinical skills and deepen the theoretical foundations on which you base your nursing care. This unique reference provides reliable and comprehensive information on a wide range of common acute illnesses, covering everything you need to know and do to manage your patient's acute illness skillfully and confidently.

The book contains eight chapters. Chapter 1 explores the unique role of *caring* in nursing, going beyond treating and stabilizing a patient to embrace a more humanistic approach that considers all of a patient's needs—physical, emotional, even spiritual. Here you'll learn how a caring approach will help you attend to the special needs of acutely ill patients, including older patients, patients in pain, and surgical patients. You can also apply the information in this chapter to patients with the acute illnesses addressed in subsequent chapters.

Chapters 2 through 8 discuss common acute illnesses. Chapter 2 focuses on acute cardiovascular problems, Chapter 3 details acute respiratory problems, and Chapter 4 discusses acute neurologic disorders.

Chapter 5 details acute gastrointestinal illnesses; Chapter 6, acute renal disorders; Chapter 7, acute endocrine and metabolic disorders; and Chapter 8, acute hematologic and immune disorders.

For your convenience, chapters 2 through 8 follow the same format. For each entry, you'll find a concise introduction that defines that particular acute disorder, discusses its causes and pathophysiology, and lists potential complications. The next section covers assessment, detailing the expected signs and symptoms and summarizing various diagnostic findings that suggest, support, or confirm the presence of the disease or disorder. A section on treatment describes the most current forms of therapy, including drug therapy and surgery, as well as other medical interventions used to treat the disorder.

The final section, on nursing care, describes the steps you must take to help your patient survive the acute illness and includes the immediate care, surgical care, and continuing care that will help him recover fully. Here you'll also find comprehensive information on medication, diet and nutrition, supportive measures, and patient teaching.

Throughout the book, you'll come upon graphic devices called logos that direct you to essential information. The *Pathophysiology* logo alerts you to a description of disease development and progression. The *Assessment insight* logo accents clues to help you determine your patient's chief problem. The *Complications* logo highlights potential complications or related conditions you'll need to watch for when caring for an acutely ill patient. The *Multiple diagnosis* logo highlights how one disease affects the course and treatment of another—for example, congestive heart failure in a patient with acute renal failure. The *Clinical preview* logo signals a detailed case study of an acutely ill patient that highlights the nurse's role in assessing the patient and resolving his illness. Finally, the *Home care* logo calls your attention to ways you can help your patient recover from illness and prevent a recurrence after discharge.

Throughout the book, you'll find useful illustrations and charts that will enhance your understanding of pathophysiology, increase the accuracy of your assessments, and clarify difficult technical topics. For instance, Chapter 2 contains illustrations of coronary atherectomy, an alternative to percutaneous transluminal coronary angioplasty, and Chapter 5 includes a depiction of ileostomy alternatives. A flow diagram in Chapter 7 tracks the development of the Somogyi phenomenon, and a chart in Chapter 6 compares the forms of acute renal failure.

Following the last chapter is a listing of books and articles on acute illnesses recommended by the authors. Then you will find the *Advanced skilltest,* a self-test containing questions on the material, some of which are based on case studies. The answers are provided along with complete rationales. Taking this self-test will help you assess what you've learned and determine which areas of acute care you need to review.

I know you'll find *Providing Expert Care for the Acutely Ill* an invaluable aid to your nursing practice—whether you're just starting your career or have many years of experience. Each chapter was written by clinical specialists in current practice, so you can be sure the information is not only the most accurate, up-to-date material available, but is also clinically relevant. With its clear writing and crisp, easy-to-follow format, *Providing Expert Care for the Acutely Ill* will enhance your effectiveness as a member of the health care team. I am pleased to recommend it.

**Edwina A. McConnell, RN, PhD**

Nurse Consultant
Madison, Wis.

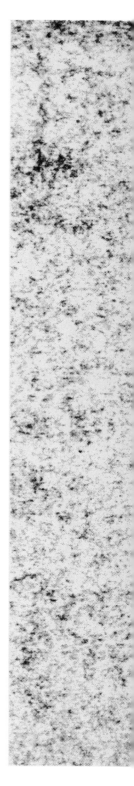

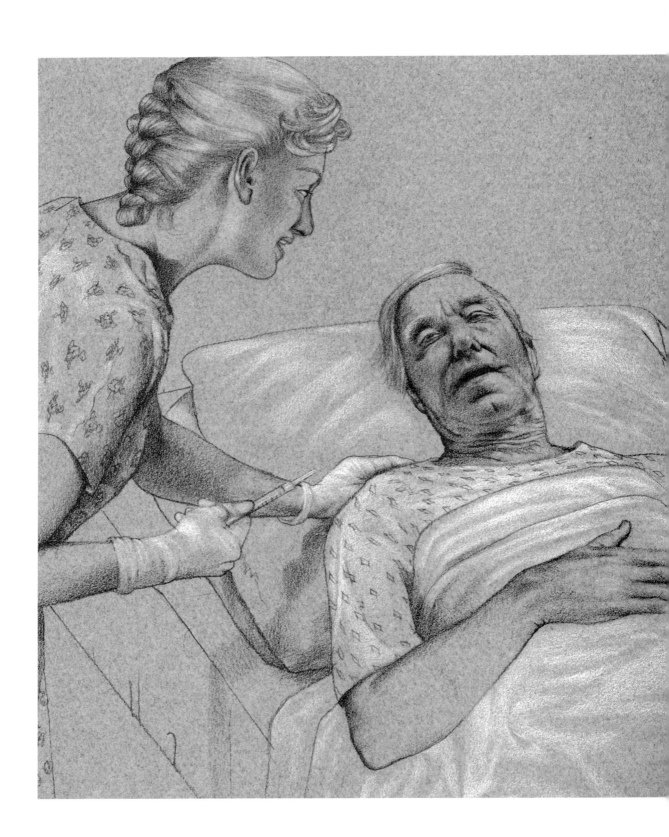

# CHAPTER 1

# Caring for the acutely ill patient

Nurses today encounter more acutely ill patients with varying needs than ever before, and *caring* for them must be one of your top priorities. But what does caring really mean?

The unifying concept—the crucial component—of nursing, caring is the ability to go beyond the technical aspects of clinical care and relate to your patients in a way that recognizes their individual worth and dignity.

Caring in nursing goes all the way back to nursing's roots, when virtually all that early religious orders could do was to minister to the sick and weary. Florence Nightingale carried on this caring tradition when she specified the character traits her nurses must possess. In modern nursing, caring became misplaced in the ongoing scientific revolution until the 1970s, when it reemerged as a major concern.

This chapter describes how a caring approach can help you attend to the special needs of acutely ill patients. It starts with how to implement caring and then focuses on caring as it relates to elderly patients, those experiencing pain, and surgical patients. Throughout, you'll read about nursing interventions that will help make caring for these patients easier — for both you and them.

### Implementing caring

One can *cure* a disease or an illness, but the practice of *caring* integrates scientific with humanistic knowledge. Make caring — not curing — your major emphasis. As health care agencies strive for efficiency, standardization, and routine, strive to prevent the health care system from dehumanizing patients. No matter how acute the patient's illness, how high the level of technology, how short the time, make sure *caring* is always present in your nursing.

You don't carry out caring directly; you accomplish it through many activities. You can convey caring in whatever you're doing — bathing a patient, measuring his blood pressure, changing his dressing, determining his cardiac output, teaching him, or discussing the patient's condition with his family. (See *How families adjust to a loved one's acute illness*.)

# Caring for the elderly patient

The population of elderly people — those over age 65 — continues to grow in the United States. Although elderly patients make up only about 10% of hospital admissions, they account for roughly 40% of all hospital costs. This major demographic and treatment shift represents a burgeoning challenge to the health care system.

Older patients don't always fare well in hospitals. They tend to have longer stays and more complications. Many take a long time to get back to their normal level of functioning; even months after successful treatment, some haven't bounced back to normal.

### Nursing considerations

• Collaborate closely with the doctor to treat elderly patients' acute problems and get them

home as soon as possible. At the same time, try to minimize deterioration, address chronic underlying problems, and prevent complications and decompensation.

• Strive to provide your elderly patients with the kind of care that will restore their previous level of functioning. If this isn't possible, try to achieve at least an optimal level of functioning, whether the patient's impairment is temporary (such as a hip fracture) or permanent (such as a major cerebrovascular deficit).

• Encourage independence. Some hospitals may foster dependence in older patients. For instance, many emergency department doctors prescribe bed rest almost universally, regardless of the admitting diagnosis. Yet most patients will recover better if you help them gain as much independence as early as possible.

A patient with pneumonia, for example, should be up, not in bed, taking deep breaths. His inactivity may set the stage for atelectasis. Patients with pelvic fractures, rib fractures, or renal calculi also fare better when they're up and moving around. Those who've had a cerebrovascular accident benefit from early mobility as soon as they're medically stable. Getting these patients up also helps ward off the complications of prolonged bed rest, such as phlebitis, incontinence, and a general loss of functioning.

• Address the patient's chronic problems, not just his acute problems. For example, suppose a patient admitted with a hip fracture has been receiving an anticonvulsant. If his anticonvulsant dosage is interrupted because no one asked the right questions about his medical history or read his chart to review his medication history, he could have a seizure and incur another injury.

Chronic conditions, such as ataxia, urinary incontinence, and bowel problems, are likely to worsen in the hospital. Mildly confused patients probably will get more confused in a new setting, and those with sensory deficits also tend to fare poorly in an unfamiliar environment. So be sure to assess the patient's chances for becoming disoriented — in the long run, this may prevent injury.

• Make anticipating and preventing complications a top priority when caring for elderly pa-

# How families adjust to a loved one's acute illness

Day after day, you meet families in varying stages of response to illness. A loved one's illness can change even the most sensible, polite members of a family into unreasonable, demanding individuals. To understand the motivations behind their behavior, remember that most families follow certain predictable stages as they try to cope with a loved one's illness. Recognizing these stages will help you better understand, assess, and interact with them.

## Stage 1: Denial

A common reaction to a harsh or painful reality, denial is a natural defense mechanism used against emotional pain and conflict. When one member of a family becomes ill, the other members typically react with shock and disbelief. This denial leads to various behaviors, such as rationalizing away symptoms.

Also, much like the patient in denial, they won't necessarily cooperate with, comprehend, or respond to you. Comprehending a diagnosis of a loved one's serious illness isn't just an intellectual process. It's an emotional trauma that may catapult the family into a major crisis.

## Stage 2: Disorganization

Out of denial comes a sense of disorganization. No longer able to deny the obvious, family members may fall into many negative behaviors. As their loved one's crisis disrupts their daily lives, some may become more demanding and irrational. Disorganization or floundering may give way to anger and blame.

## Stage 3: Anxiety

Disorganization also breeds anxiety and a sense of helplessness. For most people, the hospital is an alien environment whose unfamiliar procedures, machines, and terminology intensify their already acute emotional turmoil. Family members may be too overwhelmed to make *any* decisions about their loved one's care. Yet, because decisions must be made, and made quickly, they're forced to constantly confront critical questions.

## Stage 4: Adjustment

More information, more time, and coping with the reality of the situation help most families adjust to a loved one's illness. This final stage is a process of acceptance—not a single event, but an emotional evolution. How quickly a family reaches this stage depends a great deal on their emotional strength, both as individuals and as a family.

How can you help the family adjust? First, acknowledge their situation. They need to know, in plain language, what's happening to their loved one. Fine-tune your empathetic skills to catch not just the words spoken, but the feelings and behaviors expressed. After assessing family members' emotional status, respond appropriately.

Next, develop a plan of action. What does the family need from you? Be prepared to give specific guidance, such as explaining procedures and possible outcomes. Be prepared to repeat new or important information—perhaps many times. The most helpful thing you might offer is a realistic orientation to the hospital environment.

tients. These patients have a higher risk for complications than younger patients and they're less likely to recover. Identify patients at high risk and then intervene to reduce the risk; if the patient is at risk for respiratory distress, for example, keep an oxygen mask and other equipment on hand.
• Clarify each patient's "no-code" status. Even when admitted for elective surgical procedures or minor medical problems, some elderly patients will die in the hospital. Many patients have signed living wills, indicating they don't

want life-prolonging or lifesaving interventions if they're dying. Others haven't made a decision, so encourage them to put their wishes in writing. Determining code status is now required for all admissions. (See *What you should know about advance directives,* page 4.)
• Prepare the patient better for postdischarge living by evaluating his drug regimen, diet, and general health. Many older patients arrive at the hospital on medications they've been taking for a long time, often with unclear indications as to why they're taking them. Such

## What you should know about advance directives

Treatment decisions for a critically ill patient must often be made quickly—including decisions about life support. But the patient's loved ones may be virtually paralyzed by shock, grief, and indecision, and have no idea what to do.

The Patient Self-Determination Act of 1990 is intended to help people make these decisions for themselves before their families have to face such dilemmas. This law requires federally funded institutions (nearly all hospitals, nursing homes, health maintenance organizations, and hospices) to:
• provide, on admission, written information about state laws that cover the right to make health care decisions—including the right to accept or refuse treatment—and the right to execute advance directives (an umbrella term for documents that allow patients' decisions about their health care to be carried out if they become incapacitated)
• document in patients' medical records whether they've executed advance directives
• educate the staff and community about advance directives and applicable state laws
• maintain written policies and procedures about advance directives.

Some patients still won't want to discuss their options, however. According to the Patient Self-Determination Act, they can't be forced to sign advance directives as a condition of care. Nor can they be discriminated against if they choose not to sign.

medications typically include digoxin, metoclopramide, allopurinol, cimetidine, nonsteroidal anti-inflammatory drugs (NSAIDs), and antianxiety agents.

An elderly patient's nutritional status also can be improved while he's in the hospital. If appropriate, arrange for a nutritionist to analyze and improve his nutritional status.

Once the patient is feeling better, the doctor may check for any undiagnosed conditions and perform maintenance measures, such as overdue breast, vaginal, colon, and prostate examinations.

# Caring for the patient in pain

Nursing a patient who is experiencing severe, unmanageable pain may be one of the most emotionally trying assignments you'll have. You can deal with your patient's pain more effectively if you understand its nature and pathophysiology, as well as the latest noninvasive pain-relief methods.

## Understanding pain
Pain has both a sensory component and a reaction component. The *sensory component* involves an electrical impulse that travels to the central nervous system (CNS), where it's perceived as pain. The response to this perception is the *reaction component.*

### Responses to pain
People differ widely in their reactions to pain—mainly because pain thresholds and tolerances vary. The *pain threshold* is primarily physiologic and denotes the intensity of stimulus the patient needs to sense pain. *Pain tolerance,* in contrast, is mainly psychological and indicates the duration or intensity of pain a patient will tolerate before openly expressing his pain. Unfortunately, many nurses make highly subjective decisions about pain control without a thorough assessment—contrary to established guidelines on pain control.

The source, duration, and severity of pain are key factors in a patient's perception of pain. The source of pain is usually classified as cutaneous (or superficial), which includes skin and subcutaneous tissue; deep somatic, which includes nerve, bone, muscle, and their supporting tissues; or visceral, which includes the body's trunk organs.

### Acute vs. chronic pain
During the course of an illness, a patient may experience acute pain, chronic pain, or both. Acute pain has a sudden onset, is transient, and prompts autonomic responses, such as heavy perspiration, rising (or falling) blood pressure, and rapid pulse and respiratory rates. Usually, acute pain results from organic illness

or injury; with healing, it subsides or disappears. Acute superficial pain is usually sharp, intense, and easily localized. Acute somatic or visceral pain is heavy, aching, diffuse, and less easily localized.

Chronic pain is defined by time — it lasts 6 months or longer. It may start as acute pain, although it often has a slow, insidious onset. Typically, chronic pain is poorly localized and generates limited autonomic responses.

### Assessing pain
According to the American Pain Society (APS), pain is always subjective. Although signs of pain, such as grimacing and tachycardia, may be useful in assessing a patient's pain, these signs are often absent or misleading. That's why the APS recommends that nurses accept a patient's report of pain.

To assess your patient's pain, start by asking him to describe it. Exactly what does it feel like? When does it start? How long does it last? How often does it recur? What provokes its onset? What actions seem to relieve it? What actions seem to make it worse?

Carefully determine the pain location. Ask the patient to point to areas on his body where he feels pain. Remember that localized pain is felt only at its origin; projected pain travels along nerve pathways; radiated pain extends in several directions from the point of origin; and referred pain occurs in areas remote from the origin site.

Watch for any physiologic responses to pain, such as nausea, vomiting, and changes in vital signs; behavioral responses to pain, including facial expressions and body movements; and psychological responses, including anxiety, anger, depression, and irritability.

### Rating pain
Have the patient use a pain rating scale to describe pain intensity — for instance, a 0-to-10 scale, with 0 denoting no pain and 10 denoting extreme pain. Record on his chart the rating he gives his pain, not your personal opinion about his pain.

Remember that a simple behavior, such as smiling or grimacing, isn't strong enough evidence to conclude that a patient's pain rating is anything other than what he says it is. In fact, research has repeatedly shown that many patients with pain deliberately smile or laugh, either to help themselves cope with pain or to try to hide their pain.

## Drug therapy
The doctor may prescribe a nonnarcotic analgesic, a narcotic analgesic, or a combination of these drugs to relieve your patient's pain. Generally, the patient should receive the smallest effective dosage over the shortest period.

### Nonnarcotic analgesics
Nonnarcotic analgesics include acetaminophen and NSAIDs, such as aspirin, ibuprofen, indomethacin, naproxen, naproxen sodium, phenylbutazone, and sulindac. Most of these drugs produce analgesic and anti-inflammatory effects. They all have different chemical structures and vary in onset of action, duration of effect, and method of metabolism and excretion.

Nonnarcotic analgesics treat mild to moderate pain. Combined with narcotic analgesics, they also relieve moderate to severe pain while allowing a reduced narcotic dosage. Unlike narcotics, they don't cause physiologic dependence. They're commonly used to treat postoperative and postpartal pain, headache, myalgia, arthralgia, dysmenorrhea, and cancer pain.

NSAIDs can cause GI tract irritation, hepatotoxicity, nephrotoxicity, and headache. Acetaminophen is less likely than NSAIDS (except perhaps ibuprofen and naproxen) to cause irritation and bleeding of the GI tract. It may be used in place of aspirin and other NSAIDs in peptic ulcer or bleeding disorders. But long-term, high-dose acetaminophen use may lead to hepatic damage.

NSAIDs shouldn't be used in patients with aspirin sensitivity — especially those with the triad of allergies, asthma, and aspirin-induced nasal polyps — because bronchoconstriction or anaphylaxis may occur. NSAIDs are also contraindicated in patients with thrombocytopenia and should be used cautiously in neutropenic patients because antipyretic activity may mask the only sign of infection. Some NSAIDs also are contraindicated in renal dysfunction, hypertension, GI tract inflammation, and ulcers.

Aspirin increases prothrombin and bleeding times, so it's contraindicated in patients with hemophilia and other bleeding disorders. It shouldn't be given concomitantly with anticoagulants or other ulcerogenic drugs, such as corticosteroids, and it should be avoided in patients scheduled for surgery within 1 week.

### Narcotic analgesics

All narcotics reduce pain by binding to specific opiate receptors in the CNS, but each narcotic agent differs in potency and duration of action. Narcotic analgesics can be classified as agonists or agonist-antagonists. Agonists (such as codeine, hydromorphone, levorphanol, meperidine, methadone, morphine, and propoxyphene) produce analgesia by binding to CNS opiate receptors. Agonist-antagonists (such as buprenorphine, butorphanol, nalbuphine, and pentazocine) also produce analgesia by binding to CNS receptors. However, when another narcotic is present, they act as antagonists, blocking narcotic effects.

Many agonist-antagonists are available only in parenteral forms and may produce hallucinations and other psychotomimetic effects. In the narcotic-dependent patient, they frequently cause withdrawal symptoms.

Narcotic analgesics can be given by the oral, I.M., I.V., epidural, or intrathecal route. For most patients, oral administration is preferred. I.M. administration can result in erratic absorption, especially in debilitated patients. In severe pain, as from an anginal attack, a narcotic may be given I.V. because this route provides rapid onset of action and precise dosage control. However, I.V. narcotics may cause sudden, profound respiratory depression and hypotension. Nonetheless, continuous I.V. infusion has been used successfully. Some patients with chronic pain require long-acting narcotics, which are usually given orally. (See *Using long-acting morphine to manage chronic pain.*)

Narcotic analgesics can cause serious adverse effects, such as respiratory depression. So they're contraindicated in patients with severe respiratory depression and should be used cautiously in those with chronic obstructive pulmonary disease (COPD).

These drugs are metabolized by the liver and excreted by the kidneys, so they must be used cautiously in patients with hepatic or renal impairment. Narcotics also increase intracranial pressure (ICP) and should be used cautiously, if at all, for a head injury or for any condition that raises ICP. Also, they can induce miosis; in patients with head injuries, miosis may mask pupil dilation, an important sign of increased ICP.

The most common adverse effect of narcotics is constipation. Other adverse effects include drowsiness, dizziness, nausea, vomiting, sweating, flushing, and cough suppression. Prolonged use can lead to increased tolerance and physiologic and psychological dependence.

## Nursing considerations

• Before giving a nonnarcotic analgesic, check the patient's history for a previous hypersensitivity reaction, which may indicate hypersensitivity to a related drug in this group.
• When administering NSAIDs, ask the patient about any GI tract irritation. If irritation occurs, the doctor may reduce the dosage or discontinue the drug.
• If your patient is on long-term nonnarcotic analgesic therapy, report any abnormalities in renal and liver function studies. Monitor hematologic values and evaluate complaints of nausea or gastric burning. Stay alert for signs of iron-deficiency anemia, such as pallor, unusual fatigue, or weakness.
• Before giving a narcotic analgesic, review the patient's medication regimen for use of other CNS depressants, such as barbiturates. Concurrent use of another CNS depressant enhances respiratory depression, drowsiness, sedation, and disorientation.
• Usually, the doctor delivers a scale indicating the dosage range of pain medication, such as 5 mg of morphine for moderate pain, 10 mg of morphine for more severe pain, and 15 mg of morphine for very severe pain every 3 to 4 hours as needed. When starting narcotic therapy, give the initial recommended dose and then increase the dosage at ordered incre-

# Using long-acting morphine to manage chronic pain

The big drawback of most narcotic analgesics is their relatively short duration of action—usually 3 to 4 hours when given orally or I.M. But long-acting morphine has a longer duration—8 or more hours—without the longer half-life or the accumulation caused by repeated doses.

One form of long-acting morphine, Roxanol SR, has a duration of 8 hours. Available in 30-mg tablets, it's given mainly to adults. Another product, MS Contin, has a duration of 12 hours, although some patients require it every 8 hours for optimal pain relief. It's available in tablet strengths of 15, 30, 60, and 100 mg. Like Roxanol SR, MS Contin is used primarily in adults. Both drugs are indicated for moderate to severe pain lasting several days.

## Determining the right dosage
The dosage range for long-acting morphine varies. The dosage should be whatever amount the patient needs to relieve pain with minimal adverse effects. The average dosage for MS Contin is 120 mg every 12 hours or 240 mg/day.

As a general rule, if your patient is receiving less than 120 mg of long-acting morphine per dose, you should increase or decrease the dosage by 30 mg at a time. If his dosage is higher than 120 mg, increase it by 60 mg at a time or reduce it in 30-mg increments.

## Giving rescue doses
Patients receiving long-acting morphine may need rescue doses—immediate-release analgesics (usually short-acting morphine) for acute breakthrough pain—as needed. For instance, the patient may need a rescue dose to relieve the pain he feels when he gets out of bed or if his pain flares up when he leaves home to see the doctor.

Rescue doses are roughly 25% of the dose given every 12 hours. So a patient receiving 60 mg of MS Contin every 12 hours would receive a 15-mg rescue dose of short-acting morphine.

A word of caution: You may find a patient using rescue doses to compensate for inadequate long-acting therapy. Generally, an increased dose of long-acting morphine is indicated if the patient needs more than two rescue doses per 24-hour period.

## Giving adjuvant therapy
Even with the prescribed dose, studies show the benefits of supplementing narcotic therapy with nonnarcotic analgesics, such as aspirin or acetaminophen. Unlike narcotics, nonnarcotics don't bind at opiate receptor sites in the central nervous system. They augment the analgesia provided by narcotic agents by relieving pain at injury sites. Nonsteroidal anti-inflammatory drugs, such as choline magnesium trisalicylate, ibuprofen, indomethacin, and naproxen, are also excellent supplements to narcotic analgesics.

## Nursing considerations
• When administering long-acting morphine, *never* crush or break the tablets. They must be swallowed whole because their formulation controls medication release. When crushed or broken, the total morphine dose is released immediately. Because long-acting tablets contain more morphine than short-acting tablets, the patient would run a higher risk of overdose. Make sure that your patient is aware of this possibility.
• Respiratory depression may be a particular concern. All narcotics can cause this problem, although not to a life-threatening or even clinically significant extent in most patients. Look for it mainly when increasing the dosage.
• Also stay alert for sedation, a common adverse effect of morphine that may stem from the drug's depressant effect. Some patients who've switched to long-acting morphine report 1 to 3 days of increased sedation. When converting a patient from short-acting to long-acting morphine, make him aware of the possibility of increased sedation. Encourage him to tolerate the sedation for 2 to 3 days before you adjust his dosage, unless it becomes too distressing.

Don't confuse sedation with pain relief. A patient can become quite sedated and still be experiencing pain. Many patients sleep from exhaustion and still feel a lot of pain.

## Pain in elderly patients

Research suggests caregivers are more likely to undertreat pain in patients age 65 or older than in younger adults. The misconception that elderly patients are less sensitive to pain may contribute to undertreatment. Here are some tips on monitoring pain, especially underreported pain, and possible concurrent respiratory depression in elderly patients.

### Questioning patients' silence about pain
Question the patient to see if he's underreporting his pain. Elderly patients may be less likely to report pain, but this shouldn't be confused with the absence of pain.

Some elderly patients may assume their nurses know how much pain they're experiencing and how much medication they should receive for it. Also, elderly patients may deliberately underreport their pain because they're afraid an analgesic will make them confused and drowsy, which may lead to a bad fall or an arm or leg fracture. Or they may simply believe that pain is inevitable when you're old and that they must tolerate a certain amount of it.

For all these reasons, initiate conversations with your elderly patient about his pain.

### Monitoring for respiratory depression
Also monitor your patient closely for signs of respiratory depression during analgesic therapy. The fear of respiratory depression needn't lead to undermedication. But it does require you to monitor elderly patients more closely for early signs of this adverse effect. Remember, too, that narcotic-induced respiratory depression can be quickly reversed with naloxone, a narcotic antagonist.

ments if the patient reports he's still in pain and he's had no serious adverse reactions. Be sure to ask him if his pain relief is satisfactory; if not, discuss a higher dosage with him, subject to the doctor's approval.
• During any analgesic therapy, check the patient's vital signs and watch for respiratory depression, especially with the initial dose or a subsequent dose increase. Respiratory depres-

sion and sedation decrease with continued use at the same dose. If the respiratory rate falls to 10 breaths/minute or less, call the patient's name and touch him; then instruct him to breathe deeply. If he can't be roused or is confused or restless, notify the doctor and be prepared to provide respiratory support and oxygen. If ordered, administer a narcotic antagonist, such as naloxone.
• Encourage him to practice coughing and deep-breathing exercises to promote ventilation and prevent pooling of secretions, which could cause respiratory difficulty.
• If the patient on narcotic therapy has persistent nausea and vomiting, notify the doctor, who may change the medication. As ordered, give an antiemetic, such as chlorpromazine.
• Constipation is always a concern for the patient receiving narcotics because these drugs attach to receptors in the bowel, slowing peristalsis. To help prevent constipation, administer a stool softener and, if necessary, a stimulant laxative. Provide a high-fiber diet and encourage fluids, as permitted. Encourage regular exercise to promote intestinal motility.
• Narcotic analgesics can cause postural hypotension, so take measures to avoid accidents. For example, keep the bed's side rails raised. If the patient is mobile, help him out of bed and assist him with ambulation.
• Evaluate analgesic effectiveness. Is the patient developing a tolerance to the drug? Remember that he should receive the smallest effective dose over the shortest period. However, *don't* withhold narcotic analgesics or give ineffective doses for fear of causing dependence. Physiologic or psychological dependence occurs in fewer than 1% of hospitalized patients. In an elderly patient, take special steps to avoid undertreating pain. (See *Pain in elderly patients*.)

# Caring for the surgical patient

Because so many surgical patients are now admitted the morning of surgery, all health care team members are under pressure to work fast and effectively. You'll need to quickly and expertly practice your nursing skills — and also provide the emotional support that's so crucial for this patient. He and his family need to have confidence in your concern and compassion as well as in your clinical efficiency.

## Preoperative care
Start with a quick review of your patient's status. Most patients admitted the day of surgery need little physical care; typically, all ordered blood work and X-rays have already been done. Your unit secretary can check to make sure the laboratory reports are in the chart, but you should quickly review them yourself for anything abnormal.

Make sure that the patient has signed a surgical consent form, and note which preoperative medications have been ordered. If any information is missing, contact the doctor or the appropriate hospital department. Identify any other health problems your patient has and check for any special considerations noted on the chart. Also, spend a few moments getting acquainted with and reassuring the patient.

Typically, patients become upset because they don't know what to expect. Thorough preoperative teaching can help the patient understand the surgical procedure, alleviating many of his fears and greatly reducing his anxiety.

### Admission questions
If your hospital doesn't have a standard preoperative checklist for routine admission questions, start by asking the patient when he last ate or drank anything (including water). Although he was probably instructed not to eat or drink anything after midnight (or for at least 8 hours before surgery), you should make sure that he's followed those orders. (Some clinicians believe a small drink of water the morning of surgery *prevents* aspiration complications by speeding up gastric emptying time so that gastric acids don't remain in the stomach.)

Ask the patient whether he's currently taking any medications and when he took the last dose of each one. Make sure that his reply corresponds with what's indicated on his chart.

### Preparation
Provide a hospital gown for the patient to wear during surgery. Tell the patient to remove all clothing (including underwear), jewelry, hairpins, and barrettes. Most hospitals permit patients to wear a wedding ring during certain types of surgery as long as it's taped or tied in place. (Place a cotton ball or gauze over any stones before applying tape so a loose stone won't pull out when the tape is removed.)

Have the patient remove eyeglasses, contact lenses, or dentures (which can slip during surgery and block his airway). Tell him you'll place his belongings in a safe location or give them to a family member.

If the patient is wearing fingernail polish, explain that it must be removed because it covers the nail bed, which the surgical team must assess for color changes. Also, polish could interfere with pulse oximetry readings.

If your patient has long hair, suggest it be braided or placed in a ponytail with an elastic band to keep it away from the face. Hair also should be covered with a surgical cap.

Obtain the patient's vital signs. Start his I.V. line and administer any I.V. antibiotics or other prescription drugs. Then provide care aimed at preventing postoperative complications. (See *Preventing postoperative problems,* page 10.)

Next, assess the patient's veins for venipuncture and explain that he'll need an I.V. line for drugs and fluids. Let him know you'll administer a preoperative injection in a few minutes to help him relax.

Any caring gesture you extend to the patient may seem like a simple thing — but it will make a big difference to him. Remember, even if the scheduled surgery seems routine to you, it's anything but routine for your patient.

### Medications
Nearly every patient having surgery receives some type of preoperative medication. Such medications are given to:
• reduce anxiety
• sedate the patient (which eases anxiety, promotes anesthesia induction, and decreases intraoperative anesthetic requirements)
• ease preoperative procedures

# Preventing postoperative problems

You can help prevent postoperative complications by following these guidelines as you prepare your patient for surgery.

### Performing a preoperative assessment
Perform a preoperative assessment to establish baseline breath sounds and breathing patterns — especially if the patient has preexisting lung disease or will undergo lung surgery. Carefully document your findings. Indicate the type of breath sound and its specific location.

### Preventing respiratory complications
Before your patient goes to surgery, determine if he has any respiratory complications so you can plan accordingly. If he has a preexisting respiratory condition, such as chronic obstructive pulmonary disease, you'll need to administer bronchodilators and antibiotics, as ordered, and encourage deep breathing. If your patient smokes or has a cough producing secretions, you may need to improve secretion clearance by administering bronchodilators, chest physiotherapy, or antibiotics (if the sputum is purulent), if ordered.

### Preventing infection
To help prevent infection, the surgeon may want the patient to take a preoperative shower with antimicrobial soap. Advise him to use the bathroom before showering or before being premedicated. (After you give him the preoperative medication,

he won't be allowed to get up and will have to use a bedpan or urinal.)

For some patients, a preoperative scrub of the incisional area may take the place of a shower. Using antimicrobial soap, wash the patient's skin from approximately 5″ (13 cm) above to 5″ below the site where the incision will be made. Cover or wrap the area with sterile drapes as directed.

### Shaving or depilating the patient
Check your hospital's policy on shaving a hairy surgical site. At most hospitals, the patient is shaved in the operating room to minimize the infection risk. However, surgical teams no longer shave as large an area, and hair is sometimes clipped or a depilatory used. (The patient may have been instructed to use the depilatory the night before surgery if a skin patch test proved no allergy.) Check whether the patient used a depilatory and note his response to a patch test if he didn't.

### Performing postoperative exercises
After your patient returns from surgery, discuss postoperative exercises with him. Find out whether he's been taught how to perform coughing, deep breathing, and splinting. If he won't be allowed out of bed the day of surgery, also teach him leg exercises. To prevent postoperative complications, he'll be asked to perform these exercises for several days after surgery.

• protect the airway during surgery (an anticholinergic will dry secretions and reduce the risk of aspiration and laryngospasm)
• increase the gastric pH or gastric emptying rate, in turn reducing the risk of aspiration
• counter the postoperative nausea and vomiting that may occur as a reaction to anesthesia or to the surgery itself.

Before administering a preoperative medication, know why the anesthesiologist prescribed that particular drug for your patient. You should also be familiar with its normal dosage and potential adverse effects.

Once you've administered the preoperative injection, raise the side rails on the bed and tell the patient he's going to feel drowsy and perhaps dry-mouthed if an anticholinergic was administered. Tell him a member of the transport team will arrive shortly to take him to the preoperative holding area.

Usually, no one preoperative drug is best for your patient. Typically, the patient receives a combination of drugs, depending on the desired effects. When selecting an appropriate combination, the anesthesiologist will consider the patient's age and physiologic status, the type of surgery, goals of medication, adverse effects, as well as his own preferences.

Expect to administer preoperative drugs 1 hour before surgery or when the patient is put "on call" for surgery. This allows time for the drugs to peak and to exert their desired effects.

Document the preoperative medications on the medication administration record and, if required, on the preoperative checklist.

## Postoperative care

A patient returning from the operating room depends on you to help him through a smooth, successful recovery. You need to know how to manage his pain and administer any postoperative medications he may need.

### Postoperative pain

Pain can affect a patient's postoperative course. If he hurts, he'll balk at coughing and deep-breathing exercises — and that can lead to atelectasis, hypoxemia, and pneumonia. If he won't get out of bed, he may develop pressure sores, ileus, or thromboemboli. Constant pain can depress his spirits and appetite, depriving him of the energy and calories he needs to heal.

Some surgical procedures are more painful than others — for instance, laminectomies and surgeries involving major joints. Along with steady wound pain, the patient may have painful reflex muscle spasms when he moves. Intrathoracic, intra-abdominal, and renal procedures also can cause severe pain. Upper abdominal incisions usually are more painful than lower abdominal ones, with coughing and deep-breathing exercises making the pain worse.

Some patients experience intense pain after even minor surgical procedures. That's because fear and anxiety can heighten a patient's perception of pain.

Whatever the situation, never ignore a patient's complaint of acute pain. It's real and it always requires a thorough assessment to rule out complications, such as infection, bleeding, or compartment syndrome. Chest pain after a thoracotomy, for instance, may not be related to the incision at all, but to cardiac ischemia.

### Postoperative medications

Typically, postoperative patients report moderate to severe pain, which responds best to narcotic analgesics. For postoperative pain, the preferred administration routes are I.V., epidural, and oral. I.M. injections can be painful and cause local tissue irritation and inconsistent drug absorption.

When assessing a patient's pain and medication effectiveness, keep in mind the drug's duration of action. For instance, meperidine is generally administered every 3 to 4 hours; to ensure pain relief, you can't change the dosage to once every 2 hours because that might cause drug toxicity. Although meperidine still is frequently prescribed as a narcotic, it causes accumulation of the active metabolite normeperidine, a CNS stimulant. Substituting a drug with a longer duration of action — for instance, morphine, whose duration is 3 to 4 hours — may be preferred.

You must also consider timing when administering narcotic analgesics. Around-the-clock administration is preferred to as-needed administration because it not only treats pain but also prevents it. Any drug ordered every 4 or 8 hours should be administered around the clock.

***Supplements.*** Although narcotic analgesics are the primary drugs used to manage postoperative pain, they're usually supplemented with nonnarcotic analgesics, such as acetaminophen or NSAIDs. Unlike narcotic analgesics, which affect the CNS, nonnarcotics work peripherally. They enhance a narcotic's analgesic effects, allowing a lower narcotic dosage and reducing the risk of narcotic-related adverse effects. They're generally contraindicated in patients with bleeding problems, however.

***Patient-controlled analgesia and epidural infusion pumps.*** These devices are popular with caregivers and patients. Besides delivering a continuous narcotic infusion to keep the patient comfortable, they can provide bolus doses to control incidental pain from coughing, deep breathing, or getting out of bed.

A standard epidural catheter can be inserted into the pleural space to administer narcotics or anesthetics, such as bupivacaine. This alternative is especially helpful after chest, upper abdominal, or breast surgery. Many patients undergoing thoracotomy or cholecystectomy obtain such satisfactory pain control from this type of nerve block that they need no other analgesics.

## Nursing considerations

To help prevent and manage postoperative respiratory, cardiovascular, GI, CNS, and renal complications, follow these guidelines.

### Respiratory complications

Expect some degree of atelectasis and hypoxemia in all postoperative patients. Also watch for pneumonia, aspiration, and other respiratory complications.

• Moderate hypoxemia usually responds to supplemental oxygen at a fraction of inspired oxygen ($FIO_2$) of 0.3 to 0.4.

• If your patient can't deep-breathe on request, you can reverse narcotic-induced respiratory depression with narcotic antagonists, such as naloxone. Keep in mind, though, that these agents reverse all narcotic effects, including analgesia. So be prepared to administer a nonnarcotic analgesic to control pain.

• To detect atelectasis in patients with a preexisting respiratory disorder or who have undergone lung surgery, auscultating the affected area should reveal crackles or diminished breath sounds. In other patients, atelectasis is common at the lung bases, so carefully auscultate there. You may note dullness on percussion and decreased chest expansion. In mild atelectasis, symptoms may be absent, but as it progresses, fever, dyspnea, tachypnea, tachycardia, and coughing may occur.

• To detect pneumonia, stay alert for dyspnea, pleuritic chest pain, chills, and a cough producing purulent or bloody sputum. You also may note hypoxemia, dullness on percussion, tachypnea, fever, inspiratory crackles, and decreased breath sounds over the involved area.

• Silent aspiration is a particular risk in oversedated, obtunded, or comatose patients. Signs and symptoms of aspiration depend on the severity of aspiration. Typically, atelectatic areas become extensive within 2 minutes of aspira-

tion and respiratory distress occurs in 1 to 60 minutes. Tachypnea, dyspnea, coughing, and bronchospasm follow reflex airway closure. Noncardiac pulmonary edema may develop from damage caused by gastric aspiration.

To help prevent postoperative aspiration, remember that your patient may be drowsy for the first few hours. Monitor him closely to assess his risk for aspiration. Keep him positioned on his back or side, with the head of the bed raised. If he's lying on his side, make sure the suction catheter, emesis basin, and call button are on the side he's facing.

• Ensure proper positioning to avert respiratory complications. Semi-Fowler's position is best for matching ventilation and perfusion, reducing abdominal pressure on the diaphragm, and minimizing the risk of aspiration. Elevate the head of the bed 30 degrees unless contraindicated or unless the patient's blood pressure falls when he's in a semisitting position.

• To prevent alveolar collapse and subsequent respiratory complications, you can implement four techniques: incentive spirometry, voluntary deep breathing, sighing, and yawning. *Incentive spirometry* helps the patient take slow, deep breaths, produces high transpulmonary pressure, and increases lung volume with adequate alveolar inflation time. This method helps maintain muscle strength and promotes pulmonary hygiene.

*Voluntary deep breathing, sighing* (defined as a breath three times normal volume), and *yawning* hyperinflate the alveoli and prevent their collapse. (However, after upper abdominal surgery, a better alternative for preserving lung volumes, easing gas exchange, and preventing atelectasis may be periodic administration of continuous positive airway pressure or positive end-expiratory pressure by face mask.)

Getting the patient out of bed to walk short distances may be the most important lung expansion maneuver. Walking improves circulation and ventilation.

• Administer oxygen, as ordered, to relieve hypoxemia and prevent tissue hypoxia. However, you also must correct the underlying cause of hypoxemia. Depending on the patient's status, he may require an increase in alveolar ventilation, increased $FIO_2$, or therapy to reduce ventilation-perfusion mismatching and intrapulmonary shunting.

Oxygen therapy may be particularly helpful in patients with significant hypoxemia—for example, those with advanced COPD. In these patients, hypoxemia stems from a ventilation-perfusion mismatch. Administering continuous, low-flow (1 to 2 liters/minute) oxygen usually increases partial pressure of oxygen in arterial blood ($PaO_2$), decreases dyspnea, and improves neuropsychological function and exercise tolerance. COPD patients need supplemental oxygen when ambulating, when sitting in a chair, and perhaps even when resting in bed.

However, use caution when administering oxygen to COPD patients. Usually, you should titrate the flow rate to maintain $PaO_2$ at approximately 60 mm Hg, especially if the patient is retaining carbon dioxide ($CO_2$). Increasing the $PaO_2$ level reduces ventilatory stimulation from the patient's hypoxic drive and can lead to hypoventilation, more $CO_2$ retention and, ultimately, respiratory failure.

## Cardiovascular complications
• Tachycardia and hypertension aren't unusual in a patient who's just awaking from the effects of general anesthesia. Reassurance from the postanesthesia room staff, an I.V. analgesic, and rest can usually counteract these complications in a healthy patient.

Hypothermia may contribute to tachycardia and hypertension. If your patient is hypothermic, leave the rewarming blankets on him.
• Tachycardia with hypotension may result from anesthesia, from hypovolemia (caused by fluid loss), or from persistent pain. If your patient received isoflurane during surgery, consider this drug a possible cause of tachycardia and hypotension. Isoflurane also decreases mean arterial pressure and profoundly lowers peripheral vascular resistance.

To raise the blood pressure of a tachycardic patient with hypotension, you may simply need to stimulate him. For instance, get him to breathe more deeply and move his legs. If that doesn't work, increase the I.V. infusion rate and see if his heart rate drops and his blood pressure rises.

## GI complications
• Nausea and vomiting occur frequently, depending on the type of surgery, the patient's level of pain, and the narcotics and anesthetics administered. For the first few hours after surgery, your patient may still be drowsy and thus at risk for aspiration. Other possible causes of nausea and vomiting are pain at the incision site and blocked tubes, such as a nasogastric or tracheostomy tube.
• Abdominal surgery always carries the risk of postoperative ileus. In addition, the sympathetic nervous system's response to pain and the narcotics used to treat this pain decrease GI motility and secretions and increase sphincter tone, promoting constipation.

To help prevent ileus and constipation, monitor your patient's bowel sounds, measure his abdominal girth, and watch for such signs and symptoms as nausea, vomiting, absence of flatus, and intolerance to fluids. Try to get him out of bed and walking as soon as possible—walking stimulates peristalsis.

## CNS complications
• Postoperative somnolence stems primarily from the residual effects of nitrous oxide and isoflurane, potent inhalation agents. Keep in mind that the patient with postoperative somnolence can still hear what's going on around him, despite a decreased level of consciousness. Reassure him about where he is and what's being done for him on an ongoing basis.

## Renal complications
• The risk of urine retention depends on the type and length of surgery, the patient's age, any history of urine retention, and the amount of intraoperative I.V. fluids administered. The more I.V. fluids he received, the greater the chance that he will develop postoperative urine retention and will have to be catheterized.
• To detect urine retention early, carefully inspect, palpate, and percuss the lower abdomen over the bladder. Watch the patient for signs and symptoms of bladder distention, such as restlessness, agitation, and pain. Encourage him to go to the bathroom as soon as possible after surgery and every few hours thereafter.

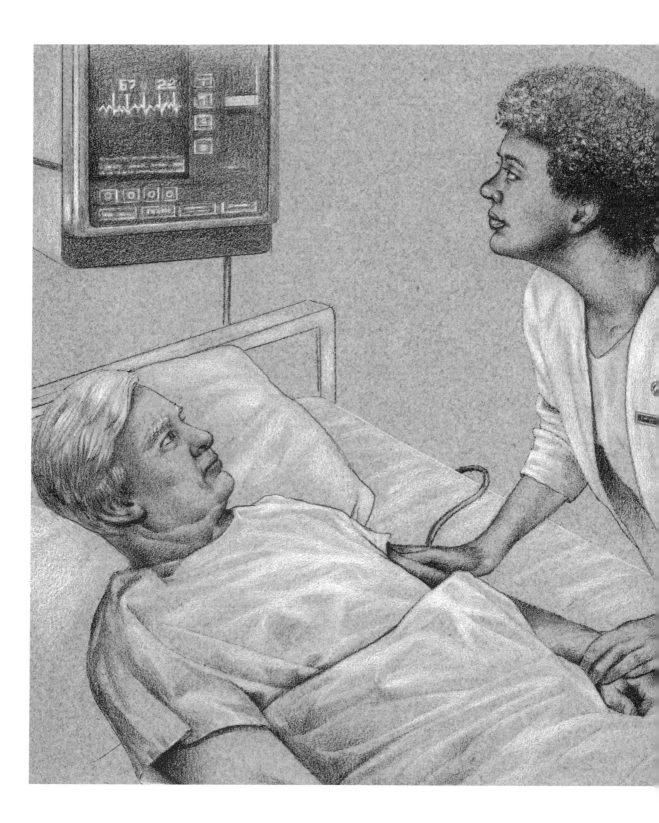

# CHAPTER 2

# Cardiovascular disorders

No matter where you practice nursing, you can expect to deal with cardiovascular patients more than any other type. Once treated almost exclusively in intensive care units (ICUs) or critical care units, patients with cardiovascular disorders are now routinely transferred to medical-surgical units and then to extended care facilities. As a result, nurses in widely varied settings must know how to provide these patients with thorough, efficient care.

Many cardiovascular disorders may be acute and even life-threatening, requiring you to intervene quickly to prevent complications or death. Others may be chronic, resulting from an insidious underlying disease, in which case you'll have to provide effective patient teaching to help the patient cope with his disorder after he leaves the hospital.

This chapter will provide you with the information you'll need to manage acutely ill cardiovascular patients. You'll find in-depth explanations of the causes and pathophysiology of unstable angina pectoris, congestive heart failure, mitral stenosis, pericarditis, and arterial occlusive disease. Then you'll learn about assessment techniques, the latest medical and surgical interventions, and thorough nursing care.

---

## Risk factors for atherosclerosis

Various risk factors have been linked to atherosclerosis. Some can't be changed, but others can be modified through medical care and life-style changes.

### Unmodifiable risk factors
• *Age.* Atherosclerosis usually occurs after age 40.
• *Sex.* Men are eight times more susceptible than premenopausal women. After menopause, however, women's atherosclerosis rates rise dramatically and heart disease becomes the leading cause of death in this group.
• *Heredity.* A family history of coronary artery disease increases the risk of atherosclerosis.
• *Race.* Blacks are more susceptible than whites because of a higher incidence of hypertension.

### Modifiable risk factors
• *Blood pressure.* A systolic pressure above 160 mm Hg or a diastolic pressure above 95 mm Hg increases the risk of atherosclerosis.
• *Serum cholesterol levels.* Increased low-density lipoprotein (LDL) levels and decreased high-density lipoprotein (HDL) levels significantly heighten the risk of atherosclerosis.
• *Smoking.* Cigarette smoking decreases HDL and increases LDL and triglyceride levels, increasing the risk of myocardial infarction and sudden death. These risks drop dramatically within 1 year after quitting.
• *Diabetes mellitus.* This disorder promotes atherosclerosis, especially in women.
• *Obesity.* Added weight increases the risk of atherosclerosis by increasing the risk of diabetes mellitus, hypertension, and an elevated serum cholesterol level.
• *Physical activity.* Lack of regular exercise increases the risk of atherosclerosis.
• *Stress.* A hostile, aggressive personality may predispose a person to atherosclerosis. New research suggests that the extremely competitive type A personality may not be as significant as previously believed.

# Unstable angina pectoris

A symptom of extensive or worsening coronary artery disease (CAD), unstable angina pectoris is a spasmodic, choking, or suffocating thoracic pain that may progress to myocardial infarction (MI). Unlike stable angina, a predictable pain that's relieved by rest or nitrates, unstable angina usually occurs at rest or with minimal exertion. This form of angina (also called preinfarction angina, crescendo angina, or intermittent coronary syndrome) increases in severity, frequency, or duration.

### Causes
Angina generally results from inadequate blood flow to the myocardium and is the classic symptom of CAD, a term that refers to a variety of pathologic conditions that obstruct blood flow through the coronary arteries.

Atherosclerosis is the most common cause of CAD and, hence, angina. Although several theories attempt to explain the pathogenesis of atherosclerosis, its etiology remains unclear. However, atherosclerosis has been linked to many risk factors, some of which can be modified. (See *Risk factors for atherosclerosis.*)

Although the precise cause of unstable angina is unknown, several hypotheses offer tentative explanations. Because unstable angina often occurs at rest, it may result from a transient decrease in coronary blood flow rather than greater myocardial oxygen demand. One theory blames unstable angina on alternating bouts of vasoconstriction and thrombus formation. Possibly, dysfunction of the coronary artery endothelium causes atherosclerosis, thrombosis, and vasoconstriction, which act together to produce unstable angina.

### Pathophysiology
The coronary arteries (especially the left one) are highly susceptible to atherosclerosis. Atherosclerotic lesions usually develop near the origin and bifurcation of the main coronary arteries. Initially, the disease process is localized, but as atherosclerosis advances, lesion formation becomes diffuse.

A fatty streak is the first lesion to form within the arterial wall. Developing as lipid-filled foam cells (xanthoma cells), the streak invades the intimal wall and may appear in the coronary vessels of individuals as young as 15.

As atherosclerosis advances, the fatty streak may develop into a calcified fibrous plaque or a complicated lesion that obstructs the vessel lumen. Such a lesion gives rise to angina. The lesion may also rupture, posing the risk of spasm, thrombus formation, and embolization. Clinical manifestations of myocardial ischemia rarely occur until the artery is about 75% occluded.

### Complications

Unstable angina carries a higher morbidity and mortality than chronic stable angina and a higher incidence of MI. The risk of MI peaks within the first 4 months after onset of unstable angina symptoms.

An estimated 5% of patients with unstable angina die within the first month, and an additional 5% within the first year. After 5 years, the cumulative mortality is about 30%.

## Assessment

### Signs and symptoms

Angina varies in severity from upper substernal pressure to agonizing pain accompanied by severe apprehension and a feeling of impending death. The patient may describe the pain as a burning, squeezing, or pressurelike substernal discomfort.

Question the patient closely about the nature of his pain, its location, and factors that aggravate or alleviate it. Investigate his history to determine the pattern and type of angina. Is the pain predictable and relieved by rest and nitrates? If so, it's probably stable angina. If the pain increases in frequency and duration and is easily induced, suspect unstable angina. (See *Comparing angina types*.)

### Diagnostic tests

Although angina can often be diagnosed from the patient's history and physical findings, several diagnostic tests help establish the diagnosis and determine the type of angina.

ASSESSMENT INSIGHT

# Comparing angina types

To help classify your patient's angina, explore his history for patterns to his pain. Use this chart as a guide.

| TYPE | CHARACTERISTICS |
|---|---|
| Unstable (preinfarction, crescendo) angina | • Occurs at rest or with minimal exertion<br>• Progressively worsens in frequency, intensity, and duration<br>• Carries an increasing risk of myocardial infarction (MI) within 3 to 18 months |
| Chronic stable angina | • Predictable, consistent pain<br>• Rarely occurs at rest |
| Nocturnal angina | • Occurs at night, usually during sleep<br>• May be relieved by sitting up<br>• Commonly results from left ventricular failure |
| Angina decubitus | • Occurs while lying down |
| Intractable or refractory angina | • Severe and incapacitating pain |
| Prinzmetal's (variant, resting) angina | • Causes spontaneous anginal pain accompanied by ST-segment elevation on electrocardiogram<br>• May result from coronary artery spasm<br>• Associated with high risk of MI |

*Electrocardiography.* Observation of electrocardiography (ECG) changes aids in diagnosing angina. ST-segment depression indicates myocardial ischemia, whose effects may be reversed through early detection and timely intervention. Without intervention, ischemia causes myocardial injury, as reflected by ST-segment elevation.

*Exercise ECG.* Also called stress testing, this noninvasive procedure evaluates the cardiovascular response to controlled physical work loads using an ECG. During this test, the patient pedals a stationary bicycle or walks on a treadmill. The speed and incline are increased gradually to measure the heart's response to an increased work load. In response to this physical exertion, he may exhibit chest pain and ECG signs of myocardial ischemia. The heart's electrical rhythm may show T-wave inversion or ST-segment depression in ischemic areas.

*Nuclear imaging.* Nuclear diagnostic procedures use radioactive isotopes, such as cardiolite or thallium, or positron emission tomography (PET) scans to visualize the heart. None of these tests should be done on patients who have had a recent or evolving MI.

In *cardiolite* testing, cardiolite is injected into the patient intravenously to determine the amount of blood flow to the myocardium. Baseline (resting) X-rays are taken 1 hour later. After a second cardiolite injection is administered, the patient exercises on a treadmill or other equipment, and a second set of X-rays is taken.

If the patient is unable to perform the exercise portion of the test (because of amputation, severe chronic obstructive pulmonary disease, or other severe disabilities), he is given dipyridamole, a vasodilator, which simulates stress to the heart. After the second injection, the second set of X-rays is taken. *Thallium* may also be used for this test, with or without dipyridamole.

A *PET scan* reveals more precise information about blood flow to the myocardium than X-ray imaging. Cardiologists use it to detect narrowing of the coronary arteries, assess collateral circulation throughout the heart's secondary vessels, and evaluate the patency of bypass grafts and the size and location of dead tissue caused by previous infarcts.

## Treatment
### Drug therapy
Treatment of unstable angina aims to stabilize the angina and prevent MI, usually with medications, and may involve various combinations of the following drugs:
• *nitrates* to dilate the coronary arteries and collateral heart vessels
• *beta blockers* to lower oxygen demand during exercise and bring the balance of oxygen supply closer to demand

• *calcium channel blockers* to decrease the heart's work load and improve oxygen supply by dilating the coronary arteries
• *antiplatelet, anticoagulant,* and *thrombolytic agents* to decrease platelet aggregation and thrombus formation.

Some doctors prescribe a calcium channel blocker along with a nitrate, while others prefer a triple-drug regimen consisting of a calcium channel blocker, a nitrate, and a beta blocker. Compared to administration of a single medication, the combined regimen reduces the likelihood of anginal symptoms and ischemia. However, it doesn't necessarily lower the incidence of MI or death.

*Nitrate therapy.* Nitrates are the drug of choice for most unstable angina patients unless contraindicated. Nitroglycerin reduces myocardial oxygen consumption, decreasing ischemia and relieving anginal pain. A vasoactive drug that dilates both arteries and veins, it causes venous pooling throughout the body. As a result, less blood returns to the heart and filling pressure declines. These effects reduce the heart's oxygen needs, creating a better balance between oxygen supply and demand.

Taken sublingually or placed in the buccal pouch, nitroglycerin usually alleviates pain within 3 minutes. The drug is also available in a lanolin-petroleum-based ointment and in sustained-release patches. (See *Teaching tips for nitroglycerin use.*)

*Beta blockers.* In stable angina, these drugs are used to reduce the heart's oxygen needs. But the rationale for their use in unstable angina is questionable because unstable angina seems to stem from a transient drop in coronary blood flow, not a greater myocardial oxygen demand. Even so, beta blockers may prevent future coronary events in the patient with unstable angina, especially if used in conjunction with a nitrate and a calcium channel blocker. However, giving a beta blocker and calcium channel blocker concomitantly to a patient with left ventricular dysfunction or a conduction disturbance calls for caution: These

# Teaching tips for nitroglycerin use

If your patient is taking nitroglycerin to prevent or relieve angina, make sure he understands how to use the medication safely and correctly. Before discharge, review the following teaching points with him.

### Using tablets
• Instruct the patient to place the tablet under his tongue at the onset of anginal pain. Explain that a burning sensation under the tongue indicates that the nitroglycerin is activated.
• Explain that if the first tablet doesn't relieve his pain, he may take a second after 5 minutes and a third after another 5 minutes. However, he should taper the dosage to avoid nitroglycerin tolerance.
• Tell the patient to call the doctor if his pain doesn't subside after the third nitroglycerin tablet. Advise him to go to the nearest emergency department—but stress that he should *never* drive himself.

### Using ointment or a patch
• Teach the patient to spread the ointment in a thin, uniform layer on any hairless body area, but *not* to rub it in. Advise him to cover the area with ordinary plastic kitchen wrap to aid drug absorption and protect his clothing.
• Advise the patient to remove all old nitroglycerin ointment using alcohol swabs before applying new ointment.
• Instruct him to follow his medication instructions to allow a nitroglycerin-free period at night to reduce the risk of tolerance.

### Storing nitroglycerin safely
• Advise the patient to keep nitroglycerin tablets or ointment in their original container or in a tightly capped, dark-colored glass bottle. Tell him to discard the cotton filler or packing because it absorbs the drug, and to place the container in a cool, dry place to avoid extremes in temperature and humidity. He should store nitroglycerin patches in sealed single-dose containers.
• Advise the patient not to carry bottles containing sublingual tablets close to his body because body heat may speed tablet decomposition. For the same reason, he should never store the medication in a closed car or in a glove compartment.
• To ensure freshness, advise the patient to replace his nitroglycerin supply every 6 months. If he's using sublingual tablets, tell him to avoid opening the bottle unnecessarily.

### Preventing adverse effects
• Tell the patient to stand up or sit down slowly after taking nitroglycerin to avoid orthostatic hypotension. This is especially important while exposed to heat—when taking a hot shower or sauna, in a hot tub, or on a hot summer day, for example.
• Inform the patient that he may have a mild headache for a few days while his body adjusts to the medication. Tell him to take a mild analgesic for relief until the headache subsides.

---

patients are at risk for congestive heart failure and severe conduction disturbances, including heart block.

The doctor may order propranolol for the patient whose chest pain persists despite lifestyle changes and nitroglycerin therapy. Propranolol reduces heart rate, blood pressure, and myocardial contractility, bringing myocardial oxygen supply more in line with demand. It also helps control chest pain and allows the patient to resume many normal activities or exercise.

*Calcium channel blockers.* These drugs enhance the heart's oxygen supply by dilating the smooth-muscle wall of coronary arterioles. They also decrease the heart's need for oxygen by reducing systemic arterial pressure, thus decreasing the left ventricle's work load.

The most commonly used calcium channel blockers are diltiazem, nifedipine, and verapamil. Their vasodilating effects, particularly on the coronary circulation, make them especially valuable in treating angina caused by coronary vasospasm (Prinzmetal's angina). However, cal-

## Understanding PTCA

In percutaneous transluminal coronary angioplasty (PTCA), a balloon catheter is repeatedly inflated within a coronary artery to split atherosclerotic plaque. If your patient will undergo this procedure, here's what to expect.

### During the procedure
A local anesthetic is administered in the groin area, and the femoral vein and artery are punctured. A bipolar pacing catheter is inserted through the femoral vein so that it's available if needed. A guide catheter is then inserted into the artery.

Once the guide catheter is in place, the doctor inserts a smaller double-lumen balloon catheter (or angioplasty catheter) through the guide catheter. Using a thin, flexible guide wire, he then threads the catheter up through the aorta into the coronary artery to the area of stenosis. An arteriogram of the diseased artery is done to confirm place-ment of the catheter and for reference during and after PTCA. The balloon is then inflated repeatedly to achieve the greatest dilatation.

During balloon inflation, monitor the patient for angina, blood pressure changes, and tachycardia or bradycardia. Check his electrocardiogram for ST-segment changes signifying ischemia. As the viable myocardium becomes hypoperfused from balloon inflation, patients normally experience chest pain and reperfusion arrhythmias.

Keep emergency drugs, such as epinephrine, atropine, lidocaine, and narcotic analgesics, available.

### After the procedure
After dilatation is completed, the doctor probably will suture the arterial and venous sheaths in place. The sites are manually compressed until bleeding stops. Usually, the patient must stay in bed for 24 hours, keeping leg movement to a minimum.

cium channel blockers must be used with the utmost caution in patients with heart failure because they block the calcium influx that promotes contractility. Also, I.V. administration may induce hypotension.

*Antiplatelet agents and anticoagulants.* Preventing thrombus formation is crucial in managing unstable angina. Drug therapy should include an antiplatelet or anticoagulant agent, such as aspirin or heparin, in addition to a nitrate, a beta blocker, and a calcium channel blocker.

Studies show that aspirin reduces the risk of MI and death from heart disease in patients with unstable angina by up to 50%. Aspirin stabilizes the patient by minimizing further platelet aggregation and preventing reocclusion. Heparin also has been shown to reduce the incidence of MI in these patients. However, combining aspirin with heparin doesn't further reduce the incidence of MI.

*Thrombolytics.* Tissue plasminogen activator is a fibrin-specific enzyme that converts plasmin-ogen to plasmin. Such conversion ultimately leads to clot dissolution. Although thrombolytic therapy is an approved treatment for acute MI, its use in unstable angina remains experimental.

### Surgery
Within 1 year after stabilization through drug therapy, one-third of patients with unstable angina require coronary artery bypass graft (CABG) surgery. This procedure is a last resort for patients who don't respond to medical therapy and, possibly, angioplasty. By circumventing an occluded coronary artery with an autogenous graft, it restores blood flow to the myocardium.

Successful CABG surgery relieves angina in about 90% of patients, improves cardiac function, and may enhance the patient's quality of life. However, its long-term effectiveness remains uncertain.

CABG surgery can be performed with internal mammary artery grafts or saphenous vein grafts. The type of graft has no effect on the early postoperative outcome. However, inernal mammary artery grafts have shown superior long-term patency and have produced better patient survival rates.

CABG surgery techniques vary with the patient's condition and the number of arteries being bypassed. The most common procedure, aortocoronary bypass, involves suturing one end of the autogenous graft to the ascending aorta and the other end to a coronary artery distal to the occlusion.

Complications include myocardial dysfunction, cardiac tamponade, bleeding, arrhythmias, neurologic dysfunction, postpericardiotomy syndrome, and wound infection. Also, this surgery requires cardiopulmonary bypass, hemodilution, hypothermia, and anticoagulation, each of which may cause postoperative sequelae.

**Other treatments**
Within 1 year after stabilization, about one-third of patients with unstable angina require percutaneous transluminal coronary angioplasty (PTCA). This procedure may be performed during cardiac catheterization to compress fatty deposits and relieve occlusion. In patients with calcification, PTCA may reduce the obstruction by fracturing the plaque. (See *Understanding PTCA.*)

PTCA is a feasible alternative to CABG surgery in older patients and those who otherwise couldn't tolerate cardiac surgery. However, patients with left main coronary artery occlusion, lesions in extremely tortuous vessels, or occlusions older than 3 months aren't candidates for PTCA. Patients with an aneurysm just proximal or distal to a significant stenosis in an artery are also not candidates because the guide wire could cause thrombus dislodgment.

Although PTCA is effective for many patients with unstable angina, it is associated with more procedural complications and an increased risk of restenosis than when used in patients with stable angina. Administering heparin or thrombolytics before and during the procedure may help minimize these complications.

The most common complication of PTCA is dissection of the artery that was dilatated. Other complications include coronary insuffi-

ciency, MI, retroperitoneal bleeding, sudden coronary occlusion, vasovagal response, arrhythmias, and death (rare). Coronary atherectomy, an investigational form of PTCA, reduces the risk of thrombosis and vessel wall dissection. (See *Coronary atherectomy: An alternative to PTCA,* pages 22 and 23.)

## Nursing care
• Administer oxygen, insert an I.V. line, and begin cardiac monitoring as ordered for the patient with unstable angina.
• Assess vital signs frequently.
• If systolic blood pressure exceeds 90 mm Hg, administer nitroglycerin (sublingual or ointment) as ordered. For pain relief, give narcotics if ordered.
• Assess the patient for eligibility for thrombolytic therapy.
• Prepare the patient for diagnostic tests, such as a 12-lead ECG and chest X-ray as ordered.
• If the diagnostic evaluation indicates the need for PTCA, prepare the patient for this procedure and answer any questions he may have.

**Surgical care**
*Preoperative care.* For the patient undergoing CABG surgery, preoperative care consists of altering his medication regimen and preparing his chest for the operation.
• Discontinue anticoagulants, such as heparin, coumadin, and other medications with anticoagulant effects, 48 hours before surgery. Discontinue digitalis glycosides and withhold diuretics on the day of surgery so that the patient is adequately hydrated.
• Have the patient shower with antimicrobial soap the night before surgery. Remove hair from his chest down to his legs by shaving or depilation, if necessary.

*Postoperative care.* The CABG patient remains in the ICU until stable. He is placed on a ventilator until he has fully recovered from anesthesia, while a continuous heart monitor watches his heart rate and rhythm.
• Connect him to a nasogastric tube (for stomach drainage or decompression), a mediastinal tube (for chest blood and fluid drainage), a

## Coronary atherectomy: An alternative to PTCA

Atherectomy is a relatively new, experimental option for patients with certain coronary artery lesions. Unlike traditional percutaneous transluminal coronary angioplasty (PTCA), atherectomy removes plaque without the risk of thrombus formation. That's because the device used to perform the procedure cuts away or pulverizes the plaque, leaving the vessel walls intact and preventing proliferation of plaque and thrombus formation.

### Avoiding PTCA complications
During traditional PTCA, a balloon catheter is repeatedly inflated to split or fracture plaque. The arterial wall is stretched, enlarging the diameter of the vessel. The media and adventitia of the wall may stretch, causing a slight tear.

For these reasons, traditional PTCA leads to restenosis within 48 hours in about 6% of patients, and within 6 months in up to 40% of patients. Abrupt closure may stem from the dissection flap occluding the vessel, thrombus formation at the site, a spasm, or a combination of these factors. Later restenosis may result from smooth-cell proliferation at the ragged edges of the vessel and from hypertrophy.

In many cases, balloon angioplasty is done with atherectomy. Preliminary studies show that vessel walls aren't damaged when the balloon catheter is used after atherectomy. But the final results aren't available yet. Researchers only know that after 6 months, the restenosis rate is the same whether balloon angioplasty is done alone or as an adjunct to atherectomy.

### Understanding atherectomy devices
Three devices are currently used for atherectomy. The *AtheroCath* has Food and Drug Administration approval. The other two—the *transluminal extraction catheter* and the *Rotablator*—have yet to be approved. Both the AtheroCath and the transluminal extraction catheter use a cutting chamber to remove the plaque. The Rotablator leaves microparticles of plaque in the circulation.

Each device may be best suited for different vessel anomalies: the AtheroCath for large vessels or grafts with eccentric lesions; the transluminal extraction catheter for smaller vessels, tight lesions, or long, diffuse lesions; and the Rotablator for smaller vessels, distal lesions, or small, discrete lesions.

The transluminal extraction catheter is introduced by a guide wire and positioned proximal to the lesion. A cutter is turned on to about 750 revolutions/minute (rpm), and the plaque removed. Suction is applied simultaneously to draw the plaque into a collection device for removal.

The Rotablator, also introduced by a guide wire and positioned proximal to the lesion, uses an elliptically shaped, abrasive burr as a cutter. Made of

pulmonary artery catheter, or a pacemaker (used as backup if the heart rate is too slow) as ordered.
• Place sterile bandages over the incision site after the metal staples have been removed.
• Gently pat the incision site dry with a towel after bathing.
• Ensure that all lines are patent, watch the monitor for any unusual activity, and record any changes. Notify the doctor immediately of any drastic change in the patient's condition or of signs of incisional infection, such as redness, swelling, or drainage.

### Continuing care
• Two hours after initial administration of propranolol, assess blood pressure and heart rate with the patient in an upright position. If his blood pressure drops significantly, you may need to administer a vasopressor. Caution the patient not to stop taking propranolol abruptly because this could worsen his angina and induce an MI.
• Emphasize the importance of healthy eating habits. Offer specific suggestions to help the patient lower his dietary fat and cholesterol intake. (See *Teaching patients to lower fat intake,* page 24.)

diamond chips, the burr rotates at speeds up to 150,000 rpm to pulverize the plaque, which is then absorbed in the circulation.

One drawback of atherectomy catheters is that they can be cumbersome, particularly the Athero-Cath. And because the AtheroCath is large, balloon angioplasty must be done first in some cases to create enough room for the AtheroCath to be passed across the lesion.

## A closer look at the AtheroCath
Here's how the AtheroCath works:

The distal end of the atherectomy catheter is positioned across the stenosis, with the lesion within the cutting chamber, as shown below.

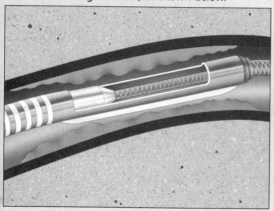

The balloon is inflated to secure the catheter. Then the cutter is advanced to shave off the plaque, below.

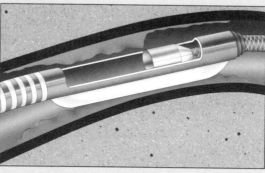

The plaque is now trapped in the cutting chamber and removed, below.

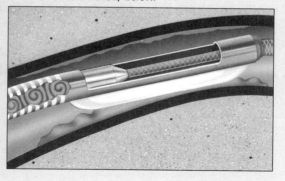

## Patient teaching
• Noncompliance with medical therapy and life-style modification is a serious problem among angina patients — one that may lead to death. To promote compliance, begin teaching early in the patient's hospitalization. Evaluate his anxiety level, readiness to learn, and support systems. Whenever possible, try to correct invalid health beliefs.
• Remind him that atherosclerosis is a progressive disease and that interventions won't have lasting effects unless he makes life-style changes.
• Teach the patient to identify events that precipitate angina attacks (such as exertion,

stress, overeating, or exposure to either cold or hot, humid conditions). Help him identify ways to minimize these events.
• Make sure the patient understands how to take prescribed medications. Teach him about nitrates, calcium channel blockers, beta blockers, and anticoagulants as needed. Review printed instructions and labels for readability.
• Suggest that he use medication compliance aids, such as pill boxes, muffin tins, egg cartons, or an ice cube tray; he may want to color-code these devices for days of the week and times of day. As necessary, help him set up the compliance aid.

## Teaching patients to lower fat intake

If fatty or fried foods are dietary staples for your patient, you'll need to motivate and encourage him to maintain his prescribed low-fat and low-cholesterol diet. Work with a dietitian and the family's primary food preparer to find ways to reduce the fat and cholesterol content of his favorite foods. To promote dietary modification and compliance, involve the whole family in making healthful dietary changes. Suggest these specific tips to lower fat and cholesterol intake:
• If a recipe calls for a greased pan, use a nonstick cooking spray.
• When roasting meat, use a rack so that meat doesn't sit in fat drippings while cooking.
• When using meat juices for gravy, first skim or pour off the fat. Baste meat with wine, fruit juice, or broth instead of fat drippings.
• Choose the leanest cuts of meat. Buy at least 85% lean ground beef, and drain off the extra fat when browning meat for spaghetti or casseroles.
• To sauté onions or other vegetables, use a small amount of broth or water instead of oil.
• Use two egg whites in place of a whole egg in scrambled eggs and baked goods.
• Use "light" mayonnaise and low-fat yogurt as a dressing for chicken or tuna salad.
• When dining out, eat at restaurants that offer "heart-healthy" menu items.

• Include the family in your teaching whenever possible.
• Be as specific as possible — patients prefer specific instructions to generalizations. For example, tell the patient why each CAD risk factor is dangerous.
• Be creative in your teaching techniques. Use the patient's peers, such as a person who has been through a cardiac rehabilitation program, to discuss realistic expectations. Remember, patients who feel capable of changing their behavior are more likely to do so.
• Make sure all caregivers provide consistent teaching.
• Evaluate the patient's learning. Be aware that

during hospitalization, recall of learning may be poor. Make sure the patient has resources to continue his learning after discharge. An outpatient cardiac rehabilitation program, for example, is an ideal setting for continued learning and provides support for risk-factor modification.
• Refer the patient to an outpatient cardiac rehabilitation center or a cardiovascular fitness program near his home or workplace. The staff can set up an exercise program that best meets his needs and limitations. To enhance his commitment to the exercise program, encourage family members or a friend to join in the physical activity.
• Refer the patient to a smoking-cessation program as needed. Acknowledge that quitting may be difficult, but urge him to make every attempt to stop smoking immediately and never restart.
• Refer the patient to a weight-control program as necessary.

# Congestive heart failure

Congestive heart failure (CHF) is a syndrome of myocardial dysfunction that causes diminished cardiac output, outright heart failure, or congestion. It occurs when the heart can't pump effectively to meet the body's metabolic needs.

CHF may result from left or right ventricular failure. However, because a properly functioning heart depends on both ventricles, failure of one ventricle almost always leads to failure of the other.

CHF is classified as left or right ventricular, high- or low-output, acute or chronic, and forward or backward. (See Classifying heart failure.)

With more patients surviving cardiac damage or living long enough to develop cardiac weakness, the incidence of CHF is increasing. CHF has become the most common diagnosis in hospitalized patients over age 65. Despite newer treatment options, the 5-year mortality from CHF remains as high as 50% even as mortality from other heart diseases declines.

# Classifying heart failure

Although heart failure is usually classified by the failure site (left ventricle, right ventricle, or even both), it can also be classified by the level of cardiac output (high or low), the stage (acute or chronic), or the direction (forward or backward). But note that these classifications represent different clinical aspects of heart failure, and not distinct diseases.

## Left and right ventricular failure

Failure of the left ventricle to pump blood to the vital organs and periphery usually results from myocardial infarction (MI). Decreased left ventricular output causes fluid to accumulate in the lungs, producing dyspnea, orthopnea, and paroxysmal nocturnal dyspnea.

In right ventricular failure, the right ventricle can't pump sufficient blood to the lungs. The typical underlying cause is a disorder that raises pulmonary vascular resistance, such as pulmonary embolism, pulmonary artery stenosis, or pulmonary hypertension. Right ventricular failure produces congestive hepatomegaly, ascites, and edema.

## High- and low-output failure

High-output failure occurs when the tissue's demands for oxygenated blood exceed the heart's ability to supply it. This may occur in arteriovenous fistula, hyperthyroidism, anemia, sickle cell anemia, beriberi, Paget's disease of the bone, thyrotoxicosis, and pregnancy. Clinical indicators include warm extremities and wide, bounding pulses.

Low-output failure, caused by impaired myocardial pumping, occurs in coronary artery disease, hypertension, primary myocardial disease, and valvular disease. It leads to impaired peripheral circulation and compensatory vasoconstriction, as reflected by pallor, cold skin, cyanotic extremities, decreased stroke volume, and narrow pulse pressure.

## Acute and chronic failure

The heart fails suddenly in acute heart failure, producing an abrupt fall in cardiac output. This causes systemic hypotension without peripheral edema and reduces organ perfusion so rapidly that the autonomic nervous system can't compensate effectively. Pulmonary edema and circulatory collapse result. Acute heart failure may occur in a chronic condition—for example, when a patient with chronic heart failure experiences acute heart failure with MI. Or it may result from any condition that stresses an already diseased heart.

Developing gradually, chronic heart failure may continue for prolonged periods. It doesn't decrease arterial blood pressure, but it does lead to peripheral edema. Chronic failure may occur in cardiomyopathy or multivalvular disease or after an extensive MI that has healed.

## Forward and backward failure

In forward heart failure, the heart can't expel enough blood into the arterial system. Diminished cardiac output compromises vital organ perfusion and leads to confusion; muscle weakness; renal, mesenteric, or hepatic insufficiency; and shock. Sodium and water are retained as a result of impaired renal perfusion and excessive distal tubular reabsorption, activating the renin-angiotensin-aldosterone system and increasing water absorption, plasma volume, cardiac output, and blood pressure.

In backward heart failure, one ventricle fails to empty its contents normally and end-diastolic ventricular pressure rises. Blood accumulates in the heart chambers and venous system, causing fluid extravasation from the capillaries into the interstitium and producing signs and symptoms of congestion. Pressures and volumes in the atrium also rise. Elevated systemic venous and capillary pressures and the resulting transudation of fluid into the interstitial space cause sodium and water retention.

**Causes**
A wide range of pathophysiologic processes can cause CHF. The syndrome commonly results from conditions that directly damage the heart—such as MI, myocarditis, myocardial fi-

brosis, or ventricular aneurysm—thus leading to decreased contractility.

Another cause of CHF is ventricular overload, caused by volume overload (increased preload) due to aortic insufficiency or a ventricular septal defect; pressure overload (increased afterload) due to aortic or pulmonic stenosis; and systemic or pulmonary hypertension. CHF may also be caused by restricted ventricular diastolic filling (characterized by too little blood for the ventricle to pump) triggered by constrictive pericarditis or cardiomyopathy, tachyarrhythmias, cardiac tamponade, or mitral stenosis.

*Precipitating factors.* Certain conditions can predispose a person to CHF, especially if he has an underlying disease. These include:
• arrhythmias, such as tachyarrhythmias, which can reduce ventricular filling time; bradycardias, which can reduce cardiac output; and arrhythmias that disrupt normal atrial and ventricular filling synchrony
• anemia, which speeds the heart rate as a compensatory mechanism to maintain tissue oxygenation
• pregnancy and thyrotoxicosis, which increase the demand for cardiac output
• infections, which increase metabolic demands and further burden the heart
• increased physical activity, emotional stress, greater sodium or water intake, or failure to comply with the prescribed treatment regimen for underlying heart disease
• pulmonary embolism, which elevates the pulmonary arterial pressures that can cause right ventricular failure.

## Pathophysiology
Normally, the pumping actions of the right and left sides of the heart complement each other, producing a synchronized and continuous blood flow. With an underlying disorder, though, one side may fail while the other continues to function normally for some time. Because of the prolonged strain, the functioning side eventually fails, resulting in total heart failure.

Usually, the heart's left side fails first. Left ventricular failure typically leads to, and is the main cause of, right ventricular failure. Here's what happens: Diminished left ventricular function allows blood to pool in the ventricle and atrium and eventually to back up into the pulmonary veins and capillaries. As the pulmonary

circulation becomes engorged, rising capillary pressure pushes sodium and water into the interstitial space, causing pulmonary edema.

When the patient lies down, fluid in the extremities moves into the systemic circulation. Because the left ventricle can't handle the increased venous return, fluid pools in the pulmonary circulation, worsening pulmonary edema. The right ventricle becomes stressed because it is pumping against greater pulmonary vascular resistance and left ventricular pressure.

As the right ventricle starts to fail, symptoms worsen. Blood pools in the right ventricle and right atrium. The backed-up blood causes pressure and congestion in the vena cava and systemic circulation. Blood also distends the visceral veins, especially the hepatic vein. As the liver and spleen become engorged, their function is impaired. Rising capillary pressure forces excess fluid from the capillaries into the interstitial space. This causes tissue edema, especially in the lower extremities and abdomen.

The chronically overloaded heart resorts to compensatory mechanisms to try to maintain adequate cardiac output. These mechanisms include hypertrophy of the heart wall, dilation of the heart chambers, and sympathetic nervous system activation. (See *Compensatory mechanisms in congestive heart failure.*)

## Complications
Pulmonary congestion can lead to pulmonary edema, a life-threatening condition. Decreased perfusion to major organs, particularly the brain and kidneys, may cause these organs to fail, necessitating dialysis for kidney failure. The patient's level of consciousness may decrease, possibly leading to coma. And MI may occur because myocardial oxygen demands can't be sufficiently met.

## Assessment
### Signs and symptoms
The patient's history usually reveals a condition that precipitated heart failure. With left ventricular failure, expect complaints of fatigue, exertional dyspnea, orthopnea, and weakness. The patient may report dyspnea that worsens at night when he lies down. He may use two

PATHOPHYSIOLOGY

# Compensatory mechanisms in congestive heart failure

When the heart begins to fail, the body responds with compensatory mechanisms to maintain blood flow to the periphery. In the short term, these mechanisms may help keep the failing heart going. But ultimately, they worsen congestive heart failure (CHF).

## Cardiac hypertrophy

When the heart is under strain, it responds by increasing its muscle mass. As the cardiac wall thickens, the heart's demand for blood and oxygen grows. The CHF patient may be unable to meet this demand, further compromising his condition.

## Cardiac dilation

When pressure inside the chambers (usually the left ventricle) rises for a sustained period, the heart compensates by dilating, or stretching. As muscle fibers stretch, their contractile force increases and they need more oxygen for contraction. Eventually, stretched muscle fibers become overstrained, reducing the heart's ability to pump.

## Sympathetic nervous system stimulation

Diminished cardiac output activates the sympathetic nervous system. Sympathetic stimulation leads to release of the catecholamines epinephrine and norepinephrine, causing an increased heart rate and myocardial contractility. Blood then shunts away from areas of low priority (such as the skin and kidneys) to areas of high priority, such as the heart and brain.

## Renin-angiotensin-aldosterone activation

Sensing the reduced renal blood flow, the kidneys activate the renin-angiotensin-aldosterone system. In the lungs, angiotensin I is converted to angiotensin II by angiotensin-converting enzyme. Angiotensin II is a potent vasoconstrictor, so afterload increases. Angiotensin II is then degraded to angiotensin III, which activates release of the hormone aldosterone. Aldosterone ultimately increases preload by promoting sodium and water uptake in the kidneys.

---

or three pillows to elevate his head to sleep, or he may have to sleep sitting up in a chair. Shortness of breath may awaken him shortly after he falls asleep, forcing him to quickly sit upright to catch his breath. He may have dyspnea, coughing, and wheezing even when he sits up (paroxysmal nocturnal dyspnea).

With right ventricular failure, the patient may complain of a slight but persistent cold and a dry cough combined with wheezing. Such symptoms may be mistaken for an allergic reaction, but inspection will reveal venous engorgement. When the patient sits upright, his neck veins may appear distended, feel rigid, and exhibit exaggerated pulsations. You may assess hepatomegaly.

Progression of CHF may lead to tachypnea, palpitations, dependent edema, unexplained steady weight gain, nausea, chest tightness, slowed mental response, anorexia, hypotension, diaphoresis, pallor, and oliguria. You may note

crackles on inspiration. The liver may be palpable and slightly tender.

In advanced CHF, pulse pressure may be diminished, reflecting reduced stroke volume. Occasionally, diastolic pressure rises from generalized vasoconstriction. Auscultation of the heart may disclose $S_3$ and $S_4$ sounds. The skin feels cool and clammy; the lips and nail beds may be cyanotic. You may note basal pulmonary crackles, hemoptysis, bronchospasm with wheezing, congestive hepatomegaly, dependent edema, ascites, confusion, and jaundice.

If pulmonary edema is present, you'll hear crackles throughout the lungs, accompanied by rhonchi and expiratory wheezing. (See *Responding to pulmonary edema*, page 29.)

## Diagnostic tests

Because the causes of CHF are so varied, many tests may be needed to pinpoint the underlying disease or condition. Diagnostic tests also help evaluate the degree of CHF and confirm the presence of coexisting diseases or complications. (See *Chronic obstructive pulmonary disease in the patient with CHF,* page 30.)

**Chest X-ray.** The most important diagnostic tool in assessing and monitoring CHF, this test reveals initial abnormalities, such as prominent and congested upper-lobe pulmonary veins. It also shows later changes, such as interstitial pulmonary edema and pulmonary effusion, as well as the degree of heart enlargement.

**ECG.** Although an ECG can't detect CHF, it can reveal arrhythmias and changes resulting from myocardial ischemia or infarction.

**Exercise ECG.** A graded exercise stress test may confirm cardiovascular disease and help assess the patient's ability to perform physical work.

**Echocardiography.** This test reveals enlargement of the heart chambers and evaluates ventricular function.

**Pulmonary artery pressure (PAP) measurement.** This test typically reveals elevated PAP and pulmonary artery wedge pressure (PAWP), increased left ventricular end-diastolic pressure in left ventricular failure, and elevated right atrial or central venous pressure (CVP) in right ventricular failure.

## Treatment
CHF is a medical emergency. Relieving dyspnea and improving arterial oxygenation are the immediate therapeutic goals. Secondary goals include minimizing or eliminating the underlying cause of CHF, reducing sodium and water retention, decreasing cardiac preload and afterload, and enhancing myocardial contractility.

### Drug therapy
Management of CHF usually requires one or more medications, such as diuretics, vasodilators, and inotropic agents.

**Diuretics.** The starting point of most CHF drug therapy, diuretic therapy increases sodium and water elimination by the kidneys. By reducing fluid overload, diuretics decrease total blood volume and relieve circulatory congestion. But for diuretics to work effectively, the patient must control his sodium intake.

Diuretic agents include thiazide diuretics, which act on the distal convoluted tubule to inhibit filtered sodium, and loop diuretics, such as furosemide or bumetanide, which act on the ascending loop of Henle. Because thiazide and loop diuretics work at different sites in the nephron, they produce a synergistic effect when given in combination.

Diuretic therapy decreases exertional dyspnea and relieves orthopnea, paroxysmal nocturnal dyspnea, and peripheral edema. It also increases urine output and reduces weight, abdominal girth, jugular vein distention, pulmonary crackles, and S$_3$ gallop. Among its important hemodynamic benefits are a decrease in PAWP and mean PAP.

Patients on diuretic therapy require careful monitoring because these drugs may disturb their electrolyte balances and lead to metabolic alkalosis or acidosis and other complications. (See *Managing adverse reactions to diuretic therapy,* page 31.)

**Vasodilators.** By decreasing arterial and venous vasoconstriction, vasodilators can reduce preload, afterload, or both. Reducing preload and afterload helps increase stroke volume and cardiac output. Vasodilator therapy is the only CHF treatment that's been proven to reduce mortality.

Vasodilators traditionally have been classified as arterial, venous, or balanced (combination). Generally, arterial dilators reduce afterload, venous dilators reduce preload, and balanced dilators reduce both preload and afterload. However, none of the current vasodilators have purely arteriodilating or venodilating properties. All vasodilators cause some reduction in both preload and afterload, and agents are classified on the basis of their major pharmacologic effects. Also, all vasodilators induce vasoconstrictive responses, which differ greatly among patients.

COMPLICATIONS

# Responding to pulmonary edema

If a patient with congestive heart failure develops pulmonary edema, a common complication, you'll need to adjust your nursing care according to the stage of the disease. Use this chart to help assess the patient and guide your responses.

| DISEASE STAGE | PATHOPHYSIOLOGY | SIGNS AND SYMPTOMS | NURSING INTERVENTIONS |
|---|---|---|---|
| Initial stage | Left ventricular failure increases pulmonary vascular bed pressure, forcing fluid and solutes from the intravascular compartment into lung interstitium. As the interstitium becomes overloaded, fluid enters peripheral alveoli, impairing gas exchange. | • Persistent, productive cough<br>• Slight dyspnea<br>• Diastolic gallop<br>• Crackles at lung bases<br>• Exercise intolerance | • Check color and amount of sputum.<br>• Position patient for comfort.<br>• Auscultate chest for crackles and $S_3$.<br>• Monitor apical and radial pulses.<br>• Assist with activities of daily living to conserve energy.<br>• Provide emotional support to patient and family. |
| Acute stage | Fluid accumulates throughout pulmonary vasculature, with further filling of the alveoli. | • Acute dyspnea<br>• Rapid, noisy respirations (wheezes)<br>• Cough producing blood-tinged sputum<br>• Cyanosis; cold, clammy skin<br>• Tachycardia, arrhythmias<br>• Hypotension | • Administer oxygen as ordered.<br>• Establish I.V. access.<br>• Suction as needed.<br>• Draw arterial blood gas sample.<br>• Apply rotating tourniquets as ordered.<br>• Give digitalis glycosides, morphine, furosemide, and vasodilators, as ordered.<br>• Insert indwelling urinary catheter; maintain adequate intake and output.<br>• Maintain cardiac monitoring.<br>• Keep resuscitation equipment available. |
| Advanced stage | Bronchial tree fills with fluid, causing rapid deterioration. | • Decreased level of consciousness<br>• Shock, ventricular arrhythmias<br>• Diminished breath sounds | • Be prepared to assist with cardioversion.<br>• Assist with intubation and mechanical ventilation, and resuscitate as necessary. |

*Angiotensin-converting enzyme (ACE) inhibitors.* ACE inhibitors, such as captopril, enalapril maleate, and lisinopril, decrease both afterload and preload by lowering angiotensin II production.

These drugs cause few adverse reactions. Hypotension, the most common problem, can be alleviated through proper dose titration. Because ACE inhibitors prevent potassium loss, hyperkalemia may develop in patients receiving concomitant potassium-sparing diuretics. For this reason, these diuretics should be discontinued when ACE inhibitor therapy begins.

*Nitrates.* Primarily venodilators, nitrates also dilate arterial smooth muscle at higher doses. Most CHF patients tolerate nitrates well. Adverse effects, such as headache, flushing, hypotension, and dizziness, usually are mild and transient.

Nitrates are available in several forms. In CHF therapy, I.V., oral, topical ointment, or patches are the most useful forms. To prevent

MULTIPLE DIAGNOSIS

# Chronic obstructive pulmonary disease in the patient with CHF

If your patient with congestive heart failure (CHF) also has chronic obstructive pulmonary disease (COPD), he'll need special care to reduce hypertension and maintain homeostasis.

## Pathophysiology
As obstructive lung disease progresses, pulmonary hypertension increases the heart's work load. To compensate, the right ventricle hypertrophies to force blood through the lungs. Eventually, as compensatory mechanisms fail, the right ventricle becomes overdilated.

   If this situation is coupled with left ventricular failure, the patient's condition worsens. Fluid backs up into the pulmonary vasculature, exacerbating COPD and potentially provoking biventricular failure.

## Interventions
• Goals of therapy are to reduce hypoxemia, increase the patient's exercise tolerance and, when possible, correct the underlying cause of heart failure or of COPD. Besides bed rest, treatment may include digitalis glycosides, a pulmonary artery vasodilator (such as diazoxide, nitroprusside, or hydralazine), and antibiotics to treat underlying respiratory tract infection. The patient probably will need oxygen therapy and, in acute cases, mechanical ventilation.
• Prevent fluid retention associated with CHF by limiting the patient's fluid intake to 1,000 to 2,000 ml/day. Clarify this need for fluid restriction, because patients with COPD are often encouraged to drink up to 10 glasses of water daily.
• Reposition a bedridden patient frequently to prevent atelectasis, but otherwise limit such procedures. Energy conservation is important in CHF.
• Evaluate your patient for complaints of chronic productive cough, exertional dyspnea, fatigue, and weakness. Expect wheezing respirations with crackles and rhonchi, tachypnea, dependent edema, distended neck veins, and an $S_3$ gallop. Depending on the severity of COPD and CHF, hepatomegaly, edema, ascites, and pleural effusions may occur.
• Provide meticulous respiratory care. Teach the patient how to perform pursed-lip breathing, and instruct him to rinse his mouth after respiratory therapy.

---

nitrate tolerance, drug-free intervals of 8 to 12 hours (while the patient is sleeping if possible) are necessary.

*Hydralazine.* This direct-acting arterial vasodilator is reserved for patients who don't respond to an adequate trial of ACE inhibitors, nitrates, or both. Adverse effects include nausea, vomiting, and exacerbation of angina or MI. Many patients can't tolerate long-term hydralazine therapy.

*Nitroprusside.* This I.V. agent has balanced vasodilating effects on arteries and veins. It is used in patients who have severe ventricular failure with adequate blood pressure and elevated PAWP.

   The major adverse effect of nitroprusside is hypotension. However, the drug has a very short duration (5 to 15 minutes) and can be titrated rapidly to minimize this problem. Nitroprusside is converted to thiocyanate in the body. Patients on prolonged therapy or those with renal dysfunction may develop thiocyanate toxicity, indicated by confusion, seizures, metabolic acidosis, and lethargy.

*Inotropic drugs.* These agents increase contractility in the failing myocardium. Digoxin is the only oral inotropic agent approved in the United States. Besides increasing contractility, digoxin slows atrioventricular (AV) node conduction and decreases systemic venous tone in CHF patients.

   Digitalis toxicity occurs in many patients, causing nausea, vomiting, anorexia, malaise, headache, and altered color vision.

*Sympathomimetics.* Dopamine, dobutamine, and amrinone may be indicated in acute CHF

COMPLICATIONS

# Managing adverse reactions to diuretic therapy

Although diuretics are the mainstay of treatment for congestive heart failure, they can cause serious electrolyte and metabolic imbalances. Here are some guidelines to help you recognize these imbalances and respond appropriately.

## Monitoring electrolyte imbalances
• Closely monitor the patient's serum electrolyte levels and arterial blood gas values.
• Stay alert for hypokalemia, which may result from increased potassium excretion. Signs and symptoms include lethargy, weakness, somnolence, muscle cramps, and arrhythmias. To correct hypokalemia, you may need to administer oral or I.V. potassium supplements.
• Assess for hypomagnesemia, which may accompany hypokalemia. Symptoms of hypomagnesemia may be neurologic (mood alterations, apathy and depression, agitation, hallucinations), neuromuscular (paresthesia, muscle tremors, weakness), GI (nausea and vomiting), and cardiac (prolonged PR and QT intervals, and a flat, wide T wave on the electrocardiogram). The patient's risk for digitalis toxicity also increases. Treatment consists of oral or parenteral magnesium replacement, followed by potassium supplements.
• To detect hyponatremia, assess your patient for lethargy, somnolence, and weakness. To combat hyponatremia, restrict fluids and temporarily discontinue diuretic therapy.

## Monitoring metabolic imbalances
• Decreased serum potassium can cause metabolic alkalosis. In metabolic alkalosis, the patient's pH and bicarbonate levels are elevated. Signs and symptoms include irritability, vertigo, muscle weakness, anorexia, nausea and vomiting, and decreased bowel motility. Treatment involves reducing the diuretic dose or adding acetazolamide for short-term therapy to restore a normal acid-base balance.
• Your patient may suffer metabolic acidosis if he receives acetazolamide continuously or if potassium-sparing diuretics induce hyperkalemia. Signs and symptoms of hyperkalemia include numbness, bradycardia, a wide QRS interval and tall, peaked T waves on the electrocardiogram.
• Chronic administration of thiazide or loop diuretics may cause hyperuricemia. This problem seldom warrants additional treatment. However, if the patient is symptomatic and does require continued diuretic therapy, the doctor may prescribe allopurinol.
• Ototoxicity may develop with high I.V. doses of loop diuretics. Signs and symptoms of ototoxicity include slight hearing loss, tinnitus, ear pain, vertigo, blurred vision, motion intolerance, nausea, and vomiting. To help prevent this complication, administer diuretics slowly.

---

to increase myocardial contractility and cardiac output.

**Morphine.** This drug is commonly used in CHF patients with acute pulmonary edema. Besides reducing anxiety, it decreases preload and afterload by dilating veins.

**Theophylline.** Also used to treat pulmonary edema, I.V. theophylline augments the diuretic action of thiazides, reduces venous filling, relieves dyspnea, and increases cardiac output. However, it has largely been replaced by diuretics.

**Surgery**
For patients with severe CHF who don't respond to drug therapy, surgery is the last resort. All candidates must have adequately functioning neuromuscular, pulmonary, hepatic, and renal systems and, for cardiomyoplasty, an intact latissimus dorsi muscle.

**Intra-aortic balloon counterpulsation (IABC).**
This procedure is indicated for selected patients with severe, acute left ventricular failure. Its goals are to increase systemic circulation, improve coronary perfusion, and reduce left ventricular work load.

The IABC device consists of a single-chamber or multichamber polyurethane balloon attached to an external pump console by a large-lumen catheter. A doctor advances the catheter up the patient's descending thoracic aorta to a point just distal to the left subclavian artery. The pump console inflates the balloon with helium or carbon dioxide during diastole and deflates it during systole. Called counterpulsation, this inflation-deflation cycle is synchronized with the patient's ECG, which appears on the console's oscilloscope.

Aortic or femoral artery dissection or perforation may occur during balloon insertion. Other complications include ischemia or loss of pulses in the extremities from compromised circulation.

*Ventricular assist devices (VADs).* These battery-powered devices replace the work of a failing ventricle by imitating the ventricle's pumping action. Left VADs are used more often than right VADs because left ventricular failure is more common than right ventricular failure. A left VAD diverts oxygenated blood from the left side of the heart (from either the atrium or the ventricle) to an artificial pump; blood returns to the arterial circulation via a catheter in the aorta.

VADs are indicated for patients who can't be weaned from cardiopulmonary bypass because of persistent ventricular failure and who will benefit from temporary circulatory assistance. If ventricular failure is reversible, VADs can provide temporary circulatory support while the myocardium rests and recovers.

*Heart transplantation.* For a select group of patients with end-stage CHF unresponsive to other treatments, heart transplantation may be considered. The advent of cyclosporine, an immunosuppressant, has dramatically increased the once-poor survival rate for heart transplant recipients. (See *Selecting candidates for heart transplantation.*)

*Cardiomyoplasty.* The use of skeletal muscle tissue to augment cardiac function is an exciting new development in cardiac surgery. In car-diomyoplasty, skeletal muscle (usually from the latissimus dorsi) is wrapped around the heart to aid ventricular contraction and pacemaker electrodes are placed in the transplanted muscle. About 2 weeks after surgery, the pacemaker is turned on to stimulate the transplanted latissimus dorsi muscle to contract simultaneously with the heart. Over the next 6 to 10 weeks, the degree of stimulation is increased gradually until the transplanted latissimus dorsi muscle contracts vigorously in time with the heart. Eventually, this muscle undergoes biochemical changes that make it biologically similar to heart muscle.

Major postoperative complications include heart failure, arrhythmias, respiratory failure, and sepsis. Care for the cardiomyoplasty patient is similar to that for other heart surgery patients. However, because the procedure doesn't involve open-heart surgery, this patient won't experience such problems as massive fluid shifts from cardiopulmonary bypass and rewarming. On the other hand, he may show symptoms of low cardiac output, such as hypotension, pulmonary edema, renal failure, and arrhythmias.

### Tourniquets
Rotating tourniquets may be used in CHF patients with pulmonary edema. These devices remove blood from the central circulation by temporarily pooling it in the extremities, decreasing venous return and blood output from the right ventricle.

Tourniquets are applied to three extremities and inflated to a pressure slightly above the patient's diastolic pressure. Every 15 minutes, the tourniquets are rotated, usually in a clockwise fashion. (If the patient is an older adult or has poor circulation, the tourniquets may have to be rotated as often as every 5 minutes to prevent tissue damage and formation of thrombi.) Keeping the cuffs inflated at diastolic pressure occludes venous flow but leaves arterial flow intact. Circulatory checks of extremities with tourniquets should reveal cool, cyanotic skin with a palpable pulse distal to the tourniquet.

## Nursing care
• Place the patient in Fowler's position and give supplemental oxygen as ordered, to help him breathe more easily.
• Administer medications as ordered. Pain control is usually managed by the patient with a patient-controlled analgesic pump.
• When administering morphine, observe the patient's respiratory status closely because the drug decreases the respiratory rate and depth.
• Obtain vital signs, checking especially for increased heart and respiratory rates and for narrowing pulse pressure. Auscultate for abnormal heart sounds, crackles, and rhonchi. Assess the patient's mental status. Report any changes in vital signs or mentation immediately.
• For the patient undergoing cardiomyoplasty, wound care involves sternotomy plus left posterior chest incision. Ensure the sterility and patency of pleural chest tubes and suction drains to promote complete drainage of the posterior wound.
• Begin latissimus dorsi stimulation 2 weeks after cardiomyoplasty. The stimulation protocol is designed to condition the patient's muscles to improve his hemodynamic response.
• Weigh the patient daily to evaluate for fluid retention, and check for peripheral edema. Monitor intake and output closely, especially if the patient is receiving diuretics.
• Frequently monitor blood urea nitrogen (BUN) and serum creatinine, potassium, sodium, chloride, and magnesium levels.
• Maintain continuous cardiac monitoring during acute and advanced disease stages to identify arrhythmias promptly.
• Encourage independent activities of daily living. Also encourage the patient's gradual use of his left arm and shoulder.
• Sodium restriction, essential in managing CHF, usually begins early in treatment to reduce preload, decrease myocardial oxygen demand, and enhance diuretic therapy. If necessary, advise the patient about ordered restrictions on fluid intake; some experts recommend limiting fluid intake to 2 liters/day to help control symptoms. In severe CHF, fluid restriction may be essential.

## Selecting candidates for heart transplantation

Although selection criteria for heart transplant recipients vary with different transplantation centers, they generally include:
• end-stage cardiomyopathy refractory to all other therapy
• expected survival of less than 1 year (without transplantation)
• upper age limit of 60
• absence of irreversible hepatic, renal, or pulmonary disease
• absence of any systemic illness that would otherwise limit life expectancy, such as Type I (insulin-dependent) diabetes mellitus
• psychological stability. Rigorous postoperative regimens, including frequent follow-up examinations and biopsies, are crucial to the success of transplantation, so all candidates must undergo extensive psychosocial evaluation.

### Patient teaching
• Emphasize the need for adequate rest. Instruct the patient to alternate activity with scheduled rest periods.
• Teach proper skin care because CHF may promote skin breakdown.
• Help the patient manage stress and anxiety, which may be exacerbated by breathing difficulty and the diagnosis of CHF. To help the patient cope with stress more effectively, identify factors that precipitate and relieve stress.
• Provide or reinforce guidelines for regular exercise. Until recently, patients with CHF weren't considered candidates for exercise training programs. Instead, they were discharged from the hospital and advised to maintain a sedentary life-style. But many experts now believe patients with moderate to severe CHF can benefit from cardiac fitness training. Refer the patient to a cardiac exercise training program near his home or workplace.
• Tell the patient to weigh himself daily on the

same scale, wearing the same amount of clothing, to check for fluid retention. Tell him to call the doctor if he gains more than 1 lb (0.45 kg) per day for 3 consecutive days.
• Instruct the patient to call the doctor if his pulse rate is irregular or measures less than 60 beats/minute or if he experiences dizziness, blurred vision, shortness of breath, a persistent dry cough, palpitations, increased fatigue, paroxysmal nocturnal dyspnea, swollen ankles, or decreased urine output.

# Mitral stenosis

In this disorder, the heart valve leaflets become thickened by fibrosis and calcification. The mitral orifice narrows, obstructing blood flow from the left atrium to the left ventricle.

## Causes
Mitral stenosis usually occurs after a long latency period ranging from 10 to 40 years after the onset of rheumatic fever. Gender is a risk factor; most patients who develop mitral stenosis as a complication of rheumatic fever are female.

## Pathophysiology
Throughout the course of rheumatic fever, large hemorrhagic and fibrinous lesions grow along the inflamed edges of the heart valves. These lesions commonly develop on adjacent valve leaflets, causing the edges to adhere together. As the disease progresses, the leaflets become scarred and permanently fuse, limiting valvular movement of the normally free-flapping edges.

As the mitral valve opening narrows, left arterial pressure (LAP) rises, which in turn elevates pulmonary venous pressure and PAWP. These pathologic changes develop gradually, and signs and symptoms of a stenotic valve usually don't emerge until many years after rheumatic fever onset.

Mitral valve disease is classified by the range of motion (ROM) of the valve leaflets:
• normal ROM — leaflet perforation and cleft mitral valve, possibly with annular dilation

• excessive ROM — elongation of the chordae or papillary muscle and billowing leaflets (prolapse refers to more than a 2-mm projection of a mitral leaflet past the annulus)
• restricted ROM — fusion of the leaflets or subvalvular mechanism and spatial displacement of the papillary muscle.

## Complications
To accommodate the increased work load required to move blood through the narrowed mitral valve orifice, the left atrium hypertrophies. The resulting increase in LAP causes further pressure on the pulmonary vasculature, resulting in pulmonary hypertension and pulmonary congestion. Eventually, these conditions lead to right ventricular failure.

Atrial fibrillation may result from structural changes in the atrial wall caused by the increased pressure. The combination of atrial fibrillation and pooling of blood in the atria heightens the risk of thrombus formation and arterial embolization. Roughly 25% of patients with atrial fibrillation develop systemic thromboemboli.

## Assessment
### Signs and symptoms
In mild mitral stenosis, the patient may be asymptomatic. In moderate to severe stenosis, she may report dyspnea on exertion, paroxysmal nocturnal dyspnea, orthopnea, weakness, fatigue, and palpitations. Inquire about a history of rheumatic fever.

Auscultation of the heart reveals a middiastolic murmur, produced by blood flowing from the left atrium into the left ventricle. This murmur is most intense when the flow is greatest, after the opening snap of the mitral valve.

As stenosis worsens, atrial contraction may force more blood across the valve and produce presystolic accentuation of the diastolic murmur. When faint or moderately loud, the murmur is low-pitched and rumbling. As it becomes louder, it sounds harsher. Exercise intensifies the murmur.

To auscultate the murmur, have the patient turn from the supine to the left lateral position. Hold the bell of the stethoscope lightly on the skin (heavy pressure may obliterate a faint middiastolic murmur). The murmur usually is audible only over a small area just medial to and above the apex, or at the point of maximal intensity.

Other auscultation findings may include an increased $S_1$ and an opening snap of the mitral valve. However, $S_1$ may be decreased and the opening snap absent if the valve and chordae tendineae are fibrotic or if the mitral valve orifice is very narrow.

### Diagnostic tests

A chest X-ray shows left atrial and ventricular enlargement (in advanced mitral stenosis), a straightened left border of the cardiac silhouette, enlarged pulmonary arteries, dilation of the upper-lobe pulmonary veins, and mitral valve calcification.

An ECG reveals hypertrophy of the left atrium or right ventricle as well as specific arrhythmias, often atrial fibrillation. Echocardiography discloses thickened mitral valve leaflets and left atrial enlargement.

Cardiac catheterization typically shows a diastolic pressure gradient across the valve, along with elevated LAP and PAWP. This technique also detects elevated right ventricular pressure, decreased cardiac output, and abnormal contraction of the left ventricle.

Because cardiac catheterization is invasive, it's usually performed only after other diagnostic studies are done. It may not be indicated in patients who have isolated mitral stenosis with mild symptoms.

## Treatment

Therapy aims to prevent complications, such as systemic embolism or infective endocarditis (a postoperative risk following valve replacement), and to treat atrial fibrillation, if present.

### Drug therapy

Initial therapy for a symptomatic patient includes oral diuretics and sodium restriction. Patients with hemoptysis from elevated pulmonary vascular resistance require sedation and aggressive diuretic therapy. Pulmonary congestion may be relieved with combined dobutamine and isosorbide dinitrate therapy.

Arrhythmias — particularly atrial fibrillation — call for digitalis glycosides to slow the ventricular rate. For the first episode of atrial fibrillation, a younger patient with mild mitral stenosis may undergo cardioversion to help restore normal sinus rhythm. If the duration of atrial fibrillation is known, anticoagulant therapy begins 4 to 6 weeks before cardioversion. Successful cardioversion is usually followed by treatment with quinidine and digitalis glycosides to maintain normal sinus rhythm. Repeat cardioversion isn't recommended if the patient reverts to atrial fibrillation while on adequate doses of quinidine or if she has significant left atrial enlargement.

A small (1% to 2%) risk of systemic embolism has been reported after electrical or chemical cardioversion using quinidine or digoxin. The risk of embolism increases in patients with paroxysmal atrial fibrillation who've undergone repeated cardioversions. In such high-risk patients, anticoagulant therapy may help prevent this complication.

Vasodilators commonly are prescribed for patients with extensive mitral lesions. The goal of vasodilator therapy is to decrease the left ventricle's size, preserve its function and, possibly, delay surgical valve replacement. ACE inhibitors are typically used for vasodilator therapy because they cause fewer adverse effects than peripheral vasodilators, such as hydralazine. In addition, newer agents, such as enalapril and lisinopril, allow once- or twice-daily dosing.

To prevent infective endocarditis, the patient requires prompt antibiotic therapy for infections and she must receive prophylactic antibiotics before surgery or other invasive procedures. Anemia also warrants prompt treatment.

### Surgery

If the patient has severe symptoms that can't be managed medically, she may undergo surgery to repair or replace the mitral valve. In mitral insufficiency, valve repair is preferred over valve replacement for several reasons. Repair is associated with a lower perioperative mortality and a lower incidence of infective endocarditis; it also allows greater retention of

# Valve repair and replacement surgery

A patient with progressive valvular disease or unmanageable symptoms or complications may require surgery to replace or repair the affected valve. Repairing a valve is preferable to replacing one. However, replacement may be necessary if the valve is calcified and immobile. The doctor selects the best procedure for each patient from the range of options described below.

### Valve repair

The doctor will perform one of three procedures to repair a valve. *Percutaneous balloon valvuloplasty* decreases valvular stenosis by cardiac catheterization and a special balloon catheter. Most commonly used to treat aortic stenosis, this procedure doesn't require cardiac surgery. It's usually performed in the cardiac catheterization laboratory.

In *annuloplasty,* the doctor tightens and sutures the annulus ring of the malfunctioning valve. This procedure requires open-heart surgery with cardiopulmonary bypass.

*Commissurotomy* dilatates the valve's commissures to enlarge the valve opening. Although sometimes performed without cardiopulmonary bypass (closed), this procedure is usually performed with bypass (open) in the United States.

### Valve replacement

Replacing a valve requires open-heart surgery with cardiopulmonary bypass to remove the diseased valve and insert a *mechanical* or *bioprosthetic valve.*

When choosing the new heart valve, the doctor evaluates its design, durability, and hemodynamic qualities. The doctor also considers the patient's ability to comply with lifelong anticoagulant therapy. That's because thrombus formation is a common complication of mechanical valves, so the patient must take anticoagulants for the rest of his life and undergo regular prothrombin time testing.

A patient who's unlikely to comply may do better with a bioprosthetic valve, which doesn't require long-term anticoagulants.

Mechanical valves are made of metal or plastic, and are designed to open and close like natural valves. Several types of mechanical valves are available, including ball-cage and tilting-disk valves.

The ball-cage mechanical valve, shown at right, is more durable than the tilting-disk valve, but can be used only in patients with a large enough annulus and chamber to accommodate the cage. The ball-cage valve is never used for tricuspid valve replacement because of the size limitations of the right ventricle.

The tilting-disk mechanical valve, also shown at right, requires less space than the ball-cage valve. This valve tilts when open and returns to a flat position when closed. The tilting-disk valve poses a high risk of clot formation.

Bioprosthetic valves, like the one shown at right, are made from specially treated, transplanted animal (including porcine) or human valves (called a homograft).

With a porcine bioprosthesis, the patient receives anticoagulants for only about 3 months after implantation. Although less durable than a mechanical valve, this valve usually doesn't cause thrombus formation after healing is complete.

A homograft is a valve removed from a human cadaver and then frozen. When a valve replacement is needed, the donor valve is thawed, trimmed, and sewn into place. For obvious reasons, such a valve isn't always readily available. Homografts aren't used for tricuspid or mitral valve replacement. They have excellent hemodynamic qualities. They're unlikely to cause hemolysis or clot formation, so anticoagulant therapy is rarely necessary.

the mitral subvalvular apparatus, helping to preserve left ventricular function. (See *Valve repair and replacement surgery.*)

*Timing of surgery.* Serial echocardiographic assessment of left ventricular size and function helps determine the best time for valve repair or replacement. Proper timing ensures the best long-term results and helps avoid the progression to irreversible left ventricular abnormalities.

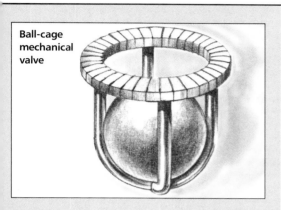

**Ball-cage mechanical valve**

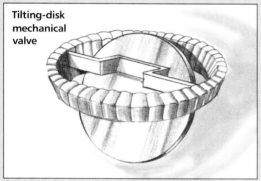

**Tilting-disk mechanical valve**

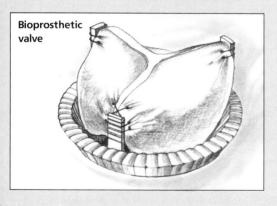

**Bioprosthetic valve**

Mitral valve repair has become the preferred operation for most patients with mitral insufficiency. Patients who are ideal candidates for valve repair are more likely to be considered for early surgery than are those who need valve replacement.

Early surgical intervention helps maintain cardiac function, lowers the risk of chronic atrial fibrillation, and increases the chance of success in patients with less advanced valvular disease. Also, with early surgery, patients are younger and healthier than they would be if surgery were delayed, so they tolerate the procedure better.

Early surgery does have certain disadvantages, including the risk of thromboembolism, endocarditis, anticoagulant complications, and the morbidity and mortality associated with any surgery. While delaying surgery may avoid multiple operations, it heightens the risk of irreversible changes in ventricular function.

### Percutaneous balloon valvuloplasty

This procedure evolved from PTCA and uses the same balloon-tipped catheters to enlarge the orifice of a heart valve. Performed in the cardiac catheterization laboratory, percutaneous balloon valvuloplasty may be indicated for young patients with no calcification or subvalvular deformity, for symptomatic pregnant women, and for older patients with end-stage disease who couldn't withstand general anesthesia.

Recent studies verify the short- and long-term efficacy of balloon valvuloplasty in patients with mitral stenosis. However, patients with advanced mitral valve disease or significant mitral insufficiency have had less than optimal results.

## Nursing care

• Evaluate the patient for indications of reduced cardiac output. These include dyspnea, angina, palpitations, syncope, peripheral edema, weight gain, and decreased ability to carry out activities of daily living.
• Auscultate the heart for rate and rhythm, presence or change in murmurs, and characteristic heart sounds at all auscultatory sites.
• Prepare the patient for ordered diagnostic tests, explaining their purpose and procedure.
• Administer medications as ordered.

## Surgical care

*Preoperative care.* To allay anxiety, listen to the patient's and family's concerns, provide teaching, and encourage them to ask questions.

• Reinforce and supplement the doctor's explanation of the procedure, as necessary. Tell the patient she'll awaken from surgery in an ICU or a postanesthesia room. Mention that she'll be connected to a cardiac monitor and have I.V. lines, an arterial line, and possibly a pulmonary artery (PA) or left atrial catheter. Explain that she'll breathe through an endotracheal tube connected to a mechanical ventilator and that she'll have a chest tube in place.

• As ordered, assist with insertion of an arterial line and possibly a PA catheter. Initiate cardiac monitoring as ordered.

• Administer medications as ordered. To decrease the risk of postoperative endocarditis, the patient may receive antibiotics. If she's been on anticoagulants, you may need to administer vitamin K to restore a normal prothrombin time (PT).

• If ordered, discontinue digitalis glycosides and diuretics before surgery to prevent arrhythmias associated with digitalis toxicity (which may be precipitated by cardiopulmonary bypass).

*Postoperative care.* After surgery, assess the patient frequently and prepare her for discharge.

• Closely monitor the patient's hemodynamic status for signs of compromise. Especially watch for severe hypotension, decreased cardiac output, and shock. Check and record vital signs every 15 minutes until her condition stabilizes. Assess heart sounds frequently; report distant sounds or new murmurs, which may indicate prosthetic valve failure. Reassure the patient that a clicking noise is normal with a prosthetic valve.

• Monitor the ECG for disturbances in heart rate and rhythm, such as bradycardia, ventricular tachycardia, and heart block. Such disturbances may indicate injury of the conduction system, which may occur during valve replacement because the atrial and mitral valves are near the AV node. Arrhythmias also may result from myocardial irritability or ischemia, fluid and electrolyte imbalance, hypoxemia, or hypothermia. If you detect abnormalities, notify the doctor and be prepared to assist with temporary epicardial pacing.

• To ensure adequate myocardial perfusion, maintain mean arterial pressure within the guidelines set by the doctor (usually between 70 and 100 mm Hg for adults). Monitor PAP and LAP as ordered.

• Frequently assess the patient's peripheral pulses, capillary refill time, skin temperature, and color. Evaluate tissue oxygenation by assessing breath sounds, chest excursion, and symmetry of chest expansion. Report any abnormalities. Check arterial blood gas values frequently, and adjust mechanical ventilator settings as needed.

• Maintain chest tube drainage at the ordered negative pressure (usually between −10 and −40 cm H$_2$O for adults). Observe for excessive drainage (more than 200 ml/hour) and a sudden decrease in or cessation of drainage.

• As ordered, administer analgesics, anticoagulants, antibiotics, antiarrhythmics, inotropic agents, and pressor drugs as well as I.V. fluids and blood products. Once anticoagulant therapy starts, evaluate its effectiveness by monitoring PT daily.

• Monitor fluid intake and output and assess for electrolyte imbalances, especially hypokalemia.

## Patient teaching

• Explain the medication regimen to the patient. She'll probably receive antibiotics for about 1 month after valve replacement.

• Identify activities of daily living that tire the patient and warrant assistance. Offer information on how to conserve energy. Instruct her to alternate periods of activity and rest. Mention that she may need supportive oxygen between activities. Counsel her to avoid activities that demand strenuous physical exertion.

• As needed, explain dietary modifications, such as sodium or fluid restrictions.

# Pericarditis

Pericarditis is an inflammation of the pericardium, the fibrous sac surrounding the heart. More common in men than in women, the disorder may be acute or chronic. Acute pericarditis, usually associated with systemic inflammation, may be fibrinous (dry) or effusive (with serous, purulent, or hemorrhagic exudate).

## Causes
Common causes of pericarditis include:
• blunt or penetrating trauma, for example, from a stab wound or rib fracture
• closed chest trauma, for example, from an automobile accident
• neoplasms, primarily lung or breast cancer, Hodgkin's disease or other lymphomas, and leukemia
• infections (viral, bacterial, or fungal)
• MI
• drugs, for example, hydralazine, procainamide, diphenylhydantoin, and isoniazid
• high-dose radiation to the chest
• hypersensitivity or autoimmune disorders, such as rheumatic fever, systemic lupus erythematosus, scleroderma, and rheumatoid arthritis
• uremia, especially now that renal dialysis is widely used in the palliative treatment of chronic renal disease
• idiopathic factors.

Early pericarditis may occur within 48 to 72 hours after myocardial damage from an MI. Dressler's syndrome (late pericarditis), an autoimmune reaction in the pericardium, may arise about 2 to 4 weeks after an MI. However, MI patients treated successfully with thrombolytic therapy rarely develop pericarditis, possibly due to reduced inflammation.

## Pathophysiology
Pericarditis can affect the serous pericardium's parietal or visceral layer. During the inflammatory process, the body sends leukocytes, fibrin, platelets, and fluid to the pericardium. Because inflamed capillaries are more permeable than usual, fluid and cellular debris may leak into surrounding tissue. If this material, or exudate,

accumulates in pericardial tissue, pain and other symptoms of pericarditis result. See *How pericarditis affects the pericardium,* page 40.)

Pericardial effusion occurs when fluid accumulates in the pericardial space. Although effusions can develop as a complication of inflammatory pericarditis, they can also occur as a primary condition — for example, from a cardiac injury that causes blood accumulation in the pericardial space.

Here's how to classify the various types of pericarditis.

*Acute inflammatory pericarditis.* Inflammation occurs in the pericardium without causing a significant increase in pericardial fluid. In some instances, thin, stringlike structures invade the pericardial sac, causing painful, fibrous adhesions. This disorder is usually associated with pericardial infection, MI, or open-heart surgery.

*Chronic constrictive or adhesive pericarditis.* After long-term fibrous invasion, the pericardium becomes abnormally thick and inflexible, constricting the heart and inhibiting ventricular filling. Possible causes include certain chronic systemic diseases (such as lupus erythematosus), prolonged therapy with certain drugs, and radiation. Pericardial adhesions can cause chronic pain.

*Acute exudative pericarditis (acute effusion).* A product of infection or inflammation, fluid accumulates rapidly in the pericardial space, compressing the heart and causing cardiac tamponade. A life-threatening emergency, this condition can be triggered by pericardial infection or MI. Acute effusion can also occur when blood accumulates rapidly in the pericardial space; possible causes include dissecting aneurysm and ventricular trauma during cardiac procedures (for example, removal of pacemaker wires).

*Chronic exudative pericarditis (chronic effusion).* Fluid accumulates gradually in the pericardial space or remains there for a prolonged time. Chronic effusion may develop as a com-

# How pericarditis affects the pericardium

In pericarditis, inflamed areas of the pericardium become permeable, and fluid and cellular debris leak into surrounding tissues and may begin to accumulate, causing pain and other symptoms. When pericarditis is long-term or chronic, adhesions begin to form and the pericardium becomes thick and inflexible.

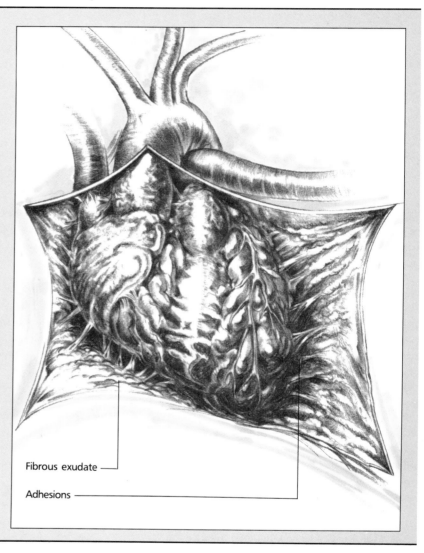

Fibrous exudate ———

Adhesions ———

plication of an inflammatory disorder or of a systemic condition, such as heart or kidney failure.

## Complications
Pericardial effusion is the major complication of acute pericarditis. Fluid accumulation in the pericardial sac may cause cardiac tamponade, which impairs ventricular filling and emptying.

Unless diagnosed and treated promptly, tamponade may severely reduce cardiac output, causing shock or death.

If pericardial constriction impedes cardiac output, pulmonary vascular pressures may increase. Fluid from the pulmonary capillary bed is pushed into the alveoli, causing pulmonary edema.

If fluid accumulates gradually, as in chronic

exudative pericarditis, the pericardium stretches to accommodate it and the patient may have only mild symptoms — even with an effusion as large as 1 to 2 liters. In contrast, rapid accumulation of a relatively small amount of fluid (150 ml) may cause cardiac tamponade.

## Assessment

### Signs and symptoms

Pericarditis typically develops during the course of another disease or disorder. So check the patient's history for an associated event, such as an MI, chest trauma, or recent infection. In acute inflammatory pericarditis, expect patient complaints of pain, fever, dyspnea, malaise, and myalgia.

*Pain assessment.* Pain associated with pericarditis is sharp and sudden, usually starting over the sternum and radiating to the neck, shoulders, back, and arms. Unlike MI pain, which is rarely affected by movement or position changes, pericardial pain is exacerbated by inspiration, coughing, swallowing, and trunk movement. Such movements bring the epicardium closer to the parietal pericardium, stimulating pain receptors in this layer. The pain may abate when the patient sits up and leans forward with forearms on legs (Mohammed's sign).

Characteristically, pain subsides or disappears when effusion develops. If pericarditis arises slowly, as after radiation therapy or with tuberculosis, neoplastic disease, or uremia, pain may be absent.

*Auscultation.* You may detect a pericardial friction rub — a rough, scratchy, grating sound resembling crunching snow or creaky leather. It's best heard at the left sternal border at the fourth intercostal space during end-expiration. Often, it's transient and variable in intensity. (See *Identifying a pericardial friction rub.*)

Occurring when the heart contracts and the inflamed pericardial layers move across each other, the friction rub may be a one-, two-, or three-component sound heard in addition to the normal sounds of atrial systole, ventricular systole, and ventricular diastole. Nor-

## Identifying a pericardial friction rub

It's easy to confuse friction rubs with other noises, such as extraneous stethoscope sounds, noise caused by hair on the chest, and murmurs. To distinguish between a pericardial friction rub and a pleural friction rub, use the diaphragm of the stethoscope and ask the patient to hold his breath during auscultation. A pleural rub is audible during each inspiration; a pericardial rub, during the heartbeat. Therefore, a pericardial rub won't stop when the patient holds his breath.

You may have to reposition the patient to hear a pericardial friction rub. If you're unsuccessful auscultating with the patient lying down, have him sit up, lean forward, and forcibly exhale.

mally, $S_1$, representing mitral and tricuspid valve closure, is louder than $S_2$, representing aortic and pulmonic valve closure. In pericarditis, however, $S_2$ may be louder because of the loud ventricular systolic component of the friction rub.

Pain typically develops before onset of the friction rub and may persist despite the absence of an audible sound. Occasionally, a pericardial friction rub lasts for several weeks.

If pericardial effusion develops, heart sounds may become distant or muffled. You may note signs and symptoms of elevated systemic venous pressure similar to those assessed in right ventricular failure (fluid retention, ascites, and hepatomegaly). $S_3$ suggests progression to constrictive pericarditis.

Watch for signs of cardiac tamponade, such as pallor, neck vein distention (secondary to increased CVP), muffled or diminished heart sounds, clammy skin, hypotension (secondary to ineffective myocardial pumping), pulsus paradoxus (a systolic pressure drop of 15 mm Hg or more during slow inspiration), narrowing pulse pressure (difference between systolic and diastolic pressures), diminished peripheral pulses, and dyspnea.

### Diagnostic tests

The ECG abnormalities observed in acute pericarditis reflect diffuse epicardial injury secondary to inflammation. The ECG also can help differentiate MI from acute pericarditis.

Cardiac catheterization can distinguish between cardiac dilation and pericardial effusion.

The following findings are consistent with pericarditis:
• elevated white blood cell count (10,000 to 20,000/μl)
• increased erythrocyte sedimentation rate
• absence of CK-MB bands (although values as high as 130 units have been reported)
• enlarged cardiac shadow on chest X-ray (with effusions of 250 ml or more)
• thickening of the pericardial sac or pericardial effusion on echocardiography (this technique can identify effusions as small as 15 ml)
• cultures and cytologic examination of pericardial fluid, which may identify the infectious organism.

## Treatment

Drug therapy for pericarditis aims to relieve pain, manage underlying systemic disease, and prevent or treat pericardial effusion and cardiac tamponade. To resolve the underlying inflammation, the doctor may prescribe nonsteroidal anti-inflammatory drugs (NSAIDs), such as high-dose salicylates (300 to 900 mg q.i.d.), indomethacin (25 to 100 mg q.i.d.), or ibuprofen (400 to 800 mg q.i.d.).

Severe cases may call for corticosteroids. To reduce the risk of adverse effects, this therapy lasts no longer than 1 week, with the dosage gradually tapered.

### Surgery

Depending on the patient's condition and the cause of pericarditis, surgery may be indicated.

*Pericardiocentesis.* To remove a pericardial effusion, the doctor may perform pericardiocentesis, a surgical procedure involving aspirating fluid from the pericardial sac through a large-bore needle inserted intercostally or using a subxiphoid approach. Possible complications include pneumothorax, laceration of the liver or another structure, and arrhythmias. If the needle lacerates a coronary artery or the epicardium, cardiac tamponade may worsen, causing cardiac arrest. Pericardiocentesis may not resolve an effusion in an inaccessible posterior area.

*Pericardiotomy or pericardial fenestration.* When pericardiocentesis fails or isn't feasible (for example, because of pericardial adhesions), the doctor must drain the pericardium by making an incision in the pericardial sac (pericardiotomy) or by cutting one or more windows out of the sac (pericardial fenestration). Both procedures can be performed via anterolateral thoracotomy, which requires entering the pleural space. Alternatively, the surgeon may use a subxiphoid approach to avoid the pleural space, although this technique may not completely correct a posterior adhesion or effusion.

*Pericardiectomy.* To treat extensive constrictive adhesions, severe tamponade, or chronic severe pericardial pain, the surgeon may remove the entire pericardium. This procedure has a 5% to 10% mortality, so it's used only if more conservative measures fail.

## Nursing care

• Periodically assess the patient's pain, using a systematic approach. Evaluate its location, radiation, frequency, and duration. Assess precipitating and alleviating factors, the effects of position changes, respiratory behavior, and presence of associated symptoms such as diaphoresis and shortness of breath. Instruct the patient to report episodes of chest pain or discomfort immediately so appropriate therapy can begin.
• Administer analgesics and NSAIDs as ordered. Give NSAIDs with food or milk to minimize adverse GI effects.
• Place the patient in an upright position to relieve dyspnea and chest pain. Auscultate for the presence of or changes in a pericardial friction rub.
• Assess vital signs every 2 to 4 hours or more often, as indicated.

ASSESSMENT INSIGHT

# Distinguishing acute pericarditis from MI

Electrocardiography (ECG) may prove indispensable in distinguishing acute pericarditis from myocardial infarction (MI) — two disorders that cause similar pain. Use these sample ECG tracings to help tell the two apart.

## Acute pericarditis
The ECG typically shows ST-segment elevation in all leads except $aV_R$ and $V_1$, reflecting the diffuse and global effects of pericarditis on the myocardium. ST-segment elevation is concave and appears in leads I and III. Q waves are absent.

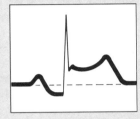

## Myocardial infarction
Expect convex ST-segment elevation specific to the injury site. The ST segment may be elevated in lead I or III and depressed in the other, depending on the myocardial region affected. Lead III changes usually mimic those in lead II, not lead I. Q waves typically are present.

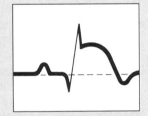

• Assess the patient's cardiovascular status frequently, watching for signs of cardiac tamponade. Monitor for arrhythmias and ST-segment and T-wave changes. Obtain an ECG if the pain origin is unclear. Remember that ECG changes may help rule out angina or MI. (See *Distinguishing acute pericarditis from MI*.)
• Anticipate the need for pericardiocentesis if CVP rises above 20 mm Hg, pulsus paradoxus exceeds 20 mm Hg, and pulse pressure measures less than 20 mm Hg.
• Emphasize the importance of bed rest, as appropriate. Assist the patient with bathing and activities of daily living as necessary.

## Surgical care
If surgery is performed, provide appropriate preoperative and postoperative care.
• Preoperative care consists of patient and family teaching, and observing the operation site for broken skin or lesions.
• Postoperative care includes cardiac monitoring, pain control, incisional care, and a gradual increase in patient activities.

## Patient teaching
• Reinforce previous teaching about heart function, the disease process, and the patient's medication regimen. Make sure the patient understands that he must take all of his discharge medication and not discontinue it if the pain subsides. Whenever possible, include his family in teaching sessions.
• Explain activity restrictions, and suggest physically undemanding activities to the patient. Tell him to resume activities slowly and to schedule rest periods into his daily routine until he has fully recuperated.
• Emphasize the importance of follow-up medical visits.

## What causes acute arterial occlusion?

Obstruction of a major artery by a clot is the most common cause of acute arterial occlusion. The occlusive mechanism may be endogenous (resulting from emboli formation, thrombosis, or plaque) or exogenous (resulting from trauma, insertion of a catheter or needle, or other causes).

### Embolism
Often the obstruction results from an embolus originating in the heart. Emboli typically lodge in the arms and legs, where blood vessels narrow or branch. In the arms, a common lodging site is the brachial artery, although emboli sometimes occlude the subclavian or axillary arteries. Common leg sites include the iliac, femoral, and popliteal arteries. Depending on their size, arterial emboli can lodge anywhere from the aortic bifurcation, disrupting arterial flow to both legs, to tiny vessels in the toes. Emboli originating in the heart can cause neurologic damage if they enter the cerebral circulation.

### Thrombosis
In a patient with atherosclerosis and marked arterial narrowing, thrombosis may cause acute intrinsic arterial occlusion. This complication typically arises in areas with severely stenotic vessels — especially in a patient who also has congestive heart failure, hypovolemia, polycythemia, or traumatic injury.

### Plaque
Plaque, or atheromatous debris from proximal arterial lesions, may intermittently obstruct small vessels (usually in the hands or feet). Plaque may also develop in the brachiocephalic vessels and travel to the cerebral circulation, where they may lead to transient cerebral ischemia or infarction.

### Exogenous causes
Acute arterial occlusion may stem from insertion of an indwelling arterial catheter, intra-arterial drug abuse, or peripheral arterial injection of foreign material.

Other exogenous causes of acute arterial occlusion are direct blunt or penetrating trauma to the artery.

# Arterial occlusive disease

An obstruction or narrowing of the lumen of the aorta and its major branches, arterial occlusive disease interrupts blood flow, usually to the legs and feet. It may affect the carotid, vertebral, innominate, subclavian, mesenteric, and celiac arteries.

### Causes
Atherosclerosis is the leading cause of arterial occlusive disease in the extremities after age 30. Modifiable risk factors for atherosclerosis include cigarette smoking, hypertension, and hyperlipidemia. Other predisposing factors include increasing age, diabetes mellitus, and a family history of MI, vascular disorders, or cerebrovascular accident.

Acute arterial occlusion usually results from a clot that blocks a major artery. (See *What causes acute arterial occlusion?*)

### Pathophysiology
When the inner wall of the artery is damaged, proteins, blood components, and other molecules move from the blood into the smooth-muscle layer of the artery, where they normally don't enter. This causes smooth-muscle cells to expand and grow into the lumen of the artery. Deposits of cholesterol, calcium, blood components, and collagen result in plaque formation. Plaque growth narrows the vessel and eventually may block it completely.

### Complications
Arterial occlusive disease can lead to severe ischemia, skin ulceration, infections, and gangrene. It may even necessitate amputation of part of the foot or leg. However, early diagnosis and treatment can prevent these complications.

### Assessment
#### Signs and symptoms
Clinical findings depend on which body part is deprived of circulation. A common complaint is intermittent claudication, a cramplike pain that develops in a muscle during exercise and

abates within 1 to 2 minutes after the exercise ends. Because the femoral artery is often involved, calf muscles are most frequently affected. (See *Claudication sites.*)

A gnawing or burning pain occurring at rest, especially at night, indicates severe arterial occlusive disease. This pain often is accompanied by other signs of impaired circulation, such as coldness, numbness, or tingling. In advanced disease, ischemia may lead to necrosis, ulceration, and gangrene, particularly of the toes and distal foot.

Acute arterial occlusion occurs suddenly, often without warning. To detect peripheral occlusion promptly, assess your patient for the six *Ps:*

• *Pain,* the most common symptom, occurs suddenly and is severe.

• *Pallor* results from vasoconstriction distal to the obstruction. With lower extremity disease, the lower leg becomes pale when the leg is elevated above heart level. (Capillary perfusion pressure isn't adequate to pump blood "uphill" to the distal limb portion.)

• *Pulselessness* arises distal to the obstruction.

• *Paralysis* occurs in the affected arm or leg as nerve endings or skeletal muscles are deprived of circulation. In severe ischemia, the patient may be unable to flex his toes.

• *Paresthesia,* a sensation of numbness or tingling caused by disturbed nerve endings, occurs in the affected arm or leg.

• *Poikilothermy,* lowered body temperature in the affected extremity distal to the occlusion, occurs because of impaired circulation. The affected limb will feel cool or cold. To assess for this sign, use the back of your fingers and hand to compare the temperature of one leg to the other.

**Pulse assessment.** Evaluate all peripheral pulses (including the carotid, brachial, radial, femoral, popliteal, dorsalis pedis, and posterior tibial pulses) for presence or absence as well as quality and symmetry. A weak or absent pulse indicates stenosis or occlusion of an artery proximal to that site. For example, presence of a femoral pulse and absence of a popliteal pulse indicates obstruction of the superficial femoral artery.

# Claudication sites

Claudication, characterized by muscle weakness and cramplike pain, frequently accompanies arterial occlusion. This illustration shows where claudication typically occurs in patients with various arterial occlusions.

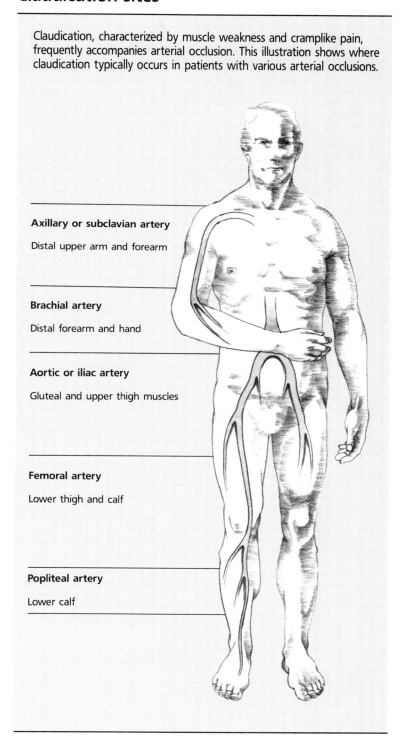

**Axillary or subclavian artery**

Distal upper arm and forearm

**Brachial artery**

Distal forearm and hand

**Aortic or iliac artery**

Gluteal and upper thigh muscles

**Femoral artery**

Lower thigh and calf

**Popliteal artery**

Lower calf

If you're not sure whether a pulse is present, document it as absent. To help differentiate the patient's pulse from the projection of your own pulse through your fingertips, ask a colleague to measure the patient's radial pulse or to check your pulse against the patient's.

When auscultating the arteries over a stenotic lesion, you may hear a *bruit.* An abnormal sound or murmur, a bruit is similar to a heart murmur but noncardiac in origin. In the presence of stenosis, bruits are audible in the carotid arteries, the abdominal aorta and its major branches, and the femoral arteries. Use the diaphragm of the stethoscope to auscultate bruits, which are medium- to high-pitched. A completely occluded artery won't project a bruit.

### Diagnostic tests

Arteriography—injection of a radiopaque contrast medium to outline the arterial circuit—demonstrates the type, location, and degree of vascular obstruction as well as the patient's collateral circulation.

Digital subtraction angiography is a special type of arteriography that uses computer technology to provide a visually enhanced image of the vascular anatomy of the lower leg. It may be used in conjunction with standard arteriography. First, an X-ray of the lower leg is taken and stored. Then a contrast medium is injected and another X-ray is taken. The stored image is digitally "subtracted," enhancing vessel resolution on the X-ray.

## Treatment

To avoid complications, the patient requires prompt treatment. He may receive thrombolytic therapy to dissolve clots and relieve the obstruction caused by a thrombus, undergo one of several surgical procedures to clear a blocked artery, or undergo nonsurgical procedures such as percutaneous transluminal angioplasty (PTA) or laser angioplasty.

A few patients with severe, life-threatening ischemia who experience pain at rest aren't surgical candidates because of coexisting medical problems that contraindicate surgery, such as severe coronary artery disease. For them, treatment consists of preventing skin break-

down, ulceration, and infection and treating any gangrenous necrosis. Gangrene is nonreversible even with adequate blood flow. If an infected limb leads to systemic septicemia, amputation may be necessary to save a patient's life.

### Drug therapy

In nontraumatic leg ischemia, heparin is given as a 5,000-unit bolus, followed by a continuous drip of 1,000 units/hour. This therapy helps prevent thrombosis to arteries distal to the occlusion.

Acute thromboembolic events or occlusion of arterial bypass grafts usually call for urokinase or streptokinase. These thrombolytic agents convert plasminogen to plasmin, leading to degradation of fibrin clots, fibrinogen, and other plasma proteins. They can be administered either I.V. or directly into an arterial occlusion via a localizing catheter. These drugs act immediately.

### Other treatments

Acute arterial occlusive disease usually calls for one of the procedures described below.

*Atherectomy.* In this procedure, the doctor uses a catheter to cut and remove the obstructive thrombus or plaque, leaving the full thickness of the artery's intimal lining. Intra-arterial urokinase may be used with atherectomy to treat lesions complicated by a thrombus.

*PTA.* A safe and effective treatment for selected patients, PTA mechanically dilatates a narrowed or occluded artery with a specially designed balloon-tipped catheter. Stenosis of the iliac artery is a common indication for peripheral PTA.

In this procedure, the doctor advances the balloon catheter to the desired anatomic site using fluoroscopic guidance. Dilatation is achieved by repeatedly inflating the balloon tip to a predetermined size, which minimizes the risk of overdistention and vessel rupture.

PTA cracks the intimal plaque. Because the procedure leaves behind a rough intimal surface that results in platelet aggregation and may induce thrombus formation, many patients receive anticoagulants or antiplatelet agents such as dipyridamole.

*Stents.* After PTA, acute artery closure or reocclusion may occur. To help prevent these problems, intravascular stents have been developed to provide internal support for the artery and prevent acute elastic recoil and possibly chronic restenosis. Clinical trials are continuing to assess the safety and efficacy of peripheral artery stents.

*Embolectomy.* In this procedure, a balloon-tipped Fogarty catheter is used to remove thrombotic material from the artery. Through an opening in the artery, the catheter is passed down the affected vascular segment with the balloon deflated. When the tip is beyond the obstruction, the balloon is inflated and the catheter and embolus are withdrawn. After the clot is removed, the artery is flushed with heparin solution and then closed.

*Fasciotomy.* The leg skin and fascia are opened surgically to allow expansion of edematous muscle fibers. This procedure is performed if the patient's leg has been severely ischemic for more than a few hours. In this situation, considerable muscle swelling and pressure (compartment syndrome) may follow circulatory restoration. Fasciotomy helps prevent permanent tissue destruction. The wound either closes slowly by itself or can be covered with skin grafts.

*Bypass graft.* This procedure bypasses an arterial obstruction resulting from atherosclerosis. After exposing the affected artery, the surgeon anastomoses a synthetic or autogenous graft to divert blood flow around the occluded arterial segment. The graft may be synthetic or it may be a vein harvested from elsewhere in the patient's body. The most commonly bypassed arterial occlusive lesions are aortoiliac, superficial femoral, and tibial.

*Laser angioplasty.* A controversial method for treating chronic arterial disease, this procedure uses a fiber-optic laser catheter with or with-out balloon angioplasty to open localized, short occlusions in the iliac artery, superficial femoral artery, and above-the-knee popliteal artery. It's especially useful for lesions that can't be bypassed using standard guide wire techniques because of total obstruction.

Complications are similar to those of conventional angioplasty. In addition, vasospasm—severe heatlike pain during the procedure—and thermal injury have been reported.

## Nursing care
• Prevent pressure on the affected limb, and avoid elevating it.
• During anticoagulant therapy, closely monitor the patient's coagulation profile.
• During and after thrombolytic therapy, monitor the patient for fever because urokinase and streptokinase are pyrogenic. Streptokinase is associated with allergic reactions, so observe for anaphylaxis. If anaphylaxis occurs, administer steroids and antihistamines as ordered. Monitor thrombin time, and withhold concurrent anticoagulants or antiplatelets. Watch for signs of hemorrhage.
• If the patient has gangrene with dry, necrotic areas of the toes or foot, leave the affected areas open to air. Assess the limb daily for evidence of gangrene progression. With purulent exudate, obtain wound cultures and administer I.V. antibiotics as ordered. Bandage the draining area with 0.9% sodium chloride wet-to-dry dressings as ordered. A foot or lower leg X-ray can identify underlying osteomyelitis.

### Procedural care
• Before any invasive or surgical procedure, obtain and record baseline pulse checks. Mark the site with a waterproof marker, and indicate if pulses were palpable or obtained using a Doppler ultrasound stethoscope. Observe the skin integrity of the extremity on which the procedure will be performed. Look for pimples, blisters, and abrasions.
• After any invasive or surgical procedure, monitor the patient's vascular status frequently, checking extremities for the six Ps. If PTA was performed, keep the line open with a heparin infusion as ordered, and monitor the insertion site for bleeding.

# Foot care for the patient with arterial occlusive disease

If your patient has arterial occlusive disease in his lower extremities, even minor foot injuries may lead to serious complications. Before discharge, stress the importance of proper foot care. To help your patient keep his feet trouble-free, include the following points in your teaching.

## Inspection
• Tell the patient to inspect his feet and toes daily. Teach him to check the plantar surface of each foot, using a mirror if necessary.
• Remind him to inspect his toes individually, including the spaces between them.

## Hygiene
• Teach the patient to bathe his feet daily with mild soap and warm water. Instruct him to check water temperature with his hand or a thermometer first because his feet may have decreased sensation.
• Teach the patient to dry his feet thoroughly, especially between his toes, because residual moisture can cause maceration or promote bacterial or fungal infection.
• Suggest a light application of skin lotion or powder to the feet, ankles, and lower leg. However,

caution the patient against using perfumed preparations, which dry the skin excessively. Tell him not to put lotion between his toes.

## Nail care
• Advise the patient to perform nail care under good lighting after the nails are softened from the bath.
• Instruct him not to trim his nails if they're badly ingrown, infected, or painful. Instead, recommend a podiatrist.

## Footwear
• Tell the patient to wear sturdy shoes made of soft, flexible leather. Instruct him to avoid man-made materials, such as patent leather and plastic, because they prevent evaporation and may contribute to fungal infections. Ideally, shoes should have low heels, a closed toe, and no front seams. Advise him not to wear sandals, especially the thong type.
• Instruct the patient to check his shoes and socks for foreign objects, torn linings, and holes before wearing them.
• Remind the patient to wear shoes at all times when he's out of bed. Explain that loose slippers can fall off, causing him to trip or fall.

---

• Observe the dressing or incision for bleeding and wound accommodation. Observe for swelling; severe swelling may signal compartment syndrome. If swelling is severe enough to threaten limb viability, it may warrant fasciotomy.
• After atherectomy, monitor the patient closely for microembolism. Immediately report sudden changes in assessment findings.
• Monitor intake and output. Expect the patient to have an indwelling urinary catheter.
• Check BUN levels, urine specific gravity, and daily weight to evaluate fluid volume status.
• Monitor vital signs for evidence of infection.
• The patient with peripheral vascular disease may have concomitant cardiopulmonary disease, so be sure to evaluate his gas exchange and maintain continuous cardiac monitoring.

• Watch blood pressure closely. A high systolic pressure may rupture the anastomosis, while excessively low systolic pressure may promote loss of graft patency. If ordered, administer nitroprusside, which controls blood pressure effectively because it has a short half-life and causes few adverse effects.
• Prevent mechanical trauma by minimizing pressure on the affected limb or foot. Use a foot cradle and heel protectors, and place lamb's wool between the patient's toes. To prevent cracking, keep the skin well lubricated using an alcohol-free emollient.
• Avoid restrictive clothing, including specialized garments such as antiembolism stockings.
• Administer analgesics as ordered, to control pain.
• Keep the affected arm or leg warm, but

never use heating pads, which can cause thermal trauma.

### Patient teaching

Remind the patient that recovery from surgery varies from individual to individual. Discuss any restrictions on activity and other guidelines established by the doctor.

Teach the patient or a family member how to change his dressing and perform wound care. Ask for a demonstration in return. Explain that sutures or staples, if present, will be removed before discharge or at the first postoperative visit.

Review the proper administration of any prescribed medications, such as anticoagulants. Instruct the patient to obtain his doctor's permission before driving a car.

Warn the patient not to wear restrictive clothing or sit with his legs crossed. To prevent an inguinal or incisional hernia, caution him not to lift anything heavier than 5 lb (2.3 kg). Discourage strenuous physical activity.

Tell the patient that he may take a shower or bath, but stress that he must pat the incision dry afterward.

Reinforce the need for proper foot care. (See *Foot care for the patient with arterial occlusive disease.*)

Stress the importance of regular exercise. Walking is an excellent activity because it increases blood flow, strengthens muscles, and promotes a sense of well-being. However, caution the patient to avoid exposure to cold, which can cause vasoconstriction.

Teach the patient to modify disease risk factors, such as hyperlipidemia. Provide him and his family with resources that can assist them with life-style changes.

Emphasize the need to quit smoking. To enhance the patient's efforts to quit, refer him to a local support group, the American Cancer Society, the American Lung Association, or the American Heart Association. Reinforce any positive efforts that show his willingness to stop smoking.

Advise the patient to avoid intense scratching of insect bites or dry skin because this may cause infection.

• If the patient has a synthetic graft, remind him to take prophylactic antibiotics before invasive tests, surgery, or extensive dental work.
• Stress the need for follow-up visits. Make sure that the patient and his family members have emergency telephone numbers for the doctor's office and hospital.

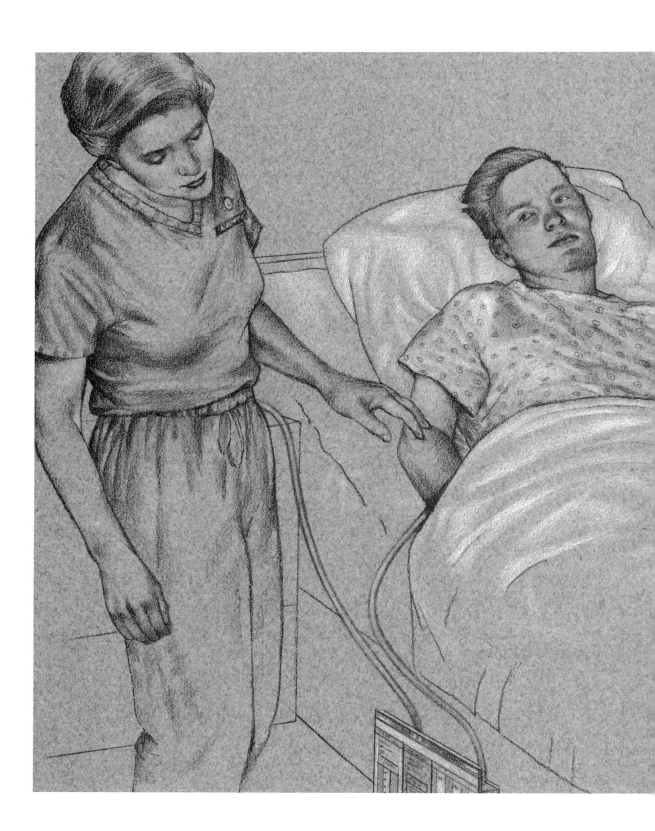

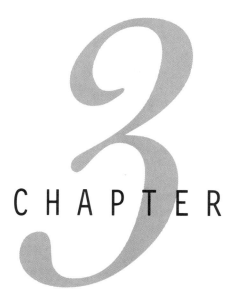

# CHAPTER 3

# Respiratory disorders

Caring for a patient with an acute respiratory disorder presents one of the most difficult challenges you'll face as a nurse. It demands sound judgment and skillful intervention, along with an ability to juggle several urgent matters at once to meet your patient's special needs.

Not only must you treat his compromised respiratory status, but you must be able to recognize and successfully manage other related complications. For example, your patient may also have ineffective airway clearance and gas exchange, and then develop alterations in cardiac output, shifts in fluid volume, and impaired thermoregulation, any of which could lead to a life-threatening situation.

This chapter will teach you how to provide the best possible care for patients with acute respiratory disorders, including acute respiratory failure in chronic obstructive pulmonary disease, cor pulmonale, pulmonary hypertension, pneumonia, pleural effusion, and lung cancer. The up-to-date clinical information contained in it will help you learn how to identify an acute respiratory condition, how to set priorities, and how to intervene with skill and confidence to avert complications.

For each disorder, you'll find causes, pathophysiology, and complications, followed by a thorough discussion of assessment and treatment, including drug therapy, surgery, and other medical treatments. Next you'll find a detailed account of the nursing care you'll need to provide for your patient—from immediate interventions to surgical care to continuing care, along with patient-teaching measures required to safeguard his well-being.

# Acute respiratory failure in COPD

Acute respiratory failure occurs when the pulmonary system can't maintain adequate gas exchange. Unchecked and untreated, it leads to tissue hypoxia and hypercapnia. In patients with normal lung tissue, acute respiratory failure usually means a partial pressure of arterial oxygen ($PaO_2$) below 50 mm Hg and a partial pressure of arterial carbon dioxide ($PaCO_2$) above 50 mm Hg. However, these values don't apply to patients who also have chronic obstructive pulmonary disease (COPD). Such patients have a low $PaO_2$ value (hypoxemia) and a consistently high $PaCO_2$ value (hypercapnia). So for them, only acute deterioration in arterial blood gas (ABG) values and corresponding clinical deterioration signal acute respiratory failure. (See *Comparing hypoxemia and hypercapnia*.)

## Causes
In a patient with COPD, acute respiratory failure may be triggered by any condition that increases the work of breathing, increases the body's oxygen needs, reduces the respiratory drive, or diminishes oxygen delivery to the lungs. Common precipitating factors include respiratory tract infection (such as bronchitis or pneumonia), increased atmospheric pollution, left ventricular heart failure, pulmonary embolism, bronchospasm, central respiratory drive depression secondary to drugs or anesthesia, and spontaneous pneumothorax related to rupture of blebs or bullae.

## Pathophysiology
In acute respiratory failure, gas exchange is diminished by any or a combination of the following factors:
- alveolar hypoventilation
- ventilation-perfusion ($\dot{V}/\dot{Q}$) mismatch
- intrapulmonary shunting
- diffusion defects. (See *What happens in acute respiratory failure*.)

The hypoxemia or hypercapnia characteristic of acute respiratory failure stimulates strong compensatory responses by all body systems, including the respiratory, cardiovascular, and central nervous systems. The most important compensatory response to hypoxemia is a rise in cardiac output. Increased heart rate and blood pressure are common early signs of hypoxemia. However, as tissue oxygenation diminishes, cardiac output drops, the heart rate and blood pressure drop, arrhythmias occur, and pulmonary vessels constrict.

ASSESSMENT INSIGHT

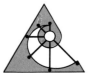

## Comparing hypoxemia and hypercapnia

Hypoxemia (a deficiency of oxygen in the arterial blood) and hypercapnia (an above-normal amount of carbon dioxide in the arterial blood) cause different signs and symptoms. Becoming familiar with them will help you assess your patient more accurately.

| HYPOXEMIA | HYPERCAPNIA |
|---|---|
| Restlessness | Headache |
| Confusion | Lethargy |
| Impaired judgment | Reduced concentration |
| Dyspnea | Irritability |
| Hypotension | Hypertension |
| Central cyanosis | Muscle twitching |

PATHOPHYSIOLOGY

# What happens in acute respiratory failure

Four major malfunctions account for impaired gas exchange and subsequent acute respiratory failure: alveolar hypoventilation, ventilation-perfusion ($\dot{V}/\dot{Q}$) mismatch, intrapulmonary (right-to-left) shunting, and diffusion defects.

### Alveolar hypoventilation
In this defect, partial pressure of arterial carbon dioxide increases, triggering a drop in partial pressure of arterial oxygen. Fatigue, central nervous system depression, retained secretions, pneumothorax, and pleural effusion are common causes of alveolar hypoventilation.

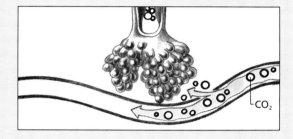

### $\dot{V}/\dot{Q}$ mismatch
The leading cause of hypoxemia, a $\dot{V}/\dot{Q}$ mismatch may result from too little ventilation with normal blood flow or from too little blood flow with normal ventilation. Causes of a $\dot{V}/\dot{Q}$ mismatch include airway obstruction, atelectasis, pulmonary embolism, and shock.

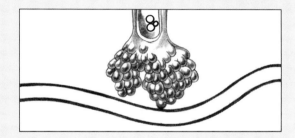

### Intrapulmonary shunting
This condition occurs when blood passes from the right to the left side of the heart without being oxygenated. Shunting can result from atelectasis, mucus plugging, pneumonia, or adult respiratory distress syndrome (ARDS). Hypoxemia secondary to shunting doesn't always respond to treatment with increased fraction of inspired oxygen.

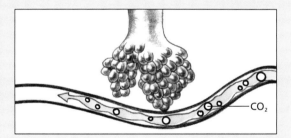

### Diffusion defects
These defects occur when the surface area available for gas exchange in the lungs decreases or when the alveolocapillary membrane thickens, diminishing gas diffusion across the membrane. Diffusion defects rarely cause hypoxemia, although they may occur in patients with chronic obstructive pulmonary disease secondary to exercise, high altitude, ARDS, or pulmonary fibrosis.

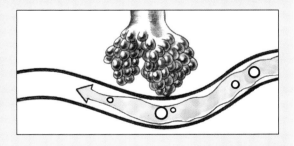

MULTIPLE DIAGNOSIS

# Managing the COPD patient with an acute MI

The patient with chronic obstructive pulmonary disease (COPD) who suffers an acute myocardial infarction (MI) needs special care. Hypoxia or hypotension may develop quickly, and hypoxia may be resistant to oxygen or drug administration. Be careful giving morphine for pain — it may trigger respiratory depression.

## Pathophysiology
Blood delivers oxygen to the tissues. Oxygen supply to the tissues depends on adequate gas exchange in the lungs and sufficient cardiac output from the heart. A patient with COPD has little reserve to compensate for the drop in cardiac output caused by an MI. This means that he may be unable to compensate for hypoxia.

## Risks
Treatment of an MI usually includes oxygen administration to correct tissue hypoxia. However, the COPD patient depends on hypoxia as the stimulus to breathe. Giving him too much oxygen may eliminate his respiratory drive. Also, the MI patient typically receives morphine to relieve pain and reduce the heart's oxygen needs. However, this drug may cause respiratory depression.

Treating COPD with a bronchodilator may cause tachycardia, which increases the heart's demand for oxygen. Treating MI with a beta blocker (to reduce the heart's oxygen demands) may lead to bronchoconstriction.

Complications of an MI may be difficult to treat in, or may worsen the respiratory status of, the COPD patient. If he develops hypotension, placing him flat in bed will increase his difficulty in breathing. If he develops heart failure, fluid may accumulate in his lungs, impeding gas exchange.

## Interventions
• Take measures to reduce the patient's oxygen needs, such as placing him on bed rest, administering prescribed nitrates, and correcting tachyarrhythmias by administering antiarrhythmics and performing vagal maneuvers and cardioversion.
• Administer oxygen at a low flow rate with nasal prongs or a Venturi mask, as ordered. Be sure to set the flow rate precisely.
• Closely monitor arterial blood gas values, and frequently assess the patient for signs of decreasing respiratory drive. Notify the doctor if his partial pressure of arterial oxygen rises above his normal level or if his partial pressure of arterial carbon dioxide starts to increase.
• After giving morphine or other narcotics, monitor the patient's respiratory status closely. Because the peak effect of I.V. morphine occurs within 7 minutes, you may titrate the drug to achieve pain relief without respiratory depression.

---

Hypoxemia also causes the brain's respiratory control center to first increase respiratory depth (tidal volume) and then speed the respiratory rate. These responses increase the work of breathing and the demand for oxygen. The body responds to hypercapnia with cerebral depression, cerebral vasodilation, and increased intracranial pressure.

## Complications
Possible complications of acute respiratory failure include tissue hypoxia, metabolic acidosis, arrhythmias, myocardial ischemia or myocardial infarction (MI), heart failure, pulmonary emboli, GI bleeding, seizures, coma, and respiratory or cardiac arrest. (See *Managing the COPD patient with an acute MI* and *Understanding the consequences of acute respiratory failure.*)

## Assessment
### Signs and symptoms
The patient in acute respiratory failure appears restless, anxious, agitated, dyspneic, confused, or lethargic. Typically, he complains that he's short of breath, and he may report a headache (from the increased $PaCO_2$). He may yawn, use accessory muscles to breathe, or exhibit pursed-lip breathing. Tachypnea signals

mpending respiratory failure.

Note the patient's position: In acute respiratory failure, the seated patient leans forward o lessen the restriction on abdominal and diaphragmatic movement. You may note cyanosis of the oral mucosa, lips, and nail beds; nasal laring; and ashen skin.

Palpation may reveal cold, clammy skin. The pulse rate may be increased and irregular. If actile fremitus is present, you'll note that it increases over consolidated lung tissue or areas of pneumonia but decreases over an obstructed bronchus or pleural effusion. Decreased actile fremitus and asymmetrical chest movement suggest pneumothorax.

Percussion may reveal hyperresonance if COPD, asthma, or pneumothorax are present. Percussion usually produces a dull or flat sound f acute respiratory failure results from atelectasis or pneumonia.

Auscultation typically discloses diminished breath sounds. You may hear such adventitious sounds as wheezes (indicating narrowing of smaller airways), crackles (signaling secretions n or reexpansion of collapsed alveoli or bronhioles), and rhonchi (revealing secretions in arger airways). In a patient with pneumothorax, expect absent breath sounds in the affected area.

### Diagnostic tests

ABG analysis is the key to diagnosis and subsequent treatment of acute respiratory failure. Usually, the patient with COPD has a chronically decreased $PaO_2$, increased $PaCO_2$, increased bicarbonate ($HCO_3^-$) level, and normal pH. ABG values that progressively deteriorate from baseline strongly suggest acute respiratory failure. In patients with essentially normal lung tissue, a pH below 7.35, $PaO_2$ less than 0 mm Hg, or $PaCO_2$ above 50 mm Hg signals acute respiratory failure. In the COPD patient, expect ABG values to deviate even more. Pulse oximetry usually shows an arterial oxygen saturation ($SaO_2$) level below 90%.

Other tests help determine what's causing or contributing to acute respiratory failure. Chest X-rays help identify underlying pulmonary disease or such conditions as emphysema, pneumonia, atelectasis, infiltrates, effusions, and

## COMPLICATIONS

## Understanding the consequences of acute respiratory failure

Acute respiratory failure can affect many body systems. This chart lists the potential complications of acute respiratory failure by body system.

| BODY SYSTEM | COMPLICATIONS |
| --- | --- |
| Cardiovascular | • Decreased venous return (from increased intrathoracic pressure)<br>• Reduced cardiac output<br>• Arrhythmias |
| Pulmonary | • Infection<br>• Oxygen toxicity<br>• Barotrauma<br>• Atelectasis<br>• Tracheal dilation and necrosis |
| Renal | • Increased antidiuretic hormone release<br>• Reduced urine output<br>• Water retention |
| Gastrointestinal | • Gastric distention<br>• Ileus<br>• Stress ulcers<br>• Bleeding<br>• Malnutrition |
| Neurologic | • Increased intracranial pressure |

pneumothorax. An elevated white blood cell count suggests an infectious process; a sputum culture can identify the pathogen. Bronchoscopy may be used to visualize the airways and obtain sputum specimens in a patient with a nonproductive cough. Electrocardiography may reveal myocardial ischemia, tachycardia, arrhythmias, right ventricular hypertrophy, or right atrial enlargement.

Other diagnostic tests that may yield abnormal results include:
• hematocrit value, which increases in patients with chronic hypoxemia
• serum potassium levels, which may decrease from COPD or increase from respiratory aci-

# Planning care for the COPD patient with acute respiratory failure

In a patient with chronic obstructive respiratory disease (COPD), acute respiratory failure can have widespread effects, typically causing hypoxemia, hypercapnia, and acidemia—dangerous conditions that affect all body organs. Consequently, you need to come up with an effective plan of care, maximizing the patient's chances for a positive outcome. But this can be difficult.

Take, for example, the case of Paul Smythe, age 69, who is placed under the care of nurse Pauline Gildea.

## Gathering the history

Mr. Smythe was admitted to the hospital with acute respiratory failure, precipitated by a respiratory infection and complicated by chronic bronchitis and emphysema.

He tells Pauline that he became ill soon after returning from a holiday with his son's family, including three children who were sick with the flu. To manage his emphysema, Mr. Smythe says he uses nebulizer treatments and takes daily bronchodilators. Occasionally, his doctor prescribes corticosteroids. Mr. Smythe also tells Pauline that his blood pressure has been high for years.

## Assessing the patient

Pauline takes Mr. Smythe's vital signs. His oral temperature is 100.2° F (37.9° C) and he's diaphoretic. His pulse rate is rapid (132 beats/minute), thready, and irregular. His respiratory rate is 48 breaths/minute, and his blood pressure registers a high 148/98 mm Hg.

On inspection, Pauline sees a thin, frail, barrel-chested man close to exhaustion from his efforts to breathe. She notes his ashen color and circumoral and capillary bed cyanosis. She notes that he uses all accessory muscles of the chest and abdomen and sees him purse his lips slightly with each exhalation.

Pauline assesses pitting edema of the feet bilaterally. She sees the patient picking at his sheets and pajamas and notes that he appears restless and cannot answer simple questions.

Chest auscultation discloses diffuse crackles and diminished breath sounds to the lung bases bilaterally. Pauline hears wheezes even without a stethoscope.

## Reviewing diagnostic findings

Pauline closely reviews the initial diagnostic results:
• arterial blood gas (ABG) values (on room air)—$Pao_2$, 40 mm Hg; $Paco_2$, 59 mm Hg; pH, 7.27; and $Sao_2$, 75%
• chest X-ray—positive for diffuse infiltrates
• red blood cell count—7.5 million/mm³
• white blood cell count—11,400/mm³
• erythrocyte sedimentation rate—elevated; thrombocytosis evident
• serum theophylline level—15.2 μg/ml
• blood urea nitrogen and serum creatinine levels—elevated
• serum glucose level—141 mg/dl
• electrocardiogram—atrial fibrillation with occasional premature ventricular contractions.

After administering oxygen and nebulizer treatments, Pauline obtains repeat ABG values. She sends a specimen of purulent, blood-tinged sputum (aspirated by nasotracheal suctioning) to the laboratory for culture and sensitivity testing.

## Formulating care goals

Pauline has identified impaired gas exchange and an inadequate breathing pattern as Mr. Smythe's primary respiratory problems, and she acts quickly to define immediate care goals. They are to:
• improve his breathing pattern, airway clearance, and gas exchange to restore optimal respiratory status
• decrease his anxiety and use coping mechanisms to minimize his fear
• increase his activity tolerance and improve his ability to perform self-care
• decrease his risk of infection.

## Carrying out proper interventions

To meet the first care goal—*improved breathing and gas exchange*—Pauline assesses Mr. Smythe's respiratory status every 15 minutes until his breathing stabilizes. She checks his respiratory rate and pattern and assesses his use of accessory muscles to breathe. She decides to use pulse oximetry to monitor his oxygenation status.

Pauline gives ordered oxygen, bronchodilators, and nebulizer treatments. When she sees that a forward-leaning position eases Mr. Smythe's breathing, she supplies an overbed table and pil-

dosis (even though intracellular potassium levels may be low).

## Treatment

Endotracheal intubation and mechanical ventilation are indicated if conservative oxygen treatment fails to raise $SaO_2$ above 90%, if acidemia continues, if the patient becomes exhausted, or if cardiorespiratory arrest occurs. Most patients, however, won't require mechanical ventilation.

Bronchodilators, especially inhalants, are used to open the airways. If the patient can't inhale effectively or is on a mechanical ventilator, he may receive a bronchodilator by nebulizer. The doctor also may order corticosteroids, theophylline, and antibiotics. He'll order heparin if he suspects pulmonary embolism as the cause of acute respiratory failure.

Bronchoscopy may be indicated to remove retained secretions. Be prepared to assist with this procedure, including obtaining sputum specimens. The doctor may order chest physiotherapy, including postural drainage, chest percussion, and chest vibration. To correct dehydration, he may order I.V. fluids, which help thin secretions.

## Nursing care
### Immediate care

• To reverse hypoxemia, administer oxygen in controlled concentrations, as ordered, via nasal prongs or Venturi mask. Maintain $PaO_2$ between 50 and 60 mm Hg and pH above 7.30. Keep in mind that the COPD patient can tolerate only small amounts of supplemental oxygen. Watch for a positive response, such as easier breathing, reduced anxiety, and improved ABG values. Monitor the patient closely for signs of respiratory depression from excessive oxygen administration. (See *Planning care for the COPD patient with acute respiratory failure.*)

• Sit the conscious patient upright in a supported, forward-leaning position to promote diaphragm movement. Supply an overbed table and pillows for support. If the patient has an acute lung disorder on one side, position him with the unimpaired lung down to improve

lows for support. She monitors chest X-ray and ABG results.

Knowing that narcotics and other central nervous system depressants may reduce the respiratory drive of a COPD patient, Pauline avoids giving these to relieve discomfort. She assesses Mr. Smythe's level of consciousness every few hours until he is stable, performs chest physiotherapy to mobilize secretions and minimize airway obstruction, and increases his fluid intake to 3,000 ml daily to help liquefy secretions.

Mr. Smythe can't mobilize secretions on his own, so Pauline places a nasopharyngeal airway in one nostril for suctioning. Throughout the acute phase of his illness, she prepares for the threat of pulmonary collapse and spontaneous pneumothorax by keeping a tracheostomy tray at the bedside.

To *reduce anxiety and promote coping,* Pauline assesses Mr. Smythe's anxiety level, staying alert for irritability, restlessness, signs of fear and frustration, and such facial expressions as grimaces.

To *increase activity tolerance and self-care,* Pauline maintains activity restrictions and promotes rest. She reinforces Mr. Smythe's use of controlled breathing techniques while he receives oxygen.

Pauline gives complete oral care and offers a bedpan and urinal when he needs them. She provides small, frequent meals that are easy to chew and swallow, keeping sherbet and gelatin handy for snacking.

To *decrease the risk of infection,* Pauline implements universal precautions and reverse isolation to avoid nosocomial infection. She prevents stasis of respiratory secretions by providing chest physiotherapy, spirometry, increased fluids, and expectorants.

## Evaluating care

She gives prescribed antibiotics and obtains sputum specimens for repeated cultures to assess treatment effectiveness. Mr. Smythe responded well to antibiotics and bronchial hygiene and was discharged within 5 days.

$\dot{V}/\dot{Q}$ matching and oxygenation.
• Maintain a patent airway. If the patient is retaining carbon dioxide, encourage slow, deep breathing with pursed lips. Urge him to cough up secretions. If he can't mobilize secretions, insert a nasopharyngeal airway and suction him when necessary.
• Administer bronchodilators using a metered-dose inhaler with an aerochamber or a nebulizer, as ordered. Administer corticosteroids and antibiotics if ordered. If you're using a metered-dose inhaler to deliver a bronchodilator or steroid, make sure the patient can inhale deeply and hold his breath for at least 3 seconds.
• Avoid giving central nervous system depressants such as narcotics to relieve discomfort in a nonventilated patient. These drugs may reduce the respiratory drive.
• Assess the patient's respiratory status every 15 minutes until his condition stabilizes. Ongoing respiratory assessment should include level of consciousness; respiratory rate, depth, and pattern; accessory muscle use; presence of or changes in adventitious breath sounds; ABG analysis; and secretion production and clearance. Notify the doctor if interventions don't improve the patient's condition.
• To prepare for intubation and mechanical ventilation, if necessary, obtain the necessary equipment and explain the procedure to the patient. Immediately after intubation and routinely thereafter, assess for correct tube position and patency. Inflate the tube cuff and fasten the tube securely.
• Make sure mechanical ventilator settings, such as fraction of inspired oxygen ($FIO_2$), tidal volume, ventilation mode, and respiratory rate, are set at the ordered parameters. Obtain ABG values 20 to 30 minutes after any change in ventilator settings, when ordered by the doctor, and with any change in the patient's condition. Monitor peak inspiratory pressure; if this increases, suspect pneumothorax, decreasing lung compliance, or the need for suctioning.
• Respond immediately to ventilator alarms. A low-pressure alarm may indicate that the ventilator has been disconnected from the patient, that the ventilator tubing is disconnected or loose, or that the endotracheal or tracheostomy tube cuff has a leak. A high-pressure alarm sounds when the patient coughs, needs to be suctioned, bites on the endotracheal tube, or has increased thoracic pressure or when the ventilator tubing is kinked or fills with fluid.

If you can't quickly identify and resolve the cause of a ventilator alarm, disconnect the patient from the ventilator and ventilate him manually with a resuscitation bag while calling for assistance.

### Continuing care
• Periodically assess the patient's respiratory status and vital signs. Monitor $SaO_2$ with a pulse oximeter. Consider taking a rectal or tympanic temperature because oxygen therapy and labored breathing may interfere with oral readings. Monitor fluid balance by recording the patient's intake and output and weighing him daily. Notify the doctor of a fever, deteriorating respiratory status, rising or falling respiratory rate, increasing pulse rate, decreasing blood pressure, or fluid imbalance. Administer antipyretics for fever, if ordered, to help reduce the patient's oxygen needs.
• Position the patient for comfort and optimal gas exchange. Place the call button within his reach. Calm and reassure him while giving care because anxiety can raise oxygen demands.
• Pace care activities to maximize the patient's energy level and provide needed rest. When he's not short of breath, perform active or passive range-of-motion exercises to help avert complications of bed rest.
• Assist the patient in mobilizing secretions, using chest physiotherapy as ordered. Reposition an immobilized patient every 1 to 2 hours.
• Unless the patient is retaining fluid or has heart failure, increase his daily fluid intake to 2 liters to liquefy secretions.
• Provide nutritional support. If the patient is intubated, give enteral feedings as ordered. Limit carbohydrates and augment protein intake because carbohydrate metabolism causes more carbon dioxide production than does protein.

• Monitor serial test results, such as ABG values, chest X-rays, sputum cultures, and electrolyte studies. Report abnormal findings. Monitor $SaO_2$ values with a pulse oximeter. Administer antibiotics and electrolyte replacements as ordered and indicated.

*Caring for the patient on a mechanical ventilator.* To ensure the patient's well-being, follow these guidelines.

• Measure and adjust cuff pressure every 8 hours, using the minimal-leak technique or a pressure-regulating valve. Cuff pressure should never exceed 18 mm Hg since this is the capillary filling pressure. This also helps prevent tracheal erosion from an overinflated cuff that compresses tracheal wall vessels.

• As ordered and indicated, administer inotropic and vasoactive drugs (to boost decreased cardiac output), diuretics and renal artery vasodilators (to increase urine output), and fluids (to correct hypovolemia).

• When breath sounds indicate the need, suction the patient using sterile technique. Administer oxygen before and after suctioning to help prevent suction-induced hypoxemia. If he's receiving high levels of positive end-expiratory pressure (PEEP), use a PEEP valve or an in-line suction catheter. Monitor the patient for suction-induced hypoxia. Observe him for any change in sputum quantity, consistency, or color.

• Periodically retape the endotracheal tube. If the patient is nasally intubated, position and maintain the tube midline within the nostril and provide meticulous tube care. When retaping an orally inserted tube, reposition the tube within the mouth to help prevent tissue breakdown. Support the tubing so that it doesn't pull on the tube.

• Instruct the patient not to pull at the tube. If necessary, restrain or sedate him to maintain a patent airway.

• Monitor for complications of mechanical ventilation, such as decreased cardiac output and pneumothorax, and take appropriate measures to prevent or correct them. Report complications to the doctor.

• Help prevent infection by using good hand-washing technique, using sterile technique when suctioning, and performing frequent oral hygiene. Change the ventilator tubing every 24 to 48 hours.

• Monitor for signs of stress ulcers, including blood in gastric secretions or stools and decreasing hemoglobin and hematocrit values. To help reduce the risk of GI bleeding, give enteral feedings and administer antacids or histamine-receptor antagonists, as ordered.

• Insert a nasogastric tube to allow gastric decompression, as ordered and indicated.

• Maintain adequate hemodynamic measurements and fluid balance to prevent decreased cardiac output. Assess intake and output and weigh the patient daily. If a pulmonary artery (PA) catheter is in place, monitor pulmonary artery pressure (PAP) and mixed venous oxygen saturation ($S\bar{v}O_2$).

• Keep in mind that the intubated patient can't speak. Provide alternative ways to communicate — for instance, a pencil and paper, a word chart, or an alphabet board.

*Weaning the patient from a mechanical ventilator.* Weaning should begin once the cause of respiratory failure is corrected and ABG values return to baseline. Weaning the patient with COPD commonly proves difficult. Help the doctor assess the patient's readiness.

• Make sure the patient is awake, alert, well rested, pain-free, and psychologically prepared for weaning. He should be able to maintain baseline ABG values on an $FIO_2$ of 0.4 or lower and PEEP below 5 cm $H_2O$. Also, he should have a minute ventilation below 10 liters/minute, a respiratory rate below 30 breaths/minute, and a negative inspiratory force above $-20$ cm $H_2O$.

• If the patient has been on the ventilator only briefly, you may be able to wean him successfully by decreasing the frequency and tidal volume of ventilated breaths or by using a T-piece.

• For the patient who has received prolonged mechanical ventilation, weaning is usually accomplished through pressure support ventilation, with or without intermittent mandatory ventilation. In the final weaning stages, the doctor may order alternate periods on and off the ventilator, increasing the time off the ventilator with each trial.

• During weaning, continue to observe the patient for signs and symptoms of hypoxia and hypercapnia.

### Patient teaching

• If the patient smokes, discuss the consequences of smoking and provide information on smoking cessation programs.

• Teach him how to use medications properly, and describe potential adverse drug effects. If he's to use a metered-dose inhaler, make sure he knows the proper technique.

• Teach the patient how to recognize signs and symptoms of overexertion as well as such complications as respiratory tract infection, bronchospasm, fluid retention, and heart failure. These may include a weight gain of 2 to 3 lb/day (0.9 to 1.4 kg/day), edema of the feet or ankles, nausea, loss of appetite, or abdominal tenderness. Discuss ways he can manage these problems with medical supervision.

• Encourage the patient to pace his activities and to rest frequently. Teach him how to conserve energy.

• Instruct the patient to notify the doctor if he has a respiratory tract infection or to start taking antibiotics if they've been prescribed. Advise him to avoid environmental irritants (such as smog, pollution, and dust) and people with illnesses. Review good nutritional practices and instruct him to avoid gas-producing foods.

• Help the patient develop the knowledge and skills he needs to perform pulmonary hygiene, which may include chest physiotherapy, incentive spirometry, coughing exercises, hydration, and suctioning. Encourage adequate hydration to thin secretions — but instruct the patient to notify the doctor of any signs and symptoms of fluid retention or heart failure.

• Arrange for the patient to enter a pulmonary rehabilitation program for exercise reconditioning, inspiratory muscle training, and ongoing education. Encourage him to obtain annual influenza vaccines and to receive at least one pneumococcal vaccine.

# Cor pulmonale

The World Health Organization defines chronic cor pulmonale as right ventricular hypertrophy secondary to diseases affecting lung function, lung structure, or both (except when such pulmonary alterations result from congenital heart disease or diseases that primarily affect the left side of the heart).

Invariably, cor pulmonale follows some disorder of the lungs, pulmonary vessels, chest wall, or respiratory control center. For instance, COPD produces pulmonary hypertension, which leads to right ventricular hypertrophy and failure. Because cor pulmonale typically occurs late in the course of COPD and other irreversible diseases, it carries a poor prognosis.

About 85% of patients with cor pulmonale have COPD. Cor pulmonale eventually develops in about 25% of patients with bronchial COPD. The disorder accounts for roughly one-quarter of all types of heart failure and is most common in COPD patients who smoke. Cor pulmonale affects middle-aged and elderly men more often than women, but the incidence in women is climbing.

In children, cor pulmonale may be a complication of cystic fibrosis, hemosiderosis, upper airway obstruction, scleroderma, extensive bronchiectasis, neurologic diseases that affect respiratory muscles, or abnormalities of the respiratory control center.

### Causes

Cor pulmonale may result from disorders that affect the pulmonary parenchyma (such as pulmonary fibrosis, pneumoconiosis, cystic fibrosis, periarteritis nodosa, and tuberculosis); pulmonary diseases that affect the airways (such as COPD and bronchial asthma); vascular diseases (such as vasculitis, pulmonary emboli, or an external vascular obstruction resulting from a tumor or an aneurysm); chest wall abnormalities, including thoracic deformities (such as kyphoscoliosis and pectus excavatum); and other factors, including obesity, high altitudes, and neuromuscular disorders (such as muscular dystrophy and poliomyelitis).

## Pathophysiology

In cor pulmonale, pulmonary hypertension increases the heart's work load. To compensate, the right ventricle hypertrophies to force blood through the lungs. However, this compensatory mechanism eventually begins to fail and larger amounts of blood remain in the right ventricle at the end of diastole. The ventricle then becomes dilated.

In response to hypoxia, the bone marrow produces more red blood cells (RBCs), resulting in polycythemia. Blood becomes more viscous, aggravating pulmonary hypertension, increasing the right ventricle's work load, and causing heart failure. (See *How cor pulmonale develops.*)

## Complications

Cor pulmonale eventually may lead to biventricular failure, hepatomegaly, edema, ascites, and pleural effusion. Because of polycythemia, the risk of thromboembolism increases.

## Assessment

### Signs and symptoms

As long as the heart can compensate for increased pulmonary vascular resistance, expect signs and symptoms associated with the underlying disorder. Typically, the patient has mostly respiratory complaints, such as a chronic productive cough, exertional dyspnea, and wheezing respirations. He also may report fatigue and weakness.

As cor pulmonale progresses, it causes dyspnea (even at rest) that worsens on exertion, tachypnea, orthopnea, edema, weakness, right upper quadrant discomfort, and clubbing of the fingers. Chest examination typically discloses characteristics of the underlying lung disease.

On inspection, you may find such signs of cor pulmonale (and right ventricular failure) as dependent edema and distended neck veins. Also expect drowsiness and an altered level of consciousness (LOC). Palpation may disclose tachycardia and a weak pulse (from decreased cardiac output), an enlarged and tender liver, hepatojugular reflux, and a prominent parasternal or epigastric cardiac impulse.

# How cor pulmonale develops

This flowchart shows the chain of events leading to cor pulmonale.

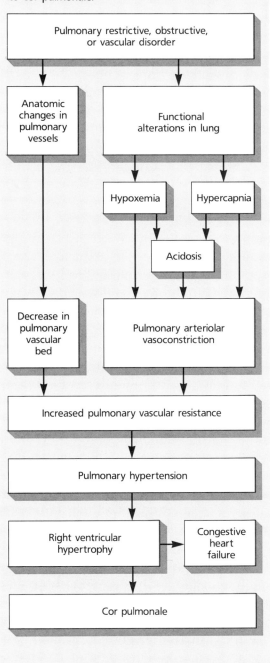

Chest auscultation findings depend on the cause of cor pulmonale. If the patient has COPD, you may detect crackles, rhonchi, and diminished breath sounds. With cor pulmonale secondary to upper airway obstruction or damage to the respiratory control center, auscultation findings may be normal except for a right ventricular heave, a gallop rhythm, and a loud pulmonic component of $S_2$.

If the patient has tricuspid insufficiency, you'll hear a pansystolic murmur at the lower left sternal border. The murmur intensifies when the patient inhales — a feature that distinguishes it from a murmur caused by mitral valve disease. Also, an early right ventricular murmur that increases on inspiration is audible at the left sternal border or over the epigastrium. You may auscultate a systolic pulmonary ejection sound.

### Diagnostic tests

PA catheterization shows increased right ventricular pressure and increased PAP secondary to increased pulmonary vascular resistance. Right ventricular systolic pressure and pulmonary artery systolic pressure (PASP) both rise above 30 mm Hg and pulmonary artery diastolic pressure (PADP) exceeds 15 mm Hg.

Echocardiography or angiography demonstrates right ventricular enlargement and ejection fraction. Chest X-rays reveal large central pulmonary arteries and right ventricular enlargement.

ABG analysis reveals decreased $PaO_2$ — usually less than 70 mm Hg and never more than 90 mm Hg. Electrocardiography (ECG) reveals arrhythmias, such as premature atrial and ventricular contractions and atrial fibrillation during severe hypoxia. It also may show right bundle-branch block, right axis deviation, prominent P waves and inverted T waves in right precordial leads, and right ventricular hypertrophy. Magnetic resonance imaging reveals right ventricular enlargement and ejection fraction.

The hematocrit value typically exceeds 50%. Serum enzyme studies show an elevated level of aspartate aminotransferase (formerly SGOT) with liver congestion and decreased liver function. If liver dysfunction and hepatomegaly are present, the serum bilirubin level may be elevated.

### Treatment

Goals of treatment for the patient with cor pulmonale include reducing hypoxemia, increasing exercise tolerance and, when possible, correcting the underlying condition. Besides bed rest, treatment may include administration of a digitalis glycoside (such as digoxin) and an antibiotic for an underlying respiratory tract infection. Usually, sputum culture and sensitivity tests determine which antibiotic the doctor prescribes. The patient with primary pulmonary hypertension may also receive a potent PA vasodilator, such as diazoxide, nitroprusside, or hydralazine.

The doctor may order oxygen by mask or cannula in concentrations ranging from 24% to 40%, depending on the patient's $PaO_2$ value. In acute disease, therapy also may include mechanical ventilation.

The patient may benefit from a low-sodium diet, restricted fluid intake, and possibly a diuretic (furosemide, for example) to reduce edema. Phlebotomy is occasionally required to decrease RBC mass. Small doses of an anticoagulant such as heparin can decrease the risk of thromboembolism.

Depending on the underlying cause of cor pulmonale, some treatment variations may be indicated. For example, the patient may need a tracheotomy if he has an upper airway obstruction, or a chest tube if he has a pneumothorax. Or he may require corticosteroids if he has vasculitis or an autoimmune disorder.

### Nursing care

• Monitor serum potassium levels closely if the patient is receiving a diuretic. Decreased serum potassium levels can potentiate arrhythmias associated with digitalis therapy.
• Be alert for complaints that signal digitalis toxicity, such as anorexia, nausea, vomiting, and seeing a yellow halo around objects. Monitor for arrhythmias.
• Prevent fluid retention by limiting the pa-

tient's daily fluid intake to 2 liters and by providing a low-sodium diet. Clarify the need for fluid restriction, especially if the patient has underlying COPD. (Usually, this patient should drink up to 10 glasses of water daily.)
• Plan a nutritious diet carefully with the patient and the staff dietitian. Because the patient may tire easily, provide small, frequent feedings rather than three heavy meals. Avoid scheduling respiratory treatments immediately before meals.
• Reposition the bedridden patient often to prevent atelectasis.
• If your patient needs oxygen, double-check his condition and watch for signs of hypercapnia and carbon dioxide narcosis. If he has underlying COPD, don't administer high oxygen concentrations because this could cause respiratory depression.
• Encourage the patient to rinse his mouth after respiratory therapy.
• Periodically obtain ABG values and watch for signs of respiratory failure: a change in the pulse rate, deep and labored respirations, and increased fatigue on exertion.
• Pace care activities to avoid patient fatigue.
• Listen to the patient's fears and concerns about his illness. Stay with him when he feels severe stress and anxiety. Encourage him to identify actions and care measures that promote comfort and relaxation. Whenever possible, include him in decisions about his care.

### Patient teaching
• Make sure the patient understands the importance of eating a low-sodium diet, weighing himself daily, and immediately reporting edema. Teach him to detect edema by pressing the skin over his shins with one finger, holding it for 1 to 2 seconds, and then checking for a finger impression. Instruct him to immediately report a weight gain of 2 to 3 lb (0.9 to 1.4 kg) over 1 to 2 days.
• Advise the patient to schedule frequent rest periods and to perform breathing exercises regularly.
• Because pulmonary infection usually exacerbates cor pulmonale (and COPD), teach the pa-

tient to watch for and immediately report early signs of infection, such as increased sputum production, change in sputum color, increased coughing or wheezing, chest pain, fever, and a feeling of tightness in the chest. Tell him to avoid crowds and people with known infections, especially during flu season.

# Pulmonary hypertension

In both the rare primary form and the more common secondary form, pulmonary hypertension is characterized by a resting PASP above 30 mm Hg and a mean PAP that is generally above 18 mm Hg. Primary, or idiopathic, pulmonary hypertension is characterized by increases in both PAP and pulmonary vascular resistance without an obvious cause. This form of the disorder, most common in women between ages 20 and 40, is usually fatal within 3 to 4 years and may not be diagnosed until autopsy. Mortality is highest in pregnant women. In secondary pulmonary hypertension, the prognosis depends on the severity of the underlying disorder.

### Causes
Although the cause of primary pulmonary hypertension remains unknown, the tendency for the disorder to occur within families points to a hereditary defect. Because this form of pulmonary hypertension occurs in association with collagen diseases, it is thought to result from altered immune mechanisms.

Secondary pulmonary hypertension is caused by hypoxemia stemming from an existing cardiac or pulmonary disease or both. The cause of hypoxemia may be:
• alveolar hypoventilation, which may result from diseases causing alveolar destruction, such as COPD (the most common cause in the United States), sarcoidosis, diffuse interstitial pneumonia, metastatic cancer, or scleroderma. Alveolar hypoventilation sometimes stems from obesity or kyphoscoliosis, which don't damage lung tissue but do prevent the chest wall from

# Identifying pulmonary hypertension on an X-ray

The chest X-ray of a patient with pulmonary hypertension typically shows prominent main pulmonary arteries, enlarged hilar vessels, reduced peripheral vessels and, in severe cases, an enlarged cardiac silhouette. The first illustration shows findings typical of mild primary pulmonary hypertension. The second depicts the changes occurring in severe pulmonary hypertension. The third shows severe pulmonary hypertension with extremely prominent main pulmonary arteries and a pruned appearance of the pulmonary vascular tree.

**Mild primary pulmonary hypertension**

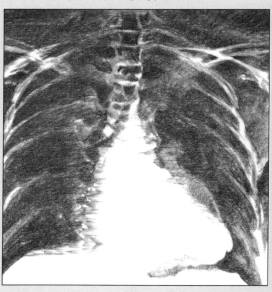

expanding sufficiently to let air into the alveoli.
• vascular obstruction from pulmonary embolism or vasculitis, and disorders that cause obstruction of small or large pulmonary veins, such as left atrial myxoma, idiopathic veno-occlusive disease, fibrous mediastinitis, or mediastinal neoplasm.
• primary congenital cardiac disease that may cause interpulmonary shunting, including patent ductus arteriosus and atrial or ventricular septal defects. Shunting into the PA reroutes blood through the lungs twice, causing pulmonary hypertension.
• acquired cardiac disease, such as rheumatic valvular disease and mitral stenosis, which leads to left ventricular failure, thereby diminishing the flow of oxygenated blood from the lungs. This increases pulmonary vascular resistance and right ventricular pressure.

### Pathophysiology

In primary pulmonary hypertension, the intimal lining of the PA thickens for no obvious reason. As the artery narrows and becomes less distensible, vascular resistance rises.

In secondary pulmonary hypertension, decreased ventilation increases pulmonary vascular resistance. Hypoxemia resulting from this $\dot{V}/\dot{Q}$ mismatch also causes vasoconstriction, further raising vascular resistance. The result is pulmonary hypertension.

### Complications

Pulmonary hypertension may lead to cor pulmonale, heart failure, and cardiac arrest.

## Assessment
### Signs and symptoms

Primary pulmonary hypertension may not cause symptoms until lung damage becomes severe. Usually, the patient with secondary pulmonary hypertension has signs and symptoms

### Severe pulmonary hypertension

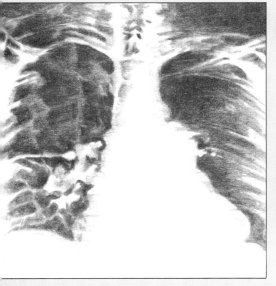

### Severe pulmonary hypertension with prominent pulmonary arteries

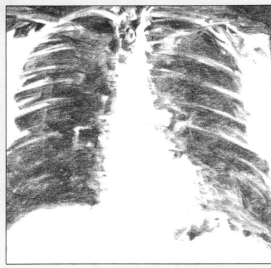

of left ventricular failure, such as increasing dyspnea on exertion, difficulty or pain on breathing, weakness, fatigue, and syncope.

Inspection may reveal signs of right ventricular failure, including ascites and neck vein distention. The patient may appear restless and agitated, with a decreased LOC, confusion, and memory loss. You may assess reduced diaphragmatic excursion and respiration along with displacement of the point of maximal impulse beyond the midclavicular line.

Palpation also may reveal signs of right ventricular failure, such as peripheral edema. Typically, the patient has an easily palpable right ventricular heave. He may also have tachycardia and a palpable, tender liver.

Auscultation findings depend on the underlying disorder but may include a systolic ejection murmur, a widely split $S_2$ sound, and $S_3$ and $S_4$ sounds. You may hear decreased breath sounds and loud tubular sounds. Blood pressure is typically low.

### Diagnostic tests

ABG studies reveal hypoxemia (decreased $PaO_2$). In right ventricular hypertrophy, the ECG shows right axis deviation and tall, peaked P waves.

Cardiac catheterization discloses a PASP above 30 mm Hg. It may show increased pulmonary artery wedge pressure (PAWP) if the underlying cause is left atrial myxoma, mitral stenosis, or left ventricular failure; otherwise, PAWP is normal. Pulmonary angiography detects filling defects in the pulmonary vasculature, such as those that develop with pulmonary emboli. Chest X-ray findings will vary with the severity of pulmonary hypertension. (See *Identifying pulmonary hypertension on an X-ray.*)

Pulmonary function tests may show decreased flow rates and increased residual volume in underlying obstructive disease and possibly reduced total lung capacity in underlying restrictive disease. Radionuclide imaging assesses right and left ventricular function. Open lung biopsy may determine the type of disorder.

Echocardiography allows assessment of ventricular wall motion and possible valvular dysfunction. It may demonstrate right ventricular enlargement, abnormal septal configuration consistent with right ventricular pressure overload, and a small left ventricular cavity. A perfusion lung scan may produce normal or abnormal results, with multiple patchy and diffuse filling defects that do not look like pulmonary thromboembolism.

## Treatment
Oxygen therapy is usually indicated to decrease hypoxemia and pulmonary vascular resistance. Treatment for a patient with right ventricular failure also includes fluid restriction, a digitalis glycoside to boost cardiac output, and a diuretic to reduce intravascular volume and extravascular fluid accumulation.

Expect the doctor to order a vasodilator or calcium channel blocker to reduce the heart's work load and oxygen consumption only if congestive heart failure is not present, because these drugs lower contractility. He also may order a bronchodilator or a pulmonary vasodilator.

For a patient with secondary pulmonary hypertension, treatment also aims to correct the underlying cause. If that's not possible and the disease progresses, the patient may require a heart and lung transplant or open-heart surgery to replace a stenotic mitral valve.

## Nursing care
### Immediate care
• Administer oxygen therapy as ordered, and observe the patient's response. Report any signs of increasing dyspnea so that the doctor can adjust therapy accordingly.
• Immediately report any change in the patient's LOC.
• Monitor vital signs, especially blood pressure and heart rate. If hypotension or tachycardia develops, notify the doctor. If the patient has a PA catheter, monitor PAP and PAWP as ordered, and report any changes.

### Continuing care
• Monitor ABG values for acidosis and hypoxemia.
• If the patient has right ventricular failure, record his weight daily and carefully measure intake and output — especially if he's receiving diuretics. Check for increasing neck vein distention, which may signal fluid overload. Explain the rationale for all medications and diet restrictions.
• Alternate periods of rest and activity to reduce the patient's oxygen needs and to prevent fatigue.
• Arrange for diversional activities. Choose the type of activity — active or passive — based on the patient's physical condition.
• Listen to the patient's fears and concerns, and stay with him during periods of extreme stress and anxiety. Answer his questions as well as you can. Encourage him to identify care measures and activities that make him comfortable and relaxed. Then try to perform these measures, and encourage him to do so, too, if appropriate.
• Encourage the patient to participate in care decisions. Include his family in all phases of his care.

### Patient teaching
• Teach the patient which signs and symptoms to report to the doctor: swelling, increasing shortness of breath, weight gain, and fatigue.
• Fully explain the prescribed medication regimen.
• If indicated, review the restrictions the patient must follow on a low-sodium diet.
• Teach the patient taking a potassium-wasting diuretic to eat plenty of foods that are high in potassium, such as apricots, bananas, cantaloupes, dried fruits, grapefruit, honeydew melons, mushrooms, nuts, oranges, peanut butter, potatoes, tomatoes, and winter squash.
• If the patient smokes, encourage him to stop. Give him the names of smoking cessation programs.
• Warn the patient not to overexert himself, and suggest frequent rest periods between activities.

• If the patient needs special equipment for home use, such as oxygen equipment, refer him to the social service department.

# Pneumonia

An acute infection of the lung parenchyma that may impair gas exchange, pneumonia can be classified in several ways. Based on *microbiological etiology,* it may be classified as viral, bacterial, fungal, protozoal, mycobacterial, mycoplasmal, or rickettsial. Based on *location,* it may be classified as bronchopneumonia, lobular pneumonia, or lobar pneumonia. Bronchopneumonia involves the distal airways and alveoli; lobular pneumonia involves part of a lobe; and lobar pneumonia involves an entire lobe.

Pneumonia is the leading cause of death from infectious disease in the United States, with more than 3 million cases annually. It affects both sexes and all age-groups. The disorder carries a good prognosis in patients with normal lungs and adequate immune systems. In debilitated patients, however, bacterial pneumonia ranks as the most common cause of death. (See *Understanding types of pneumonia,* pages 68 to 70.)

## Causes

Primary pneumonia results directly from inhalation of or contact with a pathogen, such as a bacterium or a virus. Secondary pneumonia may follow initial lung damage from a noxious material or infection, or may result from hematogenous spread of bacteria from a distant area. Aspiration pneumonia results from inhalation of foreign matter, such as vomitus or food particles, into the bronchi.

Certain predisposing factors increase the risk of pneumonia. For bacterial and viral pneumonia, these include chronic illness and debilitation, cancer (particularly of the lung), human immunodeficiency virus, acquired immunodeficiency syndrome, tracheotomy, abdominal or thoracic surgery, atelectasis, a common cold or other viral respiratory infection, chronic respiratory disease (COPD, asthma, bronchiectasis,

cystic fibrosis), influenza, smoking, malnutrition, alcoholism, sickle cell disease, exposure to noxious gases, and immunosuppressive therapy.

Aspiration pneumonia most commonly affects elderly or debilitated patients, those receiving nasogastric (NG) tube feedings, and those with an impaired gag reflex, poor oral hygiene, or a decreased LOC.

## Pathophysiology

In *bacterial pneumonia,* which can occur in any part of the lungs, an infection initially triggers alveolar inflammation and edema. Capillaries become engorged with blood, causing stasis. As the alveolocapillary membrane weakens, alveoli fill with blood and exudate, resulting in atelectasis. In severe bacterial infections, the lungs appear heavy and liverlike, as in adult respiratory distress syndrome (ARDS).

Viral infection leading to *viral pneumonia* first attacks bronchiolar epithelial cells, leading to interstitial inflammation and desquamation. It then spreads to the alveoli, which fill with blood and fluid. In advanced infection, a hyaline membrane may form. As with bacterial infection, severe viral infection may clinically resemble ARDS.

In *aspiration pneumonia,* aspiration of gastric juices or hydrocarbons triggers similar inflammatory changes and impairs surfactant function over a large area. Reduced surfactant leads to alveolar collapse. Acidic gastric juices may directly damage the airways and alveoli, leading to ARDS. Particles in the aspirated gastric juices may obstruct the airways and reduce airflow, which in turn can lead to secondary bacterial pneumonia.

## Complications

Without proper treatment, pneumonia can result in such life-threatening complications as septic shock, hypoxemia, and respiratory failure. Infection may spread within the lungs, causing empyema or lung abscess. Or it may spread via the bloodstream or by cross-contamination to other parts of the body, causing bacteremia, endocarditis, pericarditis, or meningitis.

*(Text continues on page 70.)*

# Understanding types of pneumonia

| CHARACTERISTICS | DIAGNOSTIC TESTS | TREATMENT |
| --- | --- | --- |
| **Viral pneumonias** | | |
| **Influenza**<br>• Prognosis poor even with treatment<br>• 50% mortality from cardiopulmonary collapse<br>• Signs and symptoms include cough (initially nonproductive; later, purulent sputum), marked cyanosis, dyspnea, high fever, chills, substernal pain and discomfort, moist crackles, frontal headache, myalgia. | • Diffuse bilateral bronchopneumonia radiating from hilus on chest X-ray<br>• Normal to slightly elevated white blood cell (WBC) count<br>• No specific organisms on sputum smears | • Supportive treatment for respiratory failure includes endotracheal intubation and ventilator assistance; for fever, hypothermia blanket or antipyretics; for influenza A, amantadine. |
| **Adenovirus**<br>• Insidious onset<br>• Generally affects young adults<br>• Good prognosis; usually clears with no residual effects<br>• Signs and symptoms include sore throat, fever, cough, chills, malaise, small amounts of mucoid sputum, retrosternal chest pain, anorexia, rhinitis, adenopathy, scattered crackles, and rhonchi. | • Patchy distribution of pneumonia on chest X-ray; more severe than indicated by physical examination<br>• Normal to slightly elevated WBC count | • Treatment aims to relieve symptoms.<br>• Supportive treatment may include mechanical ventilation. |
| **Respiratory syncytial virus**<br>• Most prevalent in infants and children<br>• Complete recovery in 1 to 3 weeks<br>• Signs and symptoms include listlessness, irritability, tachypnea with retraction of intercostal muscles, slight sputum production, fine moist crackles, fever, severe malaise and, possibly, cough or croup. | • Patchy bilateral consolidation on chest X-ray<br>• Normal to slightly elevated WBC count | • Supportive treatment includes humidified air, oxygen, and antimicrobials (often given until viral cause is confirmed). |
| **Measles (rubeola)**<br>• Signs and symptoms include fever, dyspnea, cough, small amounts of sputum, coryza, rash, and cervical adenopathy. | • Reticular infiltrates on chest X-ray; sometimes with hilar lymph node enlargement<br>• Characteristic giant cells in lung tissue specimen | • Supportive treatment includes bed rest, adequate hydration, antimicrobials and, if necessary, assisted ventilation. |
| **Chicken pox (varicella)**<br>• Uncommon in children, but present in 30% of adults with varicella<br>• Signs and symptoms include characteristic rash, cough, dyspnea, cyanosis, tachypnea, pleuritic chest pain, and hemoptysis and rhonchi 1 to 6 days after onset of rash. | • More extensive pneumonia on chest X-ray than indicated by physical examination; also bilateral, patchy, diffuse, nodular infiltrates evident<br>• Predominant mononuclear cells and characteristic intranuclear inclusion bodies from sputum analysis | • Supportive treatment includes adequate hydration and, in critically ill patients, oxygen therapy. |
| **Cytomegalovirus**<br>• Difficult to distinguish from other nonbacterial pneumonias<br>• In adults with healthy lung tissue, resembles mononucleosis and is generally benign; in neonates, occurs as devastating multisystem infection; in immunocompromised hosts, varies from clinically inapparent to fatal infection<br>• Signs and symptoms include fever, cough, shaking chills, dyspnea, cyanosis, weakness, and diffuse crackles. | • In early stages, variable patchy infiltrates on chest X-ray; in later stages, bilateral, nodular, and more predominant infiltrates in lower lobes<br>• Typical intranuclear and cytoplasmic inclusions on microscopic examination of lung tissue from percutaneous aspiration, transbronchial biopsy, or open lung biopsy (the virus can be cultured from lung tissue) | • Supportive treatment includes adequate hydration and nutrition, oxygen therapy, and bed rest. |

# Understanding types of pneumonia (continued)

| CHARACTERISTICS | DIAGNOSTIC TESTS | TREATMENT |
|---|---|---|
| **Bacterial pneumonias** | | |
| *Streptococcus*<br>• Caused by *Streptococcus pneumoniae*<br>• Signs and symptoms include sudden onset of a single, shaking chill, and sustained temperature of 102° to 104° F (38.9° to 40° C); often preceded by upper respiratory tract infection. | • Areas of consolidation, often lobar, on chest X-ray<br>• Elevated WBC count<br>• Possibly gram-positive *S. pneumoniae* on sputum culture | • Antimicrobial therapy consists of penicillin G or, if the patient is allergic to penicillin, erythromycin; therapy begun after obtaining culture specimen but without waiting for results and continues for 7 to 10 days. |
| *Klebsiella*<br>• More likely in patients with chronic alcoholism, pulmonary disease, and diabetes<br>• Signs and symptoms include fever and recurrent chills; cough producing rusty, bloody, viscous sputum (currant jelly); cyanosis of lips and nail beds from hypoxemia; shallow, grunting respirations. | • Typically, but not always, consolidation in the upper lobe that causes bulging of fissures on chest X-ray<br>• Elevated WBC count<br>• Possibly gram-negative cocci *Klebsiella* on sputum culture and Gram stain | • Antimicrobial therapy consists of an aminoglycoside and, in serious infections, a cephalosporin. |
| *Staphylococcus*<br>• Commonly occurs in patients with viral illness, such as influenza or measles, and in those with cystic fibrosis<br>• Signs and symptoms include a temperature of 102° to 104° F, recurrent shaking chills, bloody sputum, dyspnea, tachypnea, and hypoxemia. | • Multiple abscesses and infiltrates; frequently empyema on chest X-ray<br>• Elevated WBC count<br>• Possibly gram-positive staphylococci on sputum culture and Gram stain | • Antimicrobial therapy consists of nafcillin or oxacillin for 14 days if staphylococci are penicillinase-producing.<br>• A chest tube drains empyema. |
| **Atypical pneumonia** | | |
| *Mycoplasma*<br>• Accounts for 30% to 50% of community-acquired pneumonia<br>• Transmitted by contact with infected secretions<br>• Occurs mostly in healthy adults<br>• The most common signs and symptoms are nonproductive cough, sore throat, and otologic symptoms. Low-grade fever, scattered crackles and rhonchi, pharyngeal erythema, cervical adenopathy, bulbous myringitis, and severe headache also may occur. | • Patchy infiltrates on chest X-ray<br>• Possible elevated ESR<br>• Usually normal WBC count | • Antimicrobial therapy consists of erythromycin or tetracycline for 10 to 14 days or up to 3 weeks in severe cases. |
| **Protozoal pneumonia** | | |
| *Pneumocystis carinii*<br>• Most common life-threatening opportunistic infection in people with human immunodeficiency virus or acquired immunodeficiency syndrome<br>• Signs and symptoms include low-grade fever, fatigue, weight loss, dyspnea on exertion, nonproductive to mildly productive cough, and dry crackles. | • Diffuse bilateral interstitial infiltrates on chest X-ray<br>• Increased erythrocyte sedimentation rate (ESR)<br>• Increased lactate dehydrogenase level<br>• Expectorated sputum for staining and microscopic visualization<br>• Bronchial biopsy if patient can't expectorate sputum | • Pentamidine or both trimethoprim and sulfamethoxazole may be given for 14 to 21 days.<br>• Steroids have proven effective in patients in acute respiratory failure. |

## Understanding types of pneumonia *(continued)*

| CHARACTERISTICS | DIAGNOSTIC TESTS | TREATMENT |
|---|---|---|
| **Aspiration pneumonia** | | |
| • Results from vomiting and aspiration of gastric or oropharyngeal contents into trachea and lungs<br>• Noncardiogenic pulmonary edema possible with damage to respiratory epithelium from contact with gastric acid<br>• Subacute pneumonia possible with cavity formation<br>• Lung abscess possible if foreign body present<br>• Signs and symptoms include crackles, dyspnea, cyanosis, hypotension, and tachycardia. | • Location of areas of infiltrates on chest X-ray | • Antimicrobial therapy consists of penicillin G or clindamycin.<br>• Supportive therapy includes oxygen therapy, suctioning, coughing, deep breathing, adequate hydration, and I.V. corticosteroids. |

## Assessment
### Signs and symptoms
In bacterial pneumonia, the patient may report pleuritic chest pain, chills, a fever, and a cough that yields excessive sputum. Creamy yellow sputum suggests staphylococcal pneumonia; green sputum denotes pneumonia caused by *Pseudomonas* organisms; and sputum that looks like currant jelly suggests *Klebsiella* infection. Sputum that appears rusty or resembles prune juice may indicate streptococcal pneumonia. Clear sputum indicates absence of a bacterial process.

In advanced cases of all types of pneumonia, you'll hear dullness on lung percussion. Auscultation may disclose crackles, wheezing, or rhonchi over the affected lung area as well as decreased breath sounds and vocal fremitus.

### Diagnostic tests
Chest X-rays disclose infiltrates, which usually confirm the diagnosis. A sputum specimen for Gram stain and culture and sensitivity tests shows acute inflammatory cells. (See *Collecting a sputum specimen.*)

Typically, the white blood cell (WBC) count increases in bacterial pneumonia and decreases or remains normal in viral or mycoplasmal pneumonia. Blood cultures help determine the causative organism in bacterial pneumonia.

ABG values vary with the severity of pneumonia and the underlying lung condition. Pulse oximetry may show a reduced $SaO_2$ level.

Viral cultures obtained by nasopharyngeal or pharyngeal swab may pinpoint a viral cause. Serology, rapid antigen tests, the direct fluorescence antibody test, the enzyme-linked immunosorbent assay (ELISA), and immunofluorescent antibody stains also may help identify a viral organism. The erythrocyte sedimentation rate may rise in pneumonia caused by *Mycoplasma* or *Pneumocystis carinii.*

## Treatment
Expect the doctor to prescribe antimicrobial therapy based on the causative agent, then re-evaluate therapy early in the course of treatment. Supportive measures include humidified oxygen to correct hypoxemia, bronchodilator therapy, a nocturnal antitussive as needed, analgesics to relieve pleuritic chest pain, a high-calorie diet, adequate fluid intake, and bed rest.

If the patient is in respiratory failure, he'll be mechanically ventilated. If he has severe pneumonia, he may need PEEP to maintain adequate oxygenation and should be positioned for optimal gas exchange, with the unimpaired lung down to increase perfusion and improve oxygen transport.

## Nursing care

• Maintain a patent airway and adequate oxygenation. Monitor $SaO_2$ values by pulse oximetry or ABG analysis, especially if the patient is hypoxic. Administer supplemental oxygen as ordered if his $PaO_2$ falls below 55 mm Hg. If he has a chronic lung disease, give oxygen cautiously.

• In severe pneumonia that requires endotracheal intubation or a tracheotomy (with or without mechanical ventilation), provide thorough respiratory care and suction often, using sterile technique to remove secretions.

• Obtain sputum specimens on admission and as needed. If the patient can't produce a specimen on his own, use suction to obtain one. Collect specimens in a sterile container, and deliver them to the microbiology laboratory promptly.

• Administer antibiotics and pain medication as ordered and needed. To prevent nausea, avoid giving medications right before meals.

• Administer I.V. fluids and electrolyte replacement, if needed, to manage fever and ensure adequate hydration.

• Provide a high-calorie, high-protein diet of soft foods to offset the calories the patient must use to fight the infection. If necessary, supplement oral feedings with NG tube feedings or parenteral nutrition.

• Monitor the patient's fluid intake and output.

• To control infection spread, dispose of secretions properly. Instruct the patient to sneeze and cough into a disposable tissue, and tape a waxed bag to the side of the bed for used tissues.

• Position the patient properly to promote full aeration and drainage of secretions.

• Urge a bedridden or postoperative patient to perform deep-breathing and coughing exercises frequently.

• Explain all procedures (especially intubation and suctioning) to the patient and his family, including them whenever possible in discussions and decisions about his care.

• Provide a quiet, calm environment and schedule frequent rest periods.

• Listen to the patient's fears and concerns, and stay with him during periods of severe stress and anxiety. Encourage him to identify

## Collecting a sputum specimen

Using proper technique when collecting a sputum specimen is essential. Ideally, you should collect the specimen before antibiotic therapy begins; contaminated specimens can lead to a treatment delay. To help ensure that the specimen is acceptable for laboratory analysis, follow these guidelines:

• Obtain the specimen just after the patient awakens in the morning.

• Have the patient rinse his mouth with water first. Instruct him *not* to use mouthwash.

• To maintain sterility, instruct the patient to expectorate as deeply as possible into a sterile sputum container after coughing deeply. A deep cough is important because the lower respiratory tract (lungs, bronchi, and trachea) is sterile. Make sure that the patient doesn't touch the rim or inside of the container. Instruct him to avoid mixing saliva with the sputum specimen.

• If the patient can't expectorate sputum, attempt chest physiotherapy and administer a bronchodilator as ordered. If he still can't produce a sputum specimen, nasotracheal suctioning may be necessary.

• Label the laboratory slip and specimen container with the patient's name, identification number, and room number; the doctor's name; and the date and time that the specimen was collected.

actions and care measures that promote comfort and relaxation.

### Patient teaching

• Instruct the patient about his medication regimen. Stress the need to take the entire amount of the prescribed medication, even if he feels better, to prevent a relapse.

• Teach the patient and his family about chest physiotherapy to enhance removal of lung secretions. Explain to them how to perform deep breathing, coughing exercises, and pursed-lip breathing. Discuss postural drainage and vibration.

• Teach the patient and his family about home oxygen therapy.

• Urge the patient to drink 2 to 3 qt (about 2 to 3 liters) of fluid daily. This will help him to

maintain adequate hydration and keep secretions thin for easier removal.
• Discuss ways to avoid spreading the infection to others. Remind the patient to sneeze and cough into tissues, and then dispose of them in a waxed or plastic bag. Advise him to wash his hands thoroughly after handling contaminated tissues.
• Emphasize the importance of adequate rest in achieving a complete recovery and preventing a relapse. Tell the patient that the doctor will inform him when he can resume full activity and return to work.
• Encourage the high-risk patient to consult his doctor about getting annual influenza vaccinations and a one-time pneumococcal pneumonia vaccination.
• Urge the patient to avoid irritants that stimulate secretions, such as cigarette smoke, dust, and significant environmental pollution. If indicated, refer the patient to community programs or agencies that can help him stop smoking.
• To help prevent pneumonia, you should advise all patients to avoid using antibiotics indiscriminately for minor infections because this could cause upper airway colonization with antibiotic-resistant bacteria; if pneumonia later develops, the causative organisms may require more toxic antibiotics.

# Pleural effusion

Pleural effusion occurs when excess fluid accumulates in the pleural space, for example, from increased fluid production or reduced fluid removal. Normally, the pleural space contains only a small amount of extracellular fluid, which lubricates the pleural surfaces. The five major types of pleural effusions are transudative effusion, exudative effusion, hemothorax (hemorrhagic effusion, or blood in the pleural space), chylous effusion (chyliform, or lymph in the pleural space), and empyema (pus in the pleural space).

## Causes
*Transudative pleural effusion* occurs when fluid accumulation results from increased hydrostatic pressure, decreased osmotic pressure, and greater negative intrapleural pressure. *Exudative effusion* results from pleural disease in association with increased capillary permeability or reduced lymphatic drainage.

Congestive heart failure (CHF) is the most common underlying cause of pleural effusion and accounts for most cases of transudative effusion. Bacterial pneumonia and cancer are typical underlying causes of exudative effusion.

## Pathophysiology
Fluid accumulates in the pleural space (as in any part of the body) when an imbalance occurs between fluid formation and fluid absorption. The difference between the hydrostatic pressure of parietal pleural capillaries (supplied by the systemic circulation) and that of visceral pleural capillaries (supplied mostly by the pulmonary circulation) suggests that fluid forms at the parietal pleura and is absorbed by the visceral pleura.

Disease states may upset the balance between pleural fluid formation and absorption, causing fluid accumulation and effusion. Both the fluid source and the absorption mechanism may differ from those occurring in a normal state.

## Complications
Large pleural effusions may lead to atelectasis, infection, and hypoxemia.

## Assessment
### Signs and symptoms
The patient's history typically shows underlying pulmonary disease. Large pleural effusions may cause dyspnea, particularly in a patient with underlying cardiopulmonary disease. Pleuritic chest pain and a dry cough also may occur. Pain is usually unilateral and sharp, worsening with inspiration, coughing, or rib cage movement.

Small pleural effusions rarely cause symptoms. With larger effusions, physical findings may include a decrease in tactile fremitus, dullness on percussion, and diminished breath sounds over the effusion. If a large effusion is compressing a lung, expect accentuated breath sounds and possibly egophony above the effusion. A massive pleural effusion causing high intrapleural pressure may lead to shifting of the trachea from the midline toward the affected side (tension hydrothorax).

With empyema, expect fever and subjective complaints of malaise along with other manifestations of bacterial infection such as an elevated WBC.

## Diagnostic tests

Chest X-ray, the primary test used to diagnose pleural effusion, shows radiopaque fluid in dependent regions. Lateral decubitus views are preferred over conventional posteroanterior views because they can detect smaller amounts of free pleural fluid.

If the diagnosis remains uncertain after standard X-rays, the doctor may use thoracic ultrasound, a computed tomography (CT) scan, or both to confirm and localize pleural fluid — especially when he's considering thoracentesis.

If other tests find no apparent cause for the effusion, diagnostic thoracentesis is indicated to allow analysis of aspirated pleural fluid. In exudative effusion, thoracentesis yields the following results:
- pleural fluid–to–serum ratio of 0.5 or more
- pleural fluid lactate dehydrogenase (LDH) level equal to or greater than 200 IU/liter
- ratio of pleural fluid LDH to serum LDH of 0.6 or more
- pleural fluid LDH level more than two-thirds the upper limit of normal serum LDH.

In transudative effusion, pleural fluid usually has a specific gravity below 1.015 and a protein level of less than 3 g/dl. The WBC count exceeds 1,000/μl, with mononuclear cells predominating in the differential. The pleural fluid glucose level equals the serum glucose level, and pH is normal.

The gross appearance of pleural fluid helps establish the type of effusion. (See *Identifying types of pleural effusion.*)

If careful pleural fluid examination and other studies fail to determine the cause of the effusion, pleural biopsy is the next step. In this procedure, the doctor removes small

### ASSESSMENT INSIGHT

# Identifying types of pleural effusion

Evaluating the appearance of pleural fluid helps differentiate among the less common types of pleural effusion: hemothorax (hemorrhagic effusion), chylous effusion, and empyema.

In *hemothorax,* pleural fluid appears bloody.

In *chylous effusion,* pleural fluid contains milky lymph from the thoracic duct (chyle). This type of effusion is usually associated with cancer or, less commonly, with thoracic surgery or trauma.

In *empyema,* pleural fluid is grossly purulent and contains pyogenic organisms, such as aerobic bacteria, pneumococci, staphylococci, streptococci, and certain gram-negative bacteria.

pieces of the parietal pleura and sends the specimen for histologic and bacterial analysis.

## Treatment

Management focuses on the underlying cause as well as the effusion itself. Oxygen therapy is indicated if the patient is hypoxemic. ABG values determine the concentration of oxygen to be used.

Transudative pleural effusions usually respond to treatment of the underlying condition. Therapeutic thoracentesis is warranted only if the effusion is massive and causes dyspnea. For a patient with bilateral pleural effusion and CHF, diagnostic or therapeutic thoracentesis is rarely done. Most such effusions are transudative and usually resolve with treatment of CHF.

For a pleural effusion associated with a malignant tumor that directly invades the pleural space, chemotherapy and radiation therapy are indicated (this type of tumor is inoperable). If the tumor doesn't directly invade the pleural space, surgical resection may be possible. Pleurectomy and repeated therapeutic thoracentesis are alternative approaches for selected patients with rapidly recurring malignant pleural effusion.

Parapneumonic pleural effusion usually responds to systemic antibiotic therapy. Management includes sputum for Gram stain cultures, blood cultures, diagnostic thoracentesis, and possibly closed chest drainage (or tube thoracostomy). In uncomplicated parapneumonic effusion, pleural infection usually is absent and pleural fluid glucose levels and pH are normal. Such effusions are likely to resolve spontaneously and don't require chest tube drainage. In complicated parapneumonic effusion, pleural fluid may reveal frank empyema. A pH below 7.2, a serum glucose level under 50 mg/dl, and a pleural fluid LDH level above 1,000 IU/liter help distinguish complicated from uncomplicated parapneumonic effusion.

### Surgery

Surgery for pleural effusion may involve chest tube insertion, chemical pleurodesis, or thoracentesis.

**Chest tube insertion.** In parapneumonic effusion, the doctor will perform this procedure if any of these factors are present:
• Pleural fluid resembles frank pus.
• An organism is evident on Gram stain.
• The serum glucose level exceeds 40 mg/dl.
• Arterial pH is below 7.0.

Inserting a chest tube permits drainage of fluid from the pleural space. This procedure is usually performed by a doctor with a nurse assisting. For a pleural effusion, the sixth to eighth intercostal spaces are common insertion sites because fluid settles at the lower levels of the pleural space. After insertion, the chest tube is connected to a thoracic drainage system, which removes fluid from the pleural space and prevents backflow into that space, promoting lung reexpansion.

For a hemothorax, the doctor will insert one or more large chest tubes to control bleeding by causing opposition of the pleural surfaces. Chest tube insertion also helps determine the amount of bleeding and decreases the risk of empyema and other complications. Thoracotomy is occasionally required to control bleeding, remove blood clots, or treat coexisting complications of trauma. A small hemothorax can be managed without chest tube drainage.

**Chemical pleurodesis.** This procedure obliterates the pleural space by producing fibrous adhesions between the visceral and parietal pleurae. It's recommended for selected patients with symptomatic malignant pleural effusion who don't respond to chemotherapy or mediastinal radiation.

In chemical pleurodesis, the doctor inserts an intercostal tube in a low intercostal space and connects it to suction or water-seal drainage until as much fluid as possible has been removed. The doctor then injects 500 mg to 1 g of doxycycline, dissolved in 100 to 200 ml of 0.9% sodium chloride solution, into the pleural cavity through the tube and clamps the tube. He may add lidocaine to the solution to prevent burning and irritation.

Next, the patient is moved into both lateral decubitus positions — first with his head elevated, then with his head lowered, for 5 minutes in each position to distribute doxycycline within the pleural space. Then the tube is unclamped and water-seal drainage continues until the drainage slows to less than 60 ml/24 hours. The tube is usually removed the next day.

**Thoracentesis.** In this procedure, fluid is aspirated from the pleural space, relieving pulmonary compression and respiratory distress. The doctor also may obtain a specimen of pleural fluid or tissue for analysis or may instill chemotherapeutic agents or other drugs into the pleural space.

## Nursing care
### Immediate care
• Place the patient in a position that prevents aspiration and maintains a clear airway.
• Avoid overmedication with sedatives and narcotics because oversedation and respiratory depression promote buildup of lung secretions.
• Maintain adequate hydration and oxygenation, according to doctor's orders.
• Have thoracentesis and tube thoracostomy trays available.

## Surgical care

**For chest tube insertion.** Before the procedure, tell the patient what to expect. Provide privacy, and wash your hands.

Record baseline vital signs and respiratory findings.

Position the patient so that he's firmly supported and comfortable. Although the choice of position can vary, you'll usually seat him at the edge of the bed with his legs supported and his head and folded arms resting on a pillow on the overbed table. Or you can have him straddle a chair backward and rest his head and folded arms on the back of the chair. If he can't sit, turn him on the unaffected side with the arm of the affected side raised above his head. Elevate the head of the bed 30 to 45 degrees (unless contraindicated). Proper positioning stretches the chest or back and allows easier access to the intercostal spaces.

• During the procedure, reassure the patient and assist the doctor as necessary as he inserts the chest tube.

• Using sterile technique, place two 4" × 4" drain dressings around the insertion site — one on the top and the other on the bottom. Place several 4" × 4" gauze pads on top of the drain dressings.

• Tape the chest tube to the patient's chest distal to the insertion site to help prevent accidental dislodgment. Keep petroleum gauze at the bedside in case the chest tube becomes dislodged.

• Tape the junction of the chest tube and drainage tube to prevent their separation.

• Coil the drainage tubing and secure it to the bed linens with tape and a safety pin, providing enough slack for the patient to move and turn. This prevents the drainage tubing from kinking or dropping to the floor (which would impair drainage into the bottle) and helps avert accidental chest tube dislodgment.

• Immediately after the drainage system is connected, instruct the patient to take a deep breath, hold it momentarily, and exhale slowly to promote drainage of the pleural space and lung reexpansion.

• After the procedure, arrange for a portable chest X-ray to check chest tube position.

• Take the patient's vital signs every 15 minutes for the first hour, then as his condition indicates.

• Auscultate his lungs at least every 4 hours to assess air exchange in the affected lung. Diminished or absent breath sounds indicate that the lung hasn't reexpanded.

• Provide meticulous chest tube care. Use aseptic technique when changing dressings around the tube insertion site. Ensure tube patency by watching for bubbles in the underwater seal chamber. Record the amount, color, and consistency of chest tube drainage.

• Don't clamp the chest tube because this may cause tension pneumothorax.

• Follow hospital policy regarding milking the tube.

**For thoracentesis.** Before thoracentesis, explain the procedure to the patient. Tell him to expect a stinging sensation from the local anesthetic and a feeling of pressure when the needle is inserted. Instruct him to tell you immediately if he feels uncomfortable or has trouble breathing during the procedure.

• Provide privacy and emotional support. Wash your hands.

• Administer the prescribed sedative as ordered.

• Obtain baseline vital signs and assess respiratory function.

• Position the patient appropriately, leaning him over the overbed table or straddling a chair with his arms over the back.

• Remind the patient not to cough, breathe deeply, or move suddenly during the procedure to avoid puncture of the visceral pleura or lung. If he coughs, the doctor will halt the procedure briefly and withdraw the needle slightly to prevent puncture.

• Expose the patient's entire chest or back, as appropriate.

• Shave the aspiration site as ordered.

• Wash your hands again and put on gloves before touching the sterile equipment. Then, using sterile technique, open the thoracentesis tray and assist the doctor as necessary in disinfecting the site.

• During thoracentesis, provide emotional support to the patient and keep him informed of

each step. Assess him for signs of anxiety and provide reassurance.
• Check the patient's vital signs regularly. Continually observe him for signs of distress, such as pallor, weak and rapid pulse, decreased blood pressure, dyspnea, tachypnea, diaphoresis, blood-tinged mucus, and excessive coughing, and ask him if he's experiencing faintness, vertigo, or chest pain. Alert the doctor if these signs develop because they may indicate such complications as hypovolemic shock or tension pneumothorax.
• Assist the doctor as necessary in collecting specimens, draining fluid, and dressing the site.
• After the doctor withdraws the needle or catheter, apply pressure to the puncture site, using a sterile 4″ × 4″ gauze pad. Then apply a new sterile gauze pad and secure it with tape.
• After thoracentesis, place the patient in a comfortable position, take his vital signs, and assess his respiratory status.
• Label specimens properly and send them to the laboratory.
• Discard disposable equipment. Clean nondisposable items and return them for sterilization.
• Check the patient's vital signs and assess the dressing for drainage every 15 minutes for 1 hour. Then continue to assess vital signs and respiratory status as indicated by the patient's condition.

### Continuing care
*Diet and nutrition.* Proper nutrition plays an important role in recovery for all patients. Dietary measures depend on the patient's condition and the cause of the effusion.
• To make sure your patient is receiving adequate nutrition, consult a registered dietitian about his nutritional needs.
• If the patient has underlying CHF, provide several small meals daily. Choose bland foods that are low in calories, sodium, and residue. A low-calorie diet supplemented with vitamins promotes weight loss, thereby reducing the heart's work load, cardiac output, pulse rate, and blood pressure. It also lowers the basal metabolic rate, reducing tissue demands for nourishment and oxygen. Also, gastric disten-

tion, flatulence, and heartburn are less likely to occur with bland, low-residue foods taken in small, frequent meals than with three heavy meals rich in fruits and vegetables.
• If the patient has cancer, provide a diet adequate in protein and carbohydrates. The doctor may prescribe total parenteral nutrition.

*Medication.* The doctor may prescribe medications depending on the underlying cause of pleural effusion.
• If an infection is diagnosed, expect to give systemic I.V. antibiotics. Be sure to administer them on schedule to maintain adequate blood levels.
• For malignant pleural effusion, chemotherapy is usually considered. As with all chemotherapeutic agents, these drugs must be administered with extreme care because they can be toxic to both the patient and the administering nurse. Strictly adhere to preprocedural and postprocedural chemotherapy protocols.

### Supportive care
• Administer oxygen and antibiotics as ordered.
• Use incentive spirometry to promote deep breathing. Encourage the patient to perform deep-breathing exercises to improve lung expansion.
• Offer reassurance, listen to the patient's fears and concerns, and remain with him during periods of extreme stress and anxiety. Encourage him to identify care measures and actions that make him feel comfortable and relaxed.

### Patient teaching
• Address any questions or concerns the patient may have regarding the tests or procedures.
• If the cause of pleural effusion is pneumonia or influenza, instruct the patient to seek medical attention promptly whenever he gets a chest cold.
• Teach the patient the signs and symptoms of respiratory distress. Tell him to notify his doctor if these problems arise.

## Comparing types of lung cancer

| CANCER | PREVALENCE | LOCATION | TREATMENT |
|---|---|---|---|
| Squamous cell carcinoma | Accounts for about 35% of malignant lung tumors | Usually centrally located; may cause bronchial obstruction | Limited response to chemotherapy and radiation; surgery recommended |
| Adenocarcinoma | Accounts for about 35% of malignant lung tumors | Peripherally located | Limited response to chemotherapy and radiation; surgery recommended |
| Large-cell carcinoma | Accounts for about 15% of malignant lung tumors | May arise in any lung region | Limited response to chemotherapy and radiation; surgery recommended |
| Small-cell (oat cell) carcinoma | Accounts for about 10% of malignant lung tumors | Centrally located | Grows rapidly but is highly sensitive to chemotherapy and radiation therapy |

Fully explain the prescribed drug regimen, and teach the patient about adverse drug effects. Emphasize the importance of complying with the regimen and completing the full course of medication.

If the patient smokes, urge him to stop.

# Lung cancer

Lung cancer usually develops in the bronchi and pulmonary parenchyma. The two major types of bronchogenic carcinoma are small-cell (oat cell) lung cancer (SCLC) and non-small-cell lung cancer (NSCLC). NSCLC is subdivided into squamous cell (epidermoid) carcinoma, adenocarcinoma, and large-cell carcinoma. Rarely, soft-tissue sarcomas, such as lymphomas and carcinosarcomas, develop in the chest. (See *Comparing types of lung cancer.*)

Lung cancer is the most common cause of cancer death in both men and women. Its overall 5-year survival rate is 13%—up from 7% in 1963. Despite the continuing efforts of clinicians and researchers, the long-term survival rate has increased only slightly. Late diagnosis is the main reason for the poor prognosis: Only about 20% of patients have localized disease at the time of diagnosis.

## Causes

The exact cause of lung cancer is unknown. However, the most significant risk factor for bronchogenic carcinoma is tobacco smoking. The risk increases with the number of years the person has smoked, the number of cigarettes smoked per day, cigarette length and tar content, and depth of inhalation.

Other risk factors for lung cancer include the patient's age, genetic predisposition, and exposure to carcinogenic and industrial air pollutants, such as asbestos, arsenic, chromium, coal dust, iron oxides, nickel, radon, radioactive dust, and uranium.

The interval between initial exposure to a carcinogen and lung cancer detection ranges from about 10 to 30 years. Typically, the disease is diagnosed between ages 50 and 74.

## Pathophysiology

The pathophysiology varies with the cancer cell type and the extent of metastasis at the time of diagnosis.

## Complications

When a primary tumor spreads to intrathoracic structures, complications may include tracheal obstruction, esophageal compression, nerve compression or paralysis, and hypoxemia.

## Assessment
### Signs and symptoms
Because lung cancer may not cause symptoms in its early stage, the disease may be advanced by the time the patient seeks medical attention. When taking the patient's history, be sure to assess his exposure to carcinogens. If he's a smoker, calculate his pack years (the number of packs smoked daily multiplied by the number of years smoked).

Chief complaints may include coughing (from tumor stimulation of nerve endings), hemoptysis, dyspnea (from the tumor occluding airflow), wheezing (from bronchial obstruction), fever (from pneumonitis or abscess), chest pain (from tumor invasion into the pleural or chest wall), weight loss in the preceding 6 months, and hoarseness (from the tumor or tumor-bearing lymph nodes pressing on the laryngeal nerve).

On inspection, you may note that the patient becomes short of breath when he walks or exerts himself. You may observe fatigue; finger clubbing; edema of the face, neck, upper arms, or upper torso (due to superior vena cava syndrome); and dilated chest, neck, and abdominal veins.

Palpation may reveal lymph node and liver enlargement. In a patient with pleural effusion, percussion findings may include dullness over the lung fields. Auscultation may disclose decreased breath sounds, wheezing, and pleural friction rub.

### Diagnostic tests
A chest X-ray can determine tumor size and location, identify a peripheral tumor, and reveal the effects of bronchial obstruction. It also may show diaphragmatic paralysis and invasion of the chest wall or mediastinum and can detect a lung cancer up to 2 years before signs and symptoms appear.

Cytologic sputum analysis to detect cancer cells is reliable in up to 75% of patients with a centrally located lesion. It's less reliable when the lesion is in the lung periphery. Cytologic accuracy relates directly to the specimen collection technique (expectorant from lungs and tracheobronchial tree).

Bronchoscopy can identify the tumor site, and bronchoscopic washings provide material for cytologic and histologic study. Using a flexible fiber-optic bronchoscope increases test effectiveness, yielding an 85% accuracy rate.

Needle biopsy of the lung relies on biplanar fluoroscope visual control to locate peripheral tumors to withdraw a tissue specimen for analysis. This procedure provides a definitive diagnosis in 80% of patients.

Tissue biopsy of metastatic sites (including supraclavicular and mediastinal nodes and the pleurae) helps assess disease extent. Staging, based on histologic findings, determines disease extent and prognosis and helps direct treatment. (See Staging lung cancer.)

Thoracentesis allows chemical and cytologic examination of pleural fluid. A CT scan may reveal enlarged lymph nodes and mediastinal invasion.

Additional studies include bronchography, esophagography, and angiocardiography (contrast studies of the bronchial tree, esophagus, and cardiovascular tissues). Tests used to detect metastasis include bone scans, CT scan of the brain, liver function studies, and gallium scans of the liver and spleen. Abnormal bone scan findings may warrant bone marrow biopsy, a procedure usually recommended for patients with SCLC.

## Treatment
Combinations of surgery, radiation therapy, and chemotherapy can improve the prognosis and prolong survival. But because lung cancer is usually advanced when diagnosed, most treatment is palliative.

The primary therapeutic approach differs for SCLC and NSCLC. Surgery is the main treatment for patients with stage I, stage II, or NSCLC in select cases of stage III. The primary treatment for SCLC is chemotherapy, and surgery in very selected cases.

Treatment may also include immunotherapy, laser therapy, oxygen therapy, or any combination of these.

# Staging lung cancer

Using the TNM (tumor, node, metastasis) classification system, the American Joint Committee on Cancer stages lung cancer as follows.

## Primary tumor (T)

TX—primary tumor can't be assessed; or malignant cells detected in sputum or bronchial washings but undetected by X-ray or bronchoscopy
T0—no evidence of primary tumor
Tis—carcinoma in situ
T1—tumor 3 cm or less in greatest dimension, surrounded by normal lung or visceral pleura; no bronchoscopic evidence of cancer closer to the center of the body than the lobar bronchus
T2—tumor larger than 3 cm; or one that involves the main bronchus and is 2 cm or more from the carina; or one that invades the visceral pleura; or one that's accompanied by atelectasis or obstructive pneumonitis that extends to the hilar region but doesn't involve the entire lung
T3—tumor of any size that extends into neighboring structures, such as the chest wall, diaphragm, or mediastinal pleura; or one in the main bronchus that doesn't involve but is less than 2 cm from the carina; or one that's accompanied by atelectasis or obstructive pneumonitis of the entire lung
T4—tumor of any size that invades the mediastinum, heart, great vessels, trachea, esophagus, vertebral body, or carina; or one with malignant pleural effusion

## Regional lymph nodes (N)

NX—regional lymph nodes can't be assessed
N0—no detectable metastasis to lymph nodes
N1—metastasis to the ipsilateral peribronchial or hilar lymph nodes or both
N2—metastasis to the ipsilateral mediastinal and subcarinal lymph nodes or both
N3—metastasis to the contralateral mediastinal or hilar lymph nodes, the ipsilateral or contralateral scalene lymph nodes, or the supraclavicular lymph nodes

## Distant metastasis (M)

MX—distant metastasis can't be assessed
M0—no evidence of distant metastasis
M1—distant metastasis

## Staging categories

Lung cancer progresses from mild to severe as follows:
**Occult carcinoma**—TX, N0, M0
**Stage 0**—Tis, N0, M0
**Stage I**—T1, N0, M0; T2, N0, M0
**Stage II**—T1, N1, M0; T2, N1, M0
**Stage IIIA**—T1, N2, M0; T2, N2, M0; T3, N0, M0; T3, N1, M0; T3, N2, M0
**Stage IIIB**—any T, N3, M0; T4, any N, M0
**Stage IV**—any T, any N, M1

## Surgery

Surgery may involve partial lung removal (wedge resection, segmental resection, lobectomy, radical lobectomy) or total lung removal (pneumonectomy, radical pneumonectomy).

## Radiation therapy

This therapy usually is recommended for a stage I or stage II tumor if surgery is contraindicated and for a stage III tumor confined to the involved hemithorax and ipsilateral supraclavicular lymph nodes. It's also recommended for advanced, inoperable tumors. The patient should have a good performance status with adequate pulmonary function to tolerate the potential complication of pulmonary fibrosis.

Preoperative radiation therapy may reduce tumor bulk to allow surgical resection and thus improve the patient's response to surgery. Postoperative radiation therapy usually begins about 1 month after surgery to give the wound time to heal.

## Chemotherapy

This therapy is typically used to treat SCLC or metastatic lung cancer and has been included in clinical trials of adjuvant therapy.

Combination chemotherapy is more effective than a single agent. The basic principle of combination chemotherapy is to simultaneously administer multiple drugs with no overlapping toxicity. Combinations of fluorouracil, vincristine, etoposide, cyclophosphamide, mitomycin, cisplatin, carboplatin, and vindesine produce a 30% (partial) to 70% (complete) response rate in SCLC but only a 5% to 10% response rate in NSCLC.

### Immunotherapy
This therapy is investigational. Regimens using bacille Calmette-Guérin vaccine or possibly *Corynebacterium parvum* offer the most promise.

### Laser therapy
In this procedure, largely investigational, a laser beam is directed through a bronchoscope to destroy local tumors.

### Oxygen therapy
Oxygen therapy may be indicated for a patient with dyspnea and an unacceptable $SaO_2$ level. Many patients perceive dyspnea as a sign of advancing tumor growth and become quite anxious. This symptom, which affects up to 65% of lung cancer patients, may occur throughout the course of the disease or only during the terminal stage.

### Pain management
Pain management typically requires a multidisciplinary approach, which may involve analgesics; neurosurgical interventions such as cordotomy and nerve resection; and anesthetic interventions such as bupivacaine in the pleural space. Roughly 30% to 40% of patients with early lung cancer and 60% to 90% of those with advanced disease experience pain. The health care team should identify the cause of pain, which may range from tumor infiltration and cancer treatment to another organic cause or a psychogenic source. Chronic pain from cancer progression or treatment commonly causes psychological symptoms such as depression.

## Nursing care
Most patients with lung cancer require some form of surgery, so much of your nursing care will focus on surgical care.

### Surgical care
*Preoperative care.* Provide comprehensive care before surgery in order to minimize complications and speed the patient's recovery.
• Urge the patient to voice his concerns, and allow time to answer his questions. To reduce anxiety, explain all preoperative care procedures in advance.
• Give ordered analgesics as necessary.
• Assist the patient with airway clearance measures, such as coughing, deep breathing, and postural drainage. Teach him how to use inhaled medications.
• Tell the patient what to expect after surgery, including anticipated postoperative procedures and equipment. As indicated, discuss urinary catheterization, chest tubes, endotracheal tubes, dressing changes, and I.V. therapy. Teach the patient how to cough and breathe deeply from the diaphragm and how to perform range-of-motion (ROM) exercises. Reassure him that analgesics and proper positioning will help control postoperative pain.

*Postoperative care.* Nursing responsibilities center on close monitoring to help prevent postoperative complications.
• Maintain a patent airway and monitor chest tubes to reestablish normal intrathoracic pressure and prevent complications.
• Give ordered analgesics as necessary.
• Check vital signs regularly. Watch for and report abnormal respiration and other changes.
• Suction the patient often, and encourage him to begin deep-breathing and coughing exercises as soon as possible. Check secretions frequently. Sputum initially will appear thick, dark, and bloody but should become thinner and grayish yellow within 1 day.
• Monitor and document the amount and color of closed chest drainage. Keep chest tubes patent and draining effectively. Watch for fluctuations in the water seal chamber. Check for air leaks and report them immediately. Position

the patient on the surgical side to promote drainage and lung reexpansion.
• Report any foul-smelling discharge or excessive drainage on the surgical dressing. As indicated, remove the dressing after 24 hours, unless the wound appears infected.
• Monitor intake and output. Maintain adequate hydration.
• Watch for and prepare to manage infection, shock, hemorrhage, atelectasis, dyspnea, mediastinal shift, and pulmonary emboli.
• To help prevent pulmonary emboli, apply antiembolism stockings and encourage the patient to perform ROM exercises.

## Continuing care
• For the patient receiving chemotherapy, impose reverse isolation if bone marrow suppression develops during treatment.
• Provide meticulous skin care to minimize skin breakdown if the patient is receiving radiation.
• Warn the radiation patient to avoid tight clothing, sunburn, and harsh ointments on his chest. Teach him exercises to prevent shoulder stiffness.
• Help the patient cope with adverse effects of radiation, such as anorexia, fatigue, and nausea. Be aware that complications of radiation therapy increase as the dose increases.
• Pulmonary fibrosis may occur 1 to 3 months after radiation therapy. Instruct the patient to stay alert for the symptoms: dyspnea and a nonproductive cough.
• To manage pain, select an analgesic appropriate to the patient's pain level, analgesic history, metabolic state, and the extent of disease.
• Encourage the patient to report pain.
• When giving drugs, use an administration route geared to the patient's needs. Complement narcotic agents with nonnarcotic analgesics, such as nonsteroidal anti-inflammatory drugs, as ordered.
• Anticipate adverse effects of analgesics, such as respiratory depression (unless the patient has developed a tolerance to the drug), nausea, vomiting, sedation, and constipation.
• To help evaluate analgesic effectiveness, have the patient rate his pain on a consistent scale, such as a 1-to-10 scale, with 0 denoting no

pain and 10 denoting the worst pain. Document pain relief.

*Diet and nutrition.* Take steps to prevent or manage adverse nutritional effects of cancer treatment. Be aware that malnutrition may be a consequence of anorexia, pain, taste changes, nausea, vomiting, mouth sores, bowel problems, or psychological distress.
• Administer an antiemetic 30 minutes before meals.
• Encourage the patient to drink a glass of wine or lemonade before meals to stimulate his appetite. If he declines, urge him to drink fluids 30 minutes after meals.
• Ask the dietary department to provide soft, nonirritating, protein-rich foods, avoiding those that can cause bloating or gas. Avoid high-fiber foods if the patient has diarrhea.
• Encourage the patient to eat high-calorie snacks between meals. Have snacks available at all times.
• Advise the patient to eat adequately when he feels relatively well and to experiment with different spices and textures to improve his appetite.
• Provide a dietary consult for the patient and his family to assist with nutritional planning.

## Patient teaching
• Refer smokers to the local branch of the American Cancer Society or Smokenders. Provide information about group therapy, individual counseling, and hypnosis.
• Urge all heavy smokers over age 40 to have a chest X-ray annually and a cytologic sputum analysis every 6 months.
• Encourage patients with recurring or chronic respiratory tract infections, chronic lung disease, or a nagging or changing cough to seek prompt medical evaluation.

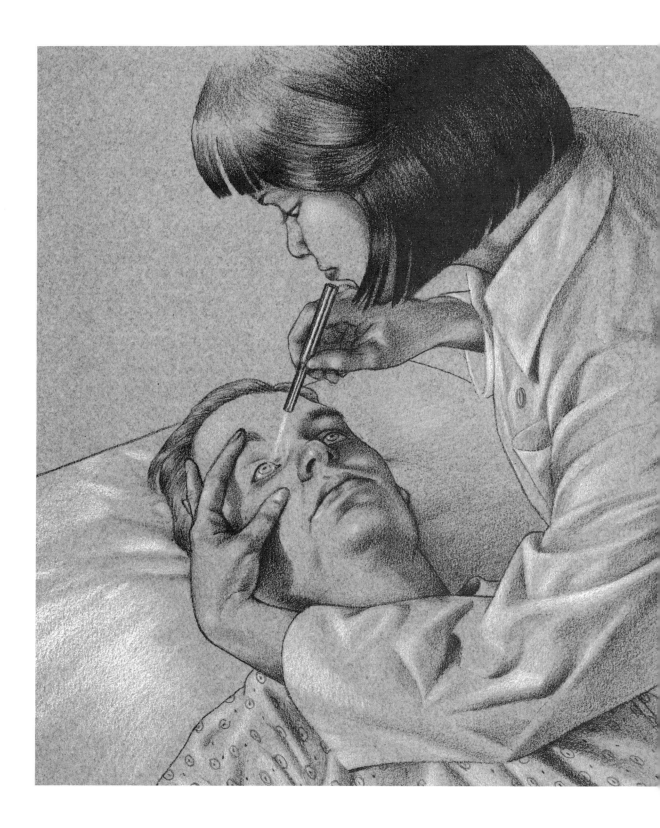

# Neurologic disorders

Acute neurologic disorders will challenge your nursing skills because of their devastating effects on the patient. Consider, for example, the mental deterioration of Alzheimer's disease or the neurologic deficits of a cerebrovascular accident. Clinical effects such as these can overwhelm the patient and his family, increasing their need for emotional support, reassurance, thorough teaching, and expert nursing care.

Aside from their psychological impact, many acute neurologic disorders produce far-reaching and sometimes life-threatening effects. For instance, disorders like Parkinson's disease, meningitis, and Guillain-Barré syndrome compromise not only the neurologic system but also the respiratory, cardiovascular, and other vital systems. Your patient's chances for recovery—or even survival—can depend on your ongoing assessment and your ability to recognize signs of deterioration early.

This chapter explains how to care for patients with acute neurologic disorders, such as those mentioned, and for patients with brain tumors. For each disorder, you'll find its causes, pathophysiology, and possible complications, followed by detailed guidelines for assessment, including characteristic signs and symptoms and pertinent diagnostic tests. You'll also find coverage of drugs and surgeries used to treat each disorder, a thorough discussion of the nursing care you must provide throughout hospitalization, and the patient-teaching directions the patient and his family must follow after discharge.

# Cerebrovascular accident

The third most common cause of death in North America, cerebrovascular accidents (CVAs) account for roughly 200,000 deaths annually. This figure doesn't include the number of patients permanently disabled by cerebrovascular disease each year.

Commonly called a stroke, a CVA is characterized by the sudden, nonconvulsant onset of neurologic deficits related to alterations in cerebral blood supply. As blood supply to the brain diminishes, so does delivery of oxygen to the tissues, resulting in tissue damage or death. The sooner circulation is restored, the better the chances for recovery.

## Causes

Possible causes of a CVA include thrombus, embolism, and hemorrhage. A *thrombotic stroke*, the most common type, is related to atherosclerosis, occurs over time, and produces progressive neurologic deficits. As the arteries narrow, the blood supply to the brain decreases.

In *transient ischemic attacks* (TIAs), recurrent episodes of neurologic deficits last from a few minutes to several hours, producing symptoms that usually disappear when the TIA concludes. The onset of the CVA varies from hours to weeks (or sometimes years) after the initial TIA. (See *Locating TIA sites*.)

In *evolving stroke syndrome*, signs and symptoms occur in a stepwise progression over

PATHOPHYSIOLOGY

## Locating TIA sites

Two types of transient ischemic attacks (TIAs) may occur. A *vertebrobasilar attack* can develop from insufficient blood flow in the vertebral artery, which extends through the cervical vertebrae to join the basilar artery. A *carotid attack* usually stems from a narrowing or partial occlusion at the bifurcation of the common carotid artery (as shown here), where it branches into the internal and external carotid arteries.

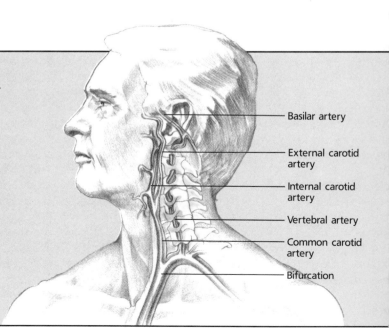

Basilar artery

External carotid artery

Internal carotid artery

Vertebral artery

Common carotid artery

Bifurcation

several hours or days, usually leading to permanent neurologic deficits. The stroke is considered complete when deficits stabilize and symptoms no longer progress.

An *embolic stroke,* usually associated with heart disease, occurs without warning when a thrombus from the heart breaks loose and is carried to the brain. Symptoms develop rapidly and neurologic deficits are complete within a few minutes.

A *hemorrhagic stroke* occurs when hypertension causes a cerebral artery to rupture, forcing blood into the brain tissue and increasing intracranial pressure. Associated symptoms occur rapidly (within minutes or hours) and persist for weeks to months until the clot absorbs.

### Pathophysiology

In a CVA, diminished cerebral perfusion deprives the brain of oxygen and glucose, leading to tissue ischemia. If oxygen deprivation lasts longer than 2 minutes, irreversible tissue necrosis occurs. The necrotic area is referred to as the infarction site.

### Complications

During a CVA, potential complications include injury and loss of vital functions. After the patient's condition stabilizes, complications may include skin breakdown, joint deformity, aspiration, deep vein thrombosis, and pulmonary embolism. (See *CVA and its effects.*)

### Assessment

#### Signs and symptoms

Obtain a history, noting any factors that might have increased the patient's risk of a CVA. Ask the patient to describe the progression of the CVA, if possible. Did he experience loss of consciousness?

Check the patient's circulation, neurologic status, and level of consciousness (LOC). Assessment findings vary with the location of the CVA (usually the middle cerebral artery), the extent of tissue damage, and the efficiency of the collateral circulation.

If the CVA occurred in the *middle cerebral artery,* your assessment may reveal contralat-

**COMPLICATIONS**

## CVA and its effects

Most complications related to cerebrovascular accident (CVA) result from the patient's inability to maintain normal body functions. They can affect virtually every body system. Some of the most common complications are listed below.

| BODY SYSTEM | COMPLICATIONS |
| --- | --- |
| Cardiovascular | • Hypertension<br>• Congestive heart failure<br>• Arrhythmias<br>• Deep vein thrombosis |
| Genitourinary | • Urinary tract infection |
| GI | • Constipation |
| Musculoskeletal | • Pressure ulcers<br>• Contractures |
| Pulmonary | • Airway obstruction<br>• Pneumonia<br>• Aspiration<br>• Embolism |

eral hemiplegia, aphasia, hemianopia, alterations in LOC ranging from confusion to coma, and inability to recognize the paralyzed side.

If the CVA occurred in the *anterior cerebral artery,* your assessment may reveal contralateral foot and leg paralysis, impaired gait, paresis of the contralateral arm, abulia, flat affect, and amnesia.

If the CVA occurred in the *posterior cerebral artery,* you may detect hemianopia, memory deficits, and visual field deficits. If the penetrating branches were affected, you may detect signs of brain stem and thalamic impairment.

#### Diagnostic tests

As ordered, prepare the patient for a computed tomography (CT) scan to detect structural abnormalities, bleeding, edema, and lesions and for magnetic resonance imaging (MRI) to evaluate the lesion's size and location (80% are visible in the first 24 hours). If the patient has suffered a hemorrhagic stroke, you may need to prepare him for a cerebral arteriogram to assess for an aneurysm or arteriovenous malformation.

Other diagnostic studies may include transcranial Doppler ultrasonography to assess blood flow through the cerebral arteries and oculoplethysmography to measure intraocular pressure and thereby assess blood flow. If the patient exhibits significant stenosis or partial occlusion of the proximal internal carotid artery, pressure in the ophthalmic artery will be reduced.

## Treatment
Interventions vary with the type of stroke. For example, a thrombotic or embolic stroke may be successfully managed with drug therapy, whereas a hemorrhagic stroke may require surgery.

### Drug therapy
If the patient has suffered a thrombotic stroke, treatment aims to manage the evolving stroke. To enhance circulation, drug therapy includes anticoagulants (heparin sodium followed by warfarin) and, if indicated, an antiplatelet (aspirin or dipyridamole). Anticoagulant dosage is calculated according to the patient's prothrombin time or his coagulation time.

A patient with an embolic stroke may also receive anticoagulants to prevent further emboli. Drug therapy doesn't affect neurologic deficits.

### Surgery
For a patient with a hemorrhagic stroke, surgery may be performed to remove the blood clot or to treat an aneurysm. Other surgical interventions, which aim to correct predisposing conditions, are controversial. These include carotid endarterectomy and, less commonly, extracranial-intracranial bypass. The best candidates for surgery include patients without major neurologic deficits or an underlying, uncontrolled systemic disease.

## Nursing care
Specific measures vary with the location and extent of brain damage and the chosen treatment. (See *How care differs by stroke site.*)

### Immediate care
During the acute phase of a stroke, direct your interventions toward helping the patient maintain vital functions and survive.
• Maintain a patent airway, and closely monitor the patient's vital and neurologic signs until his condition stabilizes.
• Once his condition has stabilized, take appropriate steps to prevent complications. Continue monitoring vital and neurologic signs. Provide skin care to prevent skin breakdown, and perform passive range-of-motion exercises to prevent joint deformity.
• Maintain good pulmonary hygiene, and assess for adequate swallow and gag reflexes to prevent aspiration and to ensure the patient's ability to eat properly.
• Institute measures to prevent deep vein thrombosis, and be alert for signs of pulmonary embolism.
• As needed, administer stool softeners and establish a regular elimination routine. Institute a bladder training program to maintain continence and to prevent urinary tract infections.
• Evaluate the need for speech, occupational, and physical therapy. If indicated, ask an occupational or physical therapist to recommend the appropriate use of splints to maintain functional position in the paralyzed extremity.

### Surgical care
*Preoperative care.* Before surgery, intervene appropriately to ensure the patient's neurologic and hemodynamic stability. Reinforce the doctor's explanation of the surgical procedure and answer any questions.

*Postoperative care.* Specific measures vary with the type of surgery.
• If the patient has undergone a vascular procedure to minimize his risk of stroke, closely monitor his neurologic status. Maintain anticoagulation therapy.
• If a blood clot has been removed from the patient's brain, provide the same care as for any craniotomy.

### Continuing care
• Be supportive of the patient and his family, and teach them how to cope with a stroke.

# How care differs by stroke site

Knowing whether a cerebrovascular accident (CVA) occurred on the left or right side of the brain can dramatically change the care your patient needs. Consider, for example, the cases of Betsy Wade and Jeff Hill.

Ms. Wade had a right CVA with a lesion in the right parietal lobe. Although alert and oriented, she can't feed or dress herself. She uses her fingers to eat — and eats food only from the right side of her tray. When she dresses herself, she sometimes puts her foot through the sleeve of her robe or doesn't dress her left side at all.

Mr. Hill, on the other hand, had a left CVA. His right side is paralyzed, not just weak like Ms. Wade's, and he has aphasia. Though it takes him a long time and he has difficulty following directions, he can eat all his food and dress himself completely without help.

Despite the fact that Mr. Hill's lesion is more extensive than Ms. Wade's, he isn't as disabled. Why?

## Behaviorial differences

The left side of the brain generally controls communication; the right side, spatial relations and perception. Thus, a left CVA can cause aphasia whereas a right CVA can cause abnormal interpretations of sensory input. Also, the resulting behavioral styles are opposite — impulsive with a right CVA and cautious with a left CVA.

Ms. Wade had a right-sided lesion. As a result, she can be impatient and impulsive. Unlike Mr. Hill,

she's steady on her feet, yet she can't get out of bed and into her wheelchair safely. She forgets to lock the wheelchair first and shows little concern about safety.

The patient with a lesion on the right side of the brain, like Ms. Wade, can be more difficult to deal with than the plodding, careful patient with a left-sided lesion, such as Mr. Hill. Although Mr. Hill is more physically disabled than Ms. Wade, he can be more independent because he's more cautious and teachable.

## Impaired perceptions

Ms. Wade is also experiencing a problem with spatial relations that's found only in patients who suffer right CVAs. For example, when she reaches for her water glass, she often knocks it over. Or if you ask her to put her call light on top of her blanket, she doesn't know what you mean.

Although Mr. Hill is more independent than Ms. Wade in performing daily activities, he hasn't escaped without a perceptual deficit. But his deficit, aphasia, interferes with communication rather than self-care.

Because CVA patients can have such different care needs, you should always know the side of the lesion before drafting a care plan. That way, you can formulate a plan that compensates for CVA losses by having the patient use motor and focal skills that haven't been impaired.

Explain that many of the behavior alterations seen after a stroke result from brain injury and can't be controlled by the patient.

Control the environment as much as possible to decrease the patient's anxiety.

Encourage the patient to relearn skills, if necessary. Divide activities into smaller tasks, allowing him to accomplish one task at a time.

## Patient teaching

Before discharge, ensure that the patient and his family fully understand the disorder and related deficits.

• Explain the medication regimen, and emphasize the need for strict compliance.

• Teach family members how to assist the patient with activities of daily living. Advise them not to perform activities the patient can perform himself, and encourage the patient to perform as many activities as possible.

• Assess the home environment for safety. As needed, suggest changes to protect the patient and to make care requirements easier for the family to meet.

• Make sure that family members recognize signs of an impending stroke and know when to notify the doctor.
• Refer the patient and his family to a local support group for stroke victims.

# Alzheimer's disease

First identified in 1907, Alzheimer's disease is a chronic, progressive neurodegenerative disorder characterized by severe premature cerebral atrophy, particularly in the frontal lobes. It occurs gradually, often beginning as forgetfulness, and progresses to severe dementia.

Alzheimer's disease affects women more often than men and occurs in people usually ages 45 and older.

## Causes

The exact cause of Alzheimer's disease is unknown, though different theories link the disorder to such factors as arteriosclerotic disease, a slow virus, or an autoimmune response. And scientists have recently discovered a genetic link related to the body's manufacture of E4 — a variant of apolipoprotein E.

## Pathophysiology

Alzheimer's disease produces distinctive pathologic changes in the brain. In the early stages, the brain's nerve cells become twisted, forming what are known as neurofibrillary tangles. Neuritic plaques (also called senile plaques) develop around the neurons. These plaques are made up of degenerated neural material and waste products, primarily amyloid. (See *Biopsy findings in Alzheimer's disease.*)

Another finding associated with Alzheimer's disease is decreased concentration of acetylcholine in the brain. Acetylcholine plays a key role in the transmission of information between brain cells.

These changes occur mainly in the cerebral cortex, limbic system, and brain stem. Because these areas of the brain control thinking, memory, behavior, mood, and sleep, the signs and symptoms of Alzheimer's disease tend to involve deficits in those specific functions.

## Complications

Related complications stem from the patient's mental deterioration, which eventually makes her unable to protect herself from environmental hazards. To prevent such complications, the patient needs constant supervision. As the disease progresses, the patient eventually becomes bedridden, and the complications of bed rest become a major concern.

## Assessment

Obtain a detailed patient history. Typically, Alzheimer's disease produces a progressive decline in cognitive function, not a stepwise decline as in multi-infarct dementia. Thoroughly review the patient's medication history to rule out the possibility of drug toxicity. Include the family in the interview; the patient's responses may not be reliable.

## Signs and symptoms

During the physical examination, try to elicit the snout reflex by tapping or stroking the patient's lips or the area right under her nose. A positive response — facial grimacing or lip puckering — suggests diffuse organic brain disease.

Also assess the patient's neurologic status, being alert for deficits commonly seen in Alzheimer's disease. These include an impaired sense of smell (often the first indicator of Alzheimer's disease), impaired stereognosis, gait disorders, tremor, loss of recent memory, and inappropriate or rambling speech.

Alzheimer's disease occurs in four stages, each marked by progressive mental deterioration.

A patient with stage 1 Alzheimer's disease experiences relatively mild memory lapses. For example, she may be unable to remember the right word for something. Associated findings include inability to concentrate, disregard for personal hygiene, lack of interest in immediate surroundings and personal affairs, and inappropriate social responses.

Stage 2 Alzheimer's disease is characterized by short-term memory loss; however, the patient's ability to recall distant past events remains undisturbed. During this stage, the patient shows a marked hesitancy in her verbal responses. Confabulation, disorientation, in-

PATHOPHYSIOLOGY

# Biopsy findings in Alzheimer's disease

These illustrations show the only physical evidence of Alzheimer's disease—the existence of neuritic plaques (near right) and neurofibrillary tangles (far right). Unfortunately, this abnormality can be discovered only through postmortem examination of a brain biopsy specimen.

**Neuritic plaques**

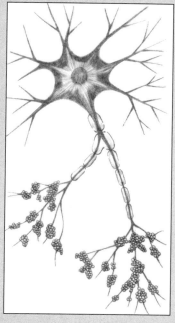

**Neurofibrillary tangles**

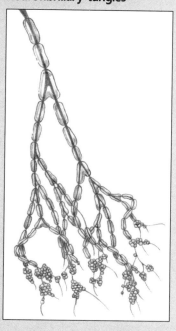

**Normal brain cell**

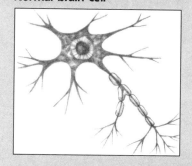

creased forgetfulness, and a tendency to misplace personal belongings may also occur.

By the time the patient reaches stage 3 Alzheimer's disease, personality disintegration is virtually complete. She'll be almost totally disoriented to person, place, and time. Holding a normal conversation will be virtually impossible for her; even if she can converse intelligently, she may forget what was said just minutes before. Motor deficits become quite apparent—apraxia, for example, may greatly interfere with her ability to carry out activities of daily living. During this stage, she may develop the habit of wandering off, especially during the early evening hours (sundown syndrome).

Stage 4—the terminal stage—is marked by severe mental and physical deterioration. The patient's gait will become ataxic; eventually, she won't be able to walk at all. She'll lose her ability to communicate; instead, she may bab-

ble incoherently for hours. She'll no longer recognize close family members. Loss of bowel and bladder control is common. The patient in this stage must be hand-fed, usually for two reasons—her eye-hand coordination will be impaired and she'll often forget to swallow.

**Diagnostic tests**
Alzheimer's disease can be confirmed only by a postmortem brain biopsy and microscopic examination for neurofibrillary tangles and neuritic plaques. The only way Alzheimer's disease can be diagnosed with any certainty is by ruling out all other possible causes of dementia.

A psychiatric interview is necessary to rule out depression. Severe depression in older adults is easily mistaken for dementia or Alzheimer's disease because it produces similar findings, including apathy, lack of responsiveness, and memory loss.

As ordered, prepare the patient for routine blood tests as well as liver and thyroid function tests. Also prepare her for chest and skull X-rays, an electrocardiogram (ECG), an electroencephalogram (EEG), a lumbar puncture, a CT scan, and positron emission tomography.

A probable diagnosis of Alzheimer's disease is based on the following criteria:
• dementia confirmed by neurologic testing (with at least two cognitive function deficits)
• progressive deterioration in memory as well as in other aspects of mentation
• onset of signs and symptoms between ages 40 and 90
• elimination of all other possible neurologic and systemic diseases.

The following factors may bolster a suspected diagnosis of Alzheimer's disease:
• aphasia, apraxia, and agnosia
• impaired activities of daily living
• a family history of Alzheimer's disease
• normal findings on lumbar puncture, EEG, and CT scan
• occasional plateaus in the progressive course of the disease
• other associated signs and symptoms, such as depression, insomnia, incontinence, delusions, hallucinations, disinhibition, and weight loss.

## Treatment
Supportive care measures are the only treatment for Alzheimer's disease. However, researchers are exploring new therapeutic options such as using tacrine, a new drug.

### Drug therapy
Tacrine acts as a chemical inhibitor, preventing the breakdown of acetylcholine. Brain cells that produce acetylcholine receive most of the damage caused by Alzheimer's disease. In correct doses, tacrine may allow these cells to function more efficiently, minimizing the severity of the patient's dementia. An earlier tacrine study was suspended when 20% of the participants showed elevated liver enzyme levels. Lower doses of this drug are currently being tested.

### Surgery
Researchers are also exploring brain tissue transplantation to treat Alzheimer's disease. This surgery has been performed with limited success in patients with advanced Parkinson's disease.

## Nursing care
After the diagnosis has been made, nursing care focuses on preparing the family for what lies ahead and planning for extended care.

### Immediate care
• Explain the disease process to the patient's family members. Describe the signs and symptoms they're likely to see as the disease progresses, and help them to develop effective coping skills.
• In the early stages of the disease, encourage the patient to participate in activities of daily living for as long as possible. Suggest ways to control the patient's activities to promote daytime wakefulness, thereby avoiding altered sleep patterns.
• Stress the need to reassess the patient's skills frequently. This helps to promote realistic expectations about the patient's abilities.
• Teach the family how to control the environment to protect the patient from injury. To minimize disorientation, advise the family not to alter the patient's daily routine and to avoid moving furniture and household items.

### Continuing care
As Alzheimer's disease progresses, many patients suffer from poor nutrition, poor personal hygiene, incontinence, and sleep disturbances. Help your patient to avoid these problems by teaching family members the following strategies.

*Diet and nutrition.* To encourage the patient to eat, try these suggestions:
• Serve meals in a calm environment so that the patient can focus on the task of eating. For example, close the door to her room so that she's not distracted by activity in the hall-

vay. Quiet music may also aid concentration.
Use plastic dishes and cups to eliminate the
sk of broken glass. Serve food in bowls in-
tead of plates whenever possible; they'll be
asier for the patient to manage. If you must
se a plate, attach a rim guard to prevent the
atient from pushing food off it.

Don't use plastic utensils because the patient
might bite through them. Choose utensils with
eavy handles to serve as a tactile reminder to
he patient that she's eating.

Make sure the food isn't too hot, especially if
has been warmed in a microwave oven. The
atient might not understand that steaming
ood is too hot to eat.

Remind her to chew her food and swallow. A
atient with late-stage Alzheimer's disease
may take food into her mouth and then forget
what to do.

If the patient plays with her food or throws
on the floor, she may be agitated because
he can't decide what to eat next. Try offering
nly one food at a time.

Keep nutritious, low-calorie finger foods avail-
ble for between-meal snacks. The patient
might forget that she has just eaten and may
sist on being given something else to eat.

Closely monitor the patient's nutritional sta-
s.

*Personal hygiene.* A patient with Alzheimer's
isease may lack interest in personal hygiene
r the skills to perform the necessary tasks.
he following suggestions may help:

Try to follow the patient's established bathing
outine. For example, if she's used to bathing
t night, honor her preference, if possible,
ather than trying to switch her to a morning
ath.

Even after the patient is in the bathtub, she
may resist the idea that she needs a bath. If
, don't argue with her. Just give her specific
structions — for example, "Now put some
oap on the washcloth" or "Now rub the
ashcloth over your chest."

Fill the tub with only 2" or 3" (5 to 8 cm) of
arm water if the patient appears to be afraid
f bathing.

Put cornstarch under skin folds instead of
erfumed powders, which can irritate the skin.

If the patient resists using an underarm de-
odorant, try baking soda instead.

*Incontinence.* Many patients with Alzheimer's
disease are incontinent because they can't find
the bathroom. To correct this and other blad-
der- and bowel-control problems, try these
suggestions:
• Set up a toileting schedule — for example,
once every 2 or 3 hours — based on the patient's voiding patterns. An older patient's
bladder capacity is only 100 to 200 ml, so frequent trips to the bathroom may be necessary.
• Leave the bathroom door open so that the
patient can see the toilet. If this isn't possible,
put an identifying symbol (like a picture of a
toilet) on the door.
• If possible, elevate the toilet seat and have
grab bars installed around it to avoid injury.
• Limit the patient's intake of fluids, especially
caffeinated beverages, after 8 p.m. to minimize
nocturnal incontinence and to help the patient
sleep well. During the rest of the day, encourage the patient to drink at least 1,500 ml of
fluids, unless contraindicated.
• Under certain circumstances, you may need
to temporarily insert an indwelling urinary
catheter — for example, if the patient has a
pressure ulcer that needs time to heal or if accurate urine output measurements are needed.
Catheters shouldn't be used routinely, though,
because patients may tug at them or pull
them out, causing urethral trauma. Long-term
catheterization may also lead to urinary tract
infections.

*Sleep disturbances.* A patient with Alzheimer's disease may wake up several times during the night and take catnaps throughout the
day. To cope with this problem, try these suggestions:
• Try to keep the patient occupied and active
during the day. A short nap in the morning
usually won't interfere with nighttime sleep,
but an afternoon nap might. Exercise, such as
a brisk walk late in the afternoon or early evening, may help promote a good night's sleep.
• Have the patient void immediately before
bedtime so that she won't be awakened during the night with a full bladder. In case she

does need to get up, provide a night-light.
• To ensure safety, keep the bed's side rails up while the patient is sleeping. Consider using a body alarm to alert you if the patient should try to crawl out of bed during the night.

***Supportive family care.*** When caring for a patient with Alzheimer's disease, don't forget her family's needs. Most family members become exhausted and distressed by the overwhelming demands of day-to-day care. (In fact, it's not uncommon for family caregivers to die before the Alzheimer's disease patient because they've neglected their own health.)
• Give family members the opportunity to express their feelings. Simply offering a sympathetic ear is the first step in helping family members cope with a loved one's illness.
• Refer the family to an Alzheimer's disease support group. Being with other people who are experiencing the same situation can help family members feel less isolated. The family may also need professional help to withstand the extreme stress. If they can no longer care for the patient and have decided to put her in a nursing home, they may need help overcoming feelings of guilt.
• Inform family members of additional resources in their community—such as Meals On Wheels, respite care, senior companion services, and home health nurses. Not every family will need to use all these resources, but just knowing they're available can alleviate some of the pressure family members may feel.
• Help the family to set realistic short- and long-term goals for the patient.

# Parkinson's disease

A progressive degenerative disorder of the basal ganglia, Parkinson's disease strikes older adults, affecting men slightly more often than women. Usually, patients first notice the characteristic tremors and gait impairment in their 60s. Parkinson's disease affects approximately 1 to 1.5 million patients, and the number is expected to grow as Americans' life span con-

tinues to lengthen. Because of its insidious onset, Parkinson's disease is commonly considered a result of the aging process. The disease is classified according to stages of progression:
• stage I—unilateral involvement
• stage II—bilateral involvement
• stage III—impaired postural and righting reflexes; mild to moderate disability
• stage IV—fully developed or severe disease; marked disability
• stage V—confinement to bed or wheelchair.

## Causes
The etiology of Parkinson's disease is unknown.

## Pathophysiology
Parkinson's disease involves progressive degeneration of the basal ganglia—the deep structures of the cortex that are primarily responsible for smooth-muscle movement. The structures involved include the striatum, globus pallidus, subthalamic nucleus, substantia nigra, and red nucleus. The pigmented cells in the substantia nigra are lost because of degenerative changes. Cell degeneration creates impairment of the extrapyramidal tracts and the coordinated movements they control.

Dopamine normally stored in the substantia nigra is greatly depleted in patients with Parkinson's disease. The reason for this is unclear.

## Complications
Possible complications of Parkinson's disease include injury (from gait instability) and aspiration. As the disease progresses, complications related to immobility may occur.

## Assessment
Because clinical findings associated with Parkinson's disease develop as the disease progresses, the diagnosis may be made several years after the first signs and symptoms appear. The patient may have difficulty remembering when symptoms began, but he should be able to identify when they became worse.

### Signs and symptoms
Resting tremors—so called because they usually occur when the hand is motionless—are a classic sign of Parkinson's disease. Muscle rigid-

ity, masklike facies, bradykinesia, akathisia, and dyskinesia may also occur. Related findings include general fatigue and muscle weakness, loss of postural reflexes, and mental depression.

Signs and symptoms associated with autonomic dysfunction include dysphagia, excessive perspiration, constipation, orthostatic hypotension, urinary hesitancy or frequency, drooling due to decreased frequency of swallowing, and seborrhea due to hypothalamic dysfunction.

### Diagnostic tests
Generally, diagnostic studies are used to rule out other disorders.

## Treatment
No known treatment can stop the degenerative process of Parkinson's disease, but drug therapy often relieves many of its symptoms.

### Drug therapy
Levodopa, the most important drug for managing Parkinson's disease, converts to dopamine in the basal ganglia, relieving muscle rigidity and bradykinesia. A peripheral decarboxylase inhibitor, such as carbidopa, is given with levodopa to ensure that the conversion takes place in the brain tissue.

The inhibitor doesn't cross the blood-brain barrier and can decrease the dosage of levodopa needed to control symptoms. The patient reaches therapeutic levels quicker when the drugs are used in combination. If the conversion takes place in the peripheral tissues instead of in the brain tissue, symptoms won't be relieved and such adverse effects as nausea, vomiting, and cardiac arrhythmias may occur.

Another drug that may be used with levodopa is selegiline. This monoamine oxidase inhibitor has the metabolites amphetamine and dextroamphetamine, which also enhance levodopa's effects.

Anticholinergics may be used if the patient's symptoms are mild or if he can't tolerate levodopa. Among the most commonly used anticholinergics are trihexyphenidyl, procyclidine, biperiden hydrochloride, and benztropine.

The correct drug and dosage are often determined by trial and error.

### Surgery
Because drug therapy controls most patients' symptoms, surgical treatment has been virtually eliminated. Although rare, surgery may be performed to destroy parts of the basal ganglia, thus eliminating tremors and rigidity.

Another surgical procedure sometimes used in patients with Parkinson's disease involves transplanting fetal adrenal tissue or autologous adrenal medulla tissue into neural tissue. However, the full benefit of tissue transplantation remains unclear. (See *Fetal adrenal tissue transplantation*, page 94.)

## Nursing care
In Parkinson's disease, the goal of nursing care is to prolong the patient's independence and to provide for his basic needs. Focus your efforts on effectively managing the patient's signs and symptoms as they progress.

### Immediate care
• After the diagnosis is made, provide the patient and his family with emotional and psychological support. Explain the disease process and treatment, and answer all questions honestly.
• Monitor the patient's response to drug therapy for effectiveness and possible adverse effects.

### Surgical care
If the patient undergoes surgery (rare), monitor him as you would any patient after craniotomy.

### Continuing care
• Because of motor impairment, the patient may have problems performing activities of daily living. Assist him as appropriate, while encouraging his independence and self-reliance.
• To ensure that the patient gets adequate nutrition, develop a plan that includes a weight chart and possibly a calorie count. Share this plan with the patient and his family.
• To decrease the risk of aspiration, serve meals with the patient in an upright position. Choose a semisolid diet.

## Fetal adrenal tissue transplantation

An investigational procedure, clinical brain grafting uses fetal adrenal or autologous adrenal medulla tissue to restore cell function. Of the two types, fetal tissue transplantation has shown some favorable results, offering new hope to patients with Parkinson's disease.

### Amelioration of Parkinson's disease
Fetal tissue transplantation has successfully ameliorated severe symptoms of Parkinson's disease, such as tremors, bradykinesia, and lead-pipe or cogwheel rigidity. Although early studies used the tissue of several fetuses, more recent studies show the same results using the tissue of only one fetus. The gestational age of the fetuses has ranged from 7 to 19 weeks.

### Ethical concerns
Although not widely available, this technique has raised ethical concerns. Some people fear that a potential increase in the need for fetal tissue may increase the frequency of abortion. The question of fetal viability also must be considered, especially as the gestational age increases and the quality of available neonatal care continues to improve. These issues will continue to pose a challenge as research helps define the role of brain grafting in treating neurologic disease.

• To manage constipation, begin the patient on a bowel elimination program that includes stool softeners. Urinary incontinence is usually related to the inability to get to the bathroom quickly enough. Encourage the patient to keep a urinal or bedpan close to the bed.
• To help prolong the patient's independence, refer him to a physical therapist for exercise therapy, gait retraining, and training to maintain balance; massage; and heat therapy.

### Patient teaching
• Teach the patient and his family how to manage daily routine care.
• Suggest ways to make the home environment safe, for example, by installing safety rails and removing throw rugs.
• Explain the need for daily hygiene to remove excess perspiration and skin oils. Warm baths also will help to relieve muscle soreness and cramps.
• When the disease progresses to the point that the patient is bedridden, teach the family or caregivers how to minimize the complications of immobility.
• Refer the family to the National Parkinson Foundation and to a local Parkinson's disease support group.

# Meningitis

An inflammation of the meninges surrounding the brain and spinal cord, meningitis may involve the three meningeal membranes — the dura mater, the arachnoid membrane, and the pia mater. The prognosis is usually good for adults, especially if the disease is recognized early and the infecting organism is isolated and responds to the prescribed antibiotics. The prognosis is poorer for infants, children, and older adults. Without treatment, an estimated 70% to 100% of patients die.

### Causes
Meningeal infections can be caused by bacteria, viruses, protozoa, or fungi. Most commonly, meningitis results from bacterial infections caused by *Neisseria meningitidis* (meningococcal meningitis), *Haemophilus influenzae*, *Streptococcus pneumoniae* (pneumococcal meningitis), or *Escherichia coli*.

Aseptic or viral meningitis is caused by enteroviruses, arboviruses, the herpes simplex virus, the mumps virus, or the lymphocytic choriomeningitis virus. Tubercular meningitis develops as an extension of a mycobacterial tuberculosis infection to the brain. Cryptococcal meningitis is the most common fungal infection of the central nervous system (CNS).

### Pathophysiology
The infecting organism enters the CNS via the bloodstream at the blood-brain barrier. Surgical procedures, traumatic injuries, or a ruptured

cerebral abscess may create direct routes of entry. The invading organisms migrate throughout the CNS by way of the subarachnoid space. This produces an inflammatory response as exudate forms in the pia mater, the arachnoid membrane, the cerebrospinal fluid (CSF), and the ventricles. Neurologic deterioration occurs when the normal flow of CSF is blocked, leading to hydrocephalus, cerebral edema, and increased intracranial pressure (ICP).

## Complications

Depending on the cause and severity of the illness, potential complications include visual impairment, optic neuritis, cranial nerve palsies, deafness, personality changes, headache, paresis or paralysis, endocarditis, coma, vasculitis, and cerebral infarction. A delay in treatment significantly increases the risk of permanent neurologic impairment and death.

# Assessment

The patient's history and a physical examination help to identify the probable cause of meningitis and the type of organism responsible. Ask the patient to describe his symptoms. Family members typically report changes in mental status, behavior, and personality. Fully explore any history of recent infection (such as respiratory tract or ear) or other predisposing conditions (such as traumatic injury, surgery, or immunosuppression).

## Signs and symptoms

Clinical manifestations may vary, depending on the type and severity of the patient's meningitis. Generally, physical findings include fever, a severe headache, photophobia, nuchal rigidity of the neck and back and, in some patients, opisthotonic posturing, vomiting, and seizures. Half of all patients with meningococcal meningitis present with a petechial, purpuric, or ecchymotic rash, usually over the lower body.

Neurologic examination shows further signs of meningeal irritation, such as a positive Brudzinski's or Kernig's sign. (See *Two telltale signs of meningitis,* page 96.)

In response to physiologic changes, the patient typically experiences varied alterations in LOC, such as memory impairment, stupor, un-

responsiveness, and coma. Intracranial physiology is altered by meningeal exudate, vasculitis, cerebral edema, and increased ICP. Signs of increased ICP include decreased LOC, pupillary changes, widened pulse pressure, bradycardia, and irregular respiratory patterns. Left untreated, increased ICP can progress to brain herniation and death.

Before meningitis is evident or diagnosed, the patient may show signs of Waterhouse-Friderichsen syndrome, a phase of meningococcemia characterized by septicemia; abrupt onset of high fever; petechial hemorrhage on the face, arms, and legs; adrenal insufficiency; shock; and disseminated intravascular coagulation.

## Diagnostic tests

If the patient's condition permits, prepare him for CSF analysis to confirm the diagnosis of meningitis. (Increased ICP may contraindicate a lumbar puncture because of the risk of herniation.) The CSF specimen is used for cell count, protein and glucose measurement, and culture and sensitivity testing.

Counterimmunoelectrophoresis may detect viruses or protozoa in the CSF. The CSF specimen commonly appears cloudy or milky white; initial pressure readings may also be elevated. The CSF glucose level is normal or slightly lower than the serum glucose level, except in viral meningitis.

Obtain samples for blood, urine, nose, and throat cultures to identify possible bacterial sources of infection. Also obtain a blood sample for a complete blood count to determine if the white blood cell count is elevated and for serum electrolyte studies to detect electrolyte abnormalities.

As ordered, prepare the patient for a CT scan to rule out cerebral edema or other neurologic disorders. Skull X-rays may help to identify inflammation of the mastoid or sinuses.

# Treatment

Medical management of meningitis includes prompt initiation of appropriate antibiotic therapy and vigorous supportive care. The choice of antibiotics — usually penicillin, ampicillin, or chloramphenicol — depends on the causative or-

# Two telltale signs of meningitis

A positive response to the following tests helps establish a diagnosis of meningitis.

### Brudzinski's sign

To test for this sign, place the patient in a dorsal recumbent position. Then put your hands behind his neck and bend it forward. Pain and resistance may indicate meningeal inflammation, neck injury, or arthritis. But if the patient also flexes his hips and knees in response to this manipulation, meningitis is a strong possibility.

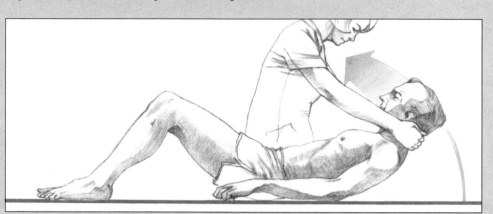

### Kernig's sign

To test for this sign, place the patient in a supine position. Flex his leg at the hip and knee, and then straighten the knee. Pain or resistance indicates meningitis.

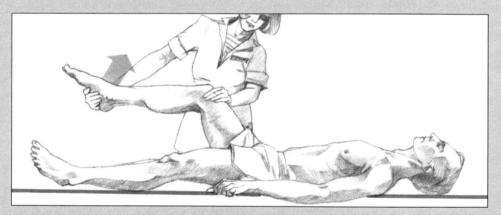

ganism. The patient is maintained on large doses of parenteral antibiotics for 2 weeks, followed by a course of oral antibiotics. For some patients, the doctor may elect intrathecal administration of antibiotic therapy. Other commonly ordered drugs may include mannitol and steroids to decrease cerebral edema, anticonvulsants to prevent seizure activity, sedatives to reduce restlessness, and acetaminophen to relieve headache and fever.

Treatment also includes appropriate therapy for any coexisting conditions, such as pneumonia or endocarditis. Supportive measures consist of bed rest, maintenance of normothermia, fluid and electrolyte replacement to prevent dehydration, and management of cerebral edema, seizures, and ICP.

Several vaccines provide immunization against meningitis. Haemophilus b conjugate vaccines are now widely used on pediatric patients to prevent invasive *Haemophilus influenzae* type B.

## Nursing care

A patient with acute meningitis is critically ill and requires ongoing assessment of his clinical status.

### Immediate care

• Unless the patient has viral meningitis, maintain respiratory isolation for 24 hours after the start of antibiotic therapy.
• Consider nasal and oral discharges infectious, and take necessary precautions. Follow strict aseptic and hand-washing techniques. Carefully dispose of all used dressings, tissues, and cotton swabs to prevent the possible spread of infection.
• Continually assess the patient's neurologic functions. Assess for pupillary changes, signs of meningeal irritation, and alterations in mental status. Test for cranial nerve involvement, watching for such signs as ptosis, strabismus, and diplopia.
• Monitor vital signs, and watch for signs of increased ICP. Frequently check the patient's temperature. Intervene appropriately to attain normothermia (for example, by using tepid baths, ice packs, antipyretics, or a cooling blanket as needed).
• Monitor the patient's respiratory effort to ensure adequate oxygenation and ventilation.
• Routinely perform vascular assessments to detect early signs of circulatory compromise from septic emboli.

### Continuing care

As you care for the patient, take steps to ensure his comfort and provide a quiet environment. Intervene appropriately to prevent the complications of immobility, to meet the patient's nutritional demands, and to prevent aspiration and any secondary infections such as pneumonia. Teach the patient and his family how to manage the illness and its treatment.
• Implement seizure precautions (padded side rails, airway and suction equipment at bedside) to prevent possible injury.
• Monitor fluid and electrolyte balance and urine output. Maintain adequate fluid intake to prevent dehydration, but avoid fluid overload because of the danger of cerebral edema.
• Carefully manage parenteral fluids to meet the patient's specific needs.
• Administer prescribed medications and note their effects. Report any adverse effects, such as gastric distress and diarrhea, to the doctor.

### Patient teaching

During convalescence, the patient's specific needs depend on his degree of disability. Most patients leave the hospital with few or no neurologic deficits.
• Inform the patient and his family of the contagion risks, and tell them to notify anyone who comes into close contact with the patient. Such people may require antimicrobial prophylaxis and immediate medical attention if fever or other signs of meningitis develop.
• Review isolation and hand-washing techniques with all persons who will come into contact with the patient.
• Provide reassurance and support. Help the patient to overcome any fear of the illness, and reassure the family that the delirium and behavior changes caused by the infection are temporary.
• If a severe neurologic deficit appears permanent, refer the patient to a rehabilitation program as soon as the acute phase of this illness has passed.
• Before discharge, make sure the patient and his family understand the medication regimen, including the correct dosage, times of administration, and possible adverse effects. Emphasize the need for strict compliance.

# Guillain-Barré syndrome

An acute condition, Guillain-Barré syndrome is a rapidly progressive, potentially fatal form of polyneuritis. It causes segmented demyelination of peripheral nerves, producing abrupt onset of paresthesia and muscle weakness. Guillain-Barré syndrome is also known as infectious polyneuritis, Landry Guillain-Barré Strohl syndrome, polyradiculoneuropathy, and acute idiopathic polyneuritis.

The clinical course of Guillain-Barré syndrome is marked by three distinct phases. The *acute phase* begins with the onset of the first definitive symptom and ends 1 to 3 weeks later, when no further deterioration is noted. The *plateau phase* lasts from several days to 2 weeks. It's followed by the *recovery phase,* a period of axonal regeneration and remyelination. This phase extends from 4 to 6 months to several years.

Supportive care advancements have greatly enhanced the prognosis. Currently, about 10% of patients suffer permanent residual disability.

### Causes
Although the etiology of Guillain-Barré syndrome remains unclear, most evidence indicates a cell-mediated immune response to a viral infection. Most patients have a history of a recent acute illness, trauma, surgery, or immunization within 2 to 4 weeks of the onset of neurologic symptoms. Other risk factors include an upper respiratory tract infection or GI illness. These prodromal events may cause a malfunction of the immune system.

### Pathophysiology
The major pathologic effect in Guillain-Barré syndrome is a segmental demyelination of the peripheral nerves, which prevents normal transmission of impulses along the sensorimotor nerve roots. Edema and inflammation accompany this demyelination process, as does a loss of nerve conduction. Although the axons remain intact, the cell body or the neurilemma sustain damage, causing a delayed recovery or permanent deficits.

Demyelination begins distally and ascends symmetrically. Function returns slowly during the remyelination process in a proximal-to-distal pattern. (See *Nerve degeneration in Guillain-Barré syndrome.*)

### Complications
The patient's inability to use his muscles leads to most complications associated with Guillain-Barré syndrome. These include thrombophlebitis, pressure ulcers, contractures, muscle wasting, aspiration, respiratory tract infections, and life-threatening respiratory and cardiac compromise.

## Assessment
Ask the patient to describe the character and onset of his signs and symptoms. Obtain a medical and surgical history. Fully explore any report of recent acute illness, trauma, surgery, or immunization.

Focus the physical examination on the patient's neurologic status. Test muscle strength and deep tendon reflexes in affected limbs. Assess the patient's LOC and cranial nerve involvement. Guillain-Barré syndrome usually doesn't alter the patient's LOC, pupillary signs, or cognitive functioning, but it commonly affects the cranial nerves.

### Signs and symptoms
Guillain-Barré syndrome may present in several variations. (See *Recognizing variations in Guillain-Barré syndrome,* page 100.) Typically, patients report an abrupt onset of symptoms. These may include paresthesia of the legs, progressing to the trunk and arms; pain (mild to severe cramping) in the hands and feet; facial weakness; and, occasionally, bladder and bowel dysfunction.

Neurologic examination typically reveals motor weakness and areflexia. Motor weakness tends to be symmetrical, beginning in the lower extremities and progressing upward to the trunk and upper extremities. Symptoms progress rapidly and commonly lead to complete paralysis.

Cranial nerve involvement is marked by weakness, which may progress to paralysis, of the ocular, facial, and oropharyngeal muscles. Signs and symptoms of facial nerve dysfunction include difficulty talking, chewing, and swallowing. Neurologic examination may also show loss of position sense and diminished or absent deep tendon reflexes.

If the respiratory musculature is affected, related clinical features may include respiratory compromise or failure. Autonomic dysfunction may cause cardiac arrhythmias and blood pressure changes (paroxysmal hypertension or orthostatic hypotension).

### Diagnostic tests
Prepare the patient for diagnostic tests, including CSF analysis, electromyography, and elec-

PATHOPHYSIOLOGY

# Nerve degeneration in Guillain-Barré syndrome

As the cells in the myelin sheath degenerate during Guillain-Barré syndrome, inflammation and edema occur. Later, patchy demyelination causes Schwann cell loss, leaving widened nodes of Ranvier. Because both dorsal and ventral nerve roots are affected, signs of both sensory and motor impairment appear, such as tingling, numbness, and paralysis.

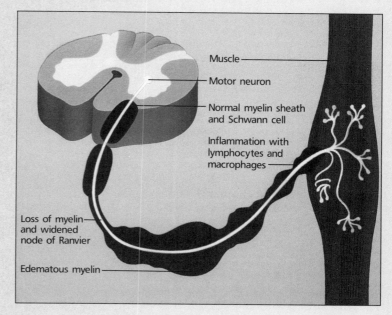

trophysiologic testing. The patient's clinical presentation, a history of a recent viral infection, and an elevated CSF protein level with a normal cell count indicate a diagnosis of Guillain-Barré syndrome.

Electromyography may demonstrate repeated firing of the same motor unit, instead of widespread sectional stimulation. Electrophysiologic testing may reveal marked slowing of nerve conduction velocities; in some patients, nerve conduction slowing develops later in the illness.

## Treatment
Medical management of Guillain-Barré syndrome includes ventilatory support, the administration of steroids, and supportive therapy. It may also include plasmapheresis.

### Procedures
Most patients with Guillain-Barré syndrome require hospitalization in the intensive care unit,

where they undergo continuous monitoring of respiratory and neurologic functioning. Many patients need endotracheal intubation and mechanical ventilation. Serial measurements of the patient's vital capacity are compared to a predetermined optimal level (12 to 15 ml/kg of body weight). Ventilatory support is usually short term; for those patients requiring prolonged assistance, a tracheotomy may be necessary.

Plasmapheresis produces a temporary reduction in the number of circulating antibodies. It's most effective when performed during the first few days of the illness. (See *Treating the effects of plasmapheresis,* page 101.)

Medical management focuses on supportive care and prevention of complications. In addition to respiratory problems, other complications may include autonomic dysfunction (blood pressure problems, cardiac arrhythmias, paralytic ileus, urine retention, and syndrome of inappropriate antidiuretic hormone secre-

## Recognizing variations in Guillain-Barré syndrome

Guillain-Barré syndrome occurs in four basic variations—ascending (most common), descending, pure motor, and Miller-Fischer (rare). You can recognize each type by the signs and symptoms it produces, as outlined here.

| VARIATION | SIGNS AND SYMPTOMS |
|---|---|
| Ascending | • Upward progression of weakness and numbness, starting in legs and leading to trunk, arms, and face<br>• Paresis to quadriplegia evolving over a period of hours to several days (1 to 10)<br>• Mild numbness<br>• Diminished to absent reflexes<br>• Respiratory insufficiency (in 50% of patients) |
| Descending | • Initial weakness of brain stem cranial nerves (facial, glossopharyngeal, vagus, and hypoglossal nerves) followed by downward progression of weakness<br>• Numbness affecting hands and, less often, feet<br>• Decreased or absent deep tendon reflexes<br>• Rapid respiratory involvement |
| Pure motor | • Same as for ascending type, but without sensory involvement |
| Miller-Fischer | • Triad of ophthalmoplegia, areflexia, and severe ataxia<br>• Usually no sensory involvement<br>• Rarely, respiratory complications |

tion), pain, and various psychological responses (fear, depression, anxiety).

Continuous hemodynamic monitoring allows for early intervention to correct abnormalities of blood pressure and heart rate and rhythm.

A nasogastric tube is used for gastric decompression if paralytic ileus occurs. Urine retention is relieved by instituting an intermittent catheterization program. Fluid and electrolyte monitoring detects any imbalances so that appropriate treatment can begin.

Fear, depression, and anxiety can often be treated by providing emotional support. Recognizing the immense effect that this illness has on the patient's daily life promotes awareness of his changing psychological needs.

Once the patient progresses to the recovery phase, treatment focuses on rehabilitation. As the patient's respiratory condition strengthens, he undergoes extensive physical and occupational therapy. Typically, the patient will be discharged to a rehabilitation facility for further treatment.

### Drug therapy

Drugs and dosages used to treat Guillain-Barré syndrome include corticotropin, 25 to 40 units three times a day I.M. or S.C.; azathioprine, 3 to 5 mg/kg/day initially, then a maintenance dose of 2 mg/kg/day; cyclophosphamide, 2 to 4 mg/kg/day for 10 days, then 1.5 to 3 mg/kg/day; and prednisone, 45 to 60 mg/day orally in two to four doses.

Although controversial, high doses of steroids may be ordered initially for their anti-inflammatory effect, followed by a tapered regimen. The ability of corticotropin to shorten the duration of illness is still under investigation. Other immunosuppresants, such as azathioprine and cyclophosphamide, have met with varied success.

In a patient with cardiac arrhythmias, propranolol is used to prevent tachycardia and hypertension. Atropine may be administered to prevent episodes of bradycardia during endotracheal suctioning and physical therapy. Marked hypotension may require volume replacement.

Pain can be treated with a combination of nonsteroidal agents or nonnarcotics. For some patients, a narcotic analgesic may be indicated.

### Nursing care

Nursing management begins with a comprehensive baseline assessment of the patient's respiratory and neurologic functions. Continually reevaluate respiratory effectiveness, paying special attention to the functional ability of chest muscles (intercostal and diaphragm).

## Immediate care

During the acute phase of Guillain-Barré syndrome, focus your care on preventing respiratory compromise, identifying neurologic deficits, and providing emotional support.
• Intervene appropriately to maintain adequate respirations and a patent airway and to prevent pulmonary infection. Monitor arterial blood gas measurements for signs of hypoventilation with hypoxemia and hypercapnia.
• Assess the patient's neurologic status, being alert for motor, sensory, or cranial nerve functional deficits.
• Remember, the rapid progression of symptoms can be frightening for the patient. He may feel anxious, depressed, or fearful of dying. Provide emotional support and reassurance that recovery is possible. Help the patient devise a means of communication (lipreading, flash cards, blinking eyes) to compensate if he cannot talk. During the acute phase of the illness, your attitude and the atmosphere you create can soothe your patient and make him less anxious.

## Continuing care

During the plateau and recovery phases of Guillain-Barré syndrome, the nursing focus changes to meet the patient's altered needs.
• Maintain adequate nutrition to promote healing.
• Help the patient to accept dependence, cope with deficits, and set realistic long-term goals. Involve his family in plans for rehabilitation.
• Paresthesia and paralysis place the patient at high risk for impaired skin integrity. Position him carefully and introduce physical therapy gradually to help prevent development of pressure ulcers, contractures, and palsies.
• Because of prolonged bed rest, the patient also has an increased risk of developing deep vein thrombosis and pulmonary emboli. Administer low-dose heparin as ordered. If hospital policy allows, apply compression boots; this procedure is controversial, however, because the boots may exert undue pressure on sensitive demyelinated peripheral nerves.

---

**COMPLICATIONS**

# Treating the effects of plasmapheresis

To prevent or correct complications commonly associated with plasmapheresis, follow the interventions outlined below.

| COMPLICATION | INTERVENTIONS |
| --- | --- |
| Trauma or infection at vascular access site | • Keep site clean and dry.<br>• Inspect site for redness, swelling, and drainage. |
| Signs of hypovolemia (hypotension, tachycardia, dizziness, diaphoresis) | • Monitor fluid and electrolyte balance and hemodynamic status.<br>• Administer fluids. |
| Hypokalemia and hypocalcemia | • Monitor fluid and electrolyte balance.<br>• Replace electrolytes.<br>• Monitor for cardiac arrhythmias. |
| Temporary circumoral and distal extremity paresthesia, muscle twitching, nausea and vomiting from citrated plasma | • Administer I.V. calcium gluconate or calcium chloride as ordered.<br>• Provide comfort measures. |

## Patient teaching

Because the course and severity of Guillain-Barré syndrome vary, predicting a patient's prognosis can be difficult.
• Teach the patient and his family about the disorder, its effects, and its treatment.
• Teach them how to compensate for any neurologic deficit to promote maximal return of function and independence.
• Use the patient's neurologic assessment findings to formulate a plan that meets his unique needs for care and rehabilitation. Encourage the family to participate in planning.
• Start discharge planning early in the patient's hospital stay to encourage a smooth transition from hospital to home.

## Caring for a patient with a pituitary tumor

When a patient has a pituitary tumor, surgery is performed to eliminate the mass, to stop endocrine hyperactivity, and to retain and improve existing pituitary function. To meet these objectives, the surgeon may choose one of two options: transfrontal removal of large tumors impinging on optic apparatus, or transsphenoidal resection of smaller tumors confined to the pituitary fossa. Radiation is used as an adjunct to surgery, especially when only part of the tumor can be removed.

### Postoperative drug therapy
After surgery, the patient receives replacement therapy with corticosteroids or thyroid or sex hormones. Electrolyte imbalances are corrected as well and, if necessary, insulin therapy is initiated. Postoperative drug therapy may also include bromocriptine to reduce prolactin secretion and shrink growth hormone–secreting tumors. Cyproheptadine, an antiserotonin drug, can reduce increased corticosteroid levels in Cushing's syndrome.

### Nursing care
A patient with a pituitary tumor needs much the same care as a patient with a brain tumor. Tailor your postoperative care measures to the patient's individual needs and type of surgery.
• After transsphenoidal resection, the patient will return from surgery with nasal packing and a moustache dressing. Instruct the patient not to blow his nose, sneeze, or cough forcibly.
• Provide frequent mouth care to minimize the discomfort from postnasal drip and mouth breathing.
• Monitor fluid intake and output to ensure that electrolyte abnormalities are corrected and adequate hydration is maintained.
• If the patient develops diabetes insipidus (a common postoperative complication), intervene appropriately. As ordered, administer desmopressin acetate, either by direct injection or intermittent infusion.
• Perform frequent neurologic examinations, assessing for visual changes.
• Teach the patient about ongoing hormone replacement therapy, if indicated.
• Reinforce the need for ongoing follow-up care.

# Brain tumor

A brain tumor is a localized intracranial lesion occupying space within the skull. Tumors cause CNS changes, primarily by invading and destroying tissues. A brain tumor's secondary effects—including cerebral edema, increased ICP, and compression of the brain, cranial nerves, and cerebral vessels—also produce CNS changes.

Most brain tumors occur in patients between ages 50 and 70. The most common types are gliomas and meningiomas. They usually occur above the covering of the cerebellum (supratentorial tumors).

Generally, a patient with a pituitary tumor requires much the same treatment and care as a patient with a brain tumor. (See *Caring for a patient with a pituitary tumor.*)

### Causes
The cause of brain tumors is unknown.

### Pathophysiology
Primary brain tumors result from a rapid proliferation of cells normally found within the CNS. Secondary brain tumors originate from malignant cells from tumors outside the CNS that metastasize to the brain. In either case, the tumor expands in an irregular fashion by infiltrating and ultimately compressing healthy brain tissue. The sequelae include vasogenic cerebral edema, increased ICP, focal neurologic deficits, obstruction of the normal flow of CSF, and pituitary dysfunction.

### Complications
In brain tumors, life-threatening complications from increasing ICP include coma, respiratory or cardiac arrest, and brain herniation.

### Assessment
The clinical presentation of a brain tumor depends on the tumor site, the related cerebral edema, and the presence of increased ICP. Specific assessment findings vary with the type of tumor, its location, and the degree of infiltration. (See *Differentiating among brain tumors,* pages 104 and 105.)

Obtain a history, exploring the patient's primary complaint and any related signs and symptoms. Focus the physical examination on assessing the patient's neurologic status. Be alert for signs of increased ICP—widened pulse pressure, bradycardia, altered respiratory pattern, and increased blood pressure.

### Signs and symptoms
The most common initial signs and symptoms of brain tumors include cognitive alterations, visual changes, headache, seizures, and vomiting. Neurologic findings commonly help pinpoint the tumor's location in the brain.

### Diagnostic tests
Prepare the patient for diagnostic tests, such as a CT scan and MRI, to identify the size, location, and extent of the brain tumor. If indicated, additional testing may include cerebral angiography, visual field and funduscopic examination, audiometric studies, brain scan, EEG, chest X-ray, and endocrine studies.

If the patient doesn't have clinically significant increased ICP, a lumbar puncture may be performed to obtain CSF for analysis. Typically, CSF analysis reveals increased protein levels and decreased glucose levels; cytologic examination may show malignant cells in the CSF.

Biopsy of the lesion reveals the tumor's histologic type and grade. Tumors are classified according to their histologic features. Grade 1 tumors are well differentiated; grade 2, moderately well differentiated; grade 3, poorly differentiated; and grade 4, extremely poorly differentiated.

## Treatment
The three basic brain tumor treatments—radiation, chemotherapy, and surgery—can be used alone or in any combination. The tumor's histologic type, radiosensitivity, size, and location determine the choice of treatment.

### Radiation
Radiation therapy destroys cancer cells by altering the cell membranes. The correct dosage depends on the tumor's histologic type, radiosensitivity, and location, and the patient's level of tolerance. The total dosage is usually 4,000 to 7,000 rad delivered over a 4- to 8-week period. Radiation is indicated for medulloblastomas, metastatic lesions, and deep or centrally located tumors that are inaccessible or inoperable. Postoperative radiation may be indicated for grade 2, 3, or 4 astrocytomas and for ependymomas, oligodendrogliomas, sarcomas, craniopharyngiomas, and chordomas.

Radiation therapy may produce such adverse effects as skin irritation, nausea and vomiting, anorexia, dry mouth, and transient increases in ICP and cerebral edema. Use of radiation therapy may be limited by the resistance of malignant cells, cerebral cell necrosis, and the debilitated patient's intolerance of the treatment.

New approaches to therapy that are under investigation include interstitial brachytherapy and interstitial hyperthermia. Interstitial brachytherapy involves the use of a radioactive isotope implanted stereotaxically to allow for high-dose focal irradiation. Interstitial hyperthermia involves localized application of heat to control or destroy tumor tissue.

### Chemotherapy
Chemotherapy may be offered after surgery and radiation therapy to patients with grade 2 or 3 astrocytomas who experience significant tumor regrowth.

Chemotherapeutic agents act by altering the cells' reproductive cycle. The dosage is determined by the amount of the drug that normal cells can absorb before being killed. Usually, these drugs are injected intrathecally or intraventricularly.

Intraventricular injection requires insertion of an Ommaya reservoir, a small-diameter catheter placed in the anterior horn of the lateral ventricle and attached to a small mushroom-shaped reservoir. This provides access for administering drugs, measuring CSF pressure, and aspirating CSF for analysis. Intraventricular access enhances the concentration of the chemotherapeutic agent in the brain.

Adverse effects of chemotherapy include severe nausea, vomiting, diarrhea, anorexia, alopecia, and oral mucosal irritation. Bone marrow suppression may also occur, necessitating

(Text continues on page 106.)

# Differentiating among brain tumors

| TUMOR AND CHARACTERISTICS | ASSESSMENT FINDINGS |
|---|---|
| **Glioblastoma multiforme** (spongioblastoma multiforme)<br>• Most common glioma, accounting for about 60% of all gliomas<br>• Peak incidence between ages 50 and 60; more common in men than in women<br>• Unencapsulated, highly malignant; grows rapidly and infiltrates the brain extensively; may become enormous before diagnosed<br>• Occurs most often in cerebral hemispheres, especially frontal and temporal lobes (rarely in brain stem and cerebellum)<br>• Occupies more than one lobe of affected hemisphere; may spread to opposite hemisphere by corpus callosum; may metastasize into cerebrospinal fluid (CSF), producing tumors in distant parts of the nervous system | *General*<br>• Increased intracranial pressure (ICP) symptoms (nausea, vomiting, headache, papilledema)<br>• Mental and behavioral changes<br>• Altered vital signs (increased systolic pressure, widened pulse pressure, respiratory changes)<br>• Speech and sensory disturbances<br>• In children, irritability and projectile vomiting<br>*Localized*<br>• Midline: headache (bifrontal or bioccipital) that's worse in morning and that's intensified by coughing, straining, or sudden head movements<br>• Temporal lobe: psychomotor seizures<br>• Central region: focal seizures<br>• Optic and oculomotor nerves: visual disturbances<br>• Frontal lobe: abnormal reflexes and motor responses |
| **Astrocytoma**<br>• Second most common glioma, accounting for about 10% of all gliomas<br>• Occurs at any age; incidence higher in men than in women<br>• Occurs most often in central and subcortical white matter; may originate in any part of the central nervous system<br>• Cerebellar astrocytomas usually confined to one hemisphere | *General*<br>• Headache and mental activity changes<br>• Decreased motor strength and coordination<br>• Seizures and scanning speech<br>• Altered vital signs<br>*Localized*<br>• Third ventricle: changes in mental activity and level of consciousness, nausea, pupillary dilation, and sluggish light reflex; paresis or ataxia in later stages of the disease<br>• Brain stem and pons: ipsilateral trigeminal, abducens, and facial nerve palsies in early stages; cerebellar ataxia, tremor, and other cranial nerve deficits as the disease progresses<br>• Third or fourth ventricle or aqueduct of Sylvius: secondary hydrocephalus<br>• Thalamus or hypothalamus: various endocrine, metabolic, autonomic, and behavioral changes |
| **Oligodendroglioma**<br>• Third most common glioma, accounting for less than 5% of all gliomas<br>• Most common in adults between ages 40 and 50; more common in women than in men<br>• Slow-growing | *General*<br>• Mental and behavioral changes<br>• Decreased visual acuity and other visual disturbances<br>• Increased ICP symptoms<br>*Localized*<br>• Temporal lobe: hallucinations and psychomotor seizures<br>• Central region: seizures (confined to one muscle group or unilateral)<br>• Midbrain or third ventricle: pyramidal tract symptoms (dizziness, ataxia, paresthesia of the face)<br>• Brain stem and cerebrum: nystagmus, hearing loss, dizziness, ataxia, paresthesia of the face, cranial nerve palsies, hemiparesis, suboccipital tenderness, loss of balance |
| **Ependymoma**<br>• Rare glioma<br>• Most common in children and young adults<br>• Located most often in fourth and lateral ventricles | *General*<br>• Increased ICP symptoms and obstructive hydrocephalus, depending on tumor size<br>• Other assessment findings similar to those of oligodendroglioma |

# Differentiating among brain tumors (continued)

| TUMOR AND CHARACTERISTICS | ASSESSMENT FINDINGS |
|---|---|
| **Medulloblastoma**<br>• Rare glioma<br>• Incidence highest in children ages 4 to 6<br>• Affects men more than women<br>• Frequently metastasizes by way of CSF | *General*<br>• Increased ICP symptoms<br>*Localized*<br>• Brain stem and cerebrum: papilledema, nystagmus, hearing loss, perception of flashing lights, dizziness, ataxia, paresthesia of the face, cranial nerve palsies (V, VI, VII, IX, X), hemiparesis, suboccipital tenderness; compression of supratentorial area produces other general and focal symptoms |
| **Meningioma**<br>• Most common nongliomatous brain tumor, constituting about 15% of primary brain tumors<br>• Occurs most frequently among people in their 50s; rare in children; more common in women than in men<br>• Rises from the meninges<br>• Common locations include parasagittal area, sphenoidal ridge, anterior part of the base of the skull, cerebellopontile angle, and spinal canal<br>• Benign, well-circumscribed, highly vascular tumor that compresses underlying brain tissue. | *General*<br>• Headache<br>• Seizures (in two-thirds of patients)<br>• Vomiting<br>• Changes in mental activity<br>• Other assessment findings similar to those of schwannomas<br>*Localized*<br>• Skull changes (bony bulge) over tumor<br>• Sphenoidal ridge, indenting optic nerve: unilateral visual changes and papilledema<br>• Prefrontal parasagittal: personality and behavioral changes<br>• Motor cortex: contralateral motor changes<br>• Anterior fossa compressing both optic nerves and frontal lobes: headaches and bilateral vision loss<br>• Pressure on cranial nerves, causing varying symptoms |
| **Pituitary tumor**<br>• Constitutes 10% to 15% of intracranial neoplasms<br>• Peak incidence between ages 30 and 50; affects men and women equally<br>• Originates most often in the anterior pituitary<br>• Exact cause unknown, but invasive growth categorizes it as a neoplastic condition<br>• Good prognosis | *General*<br>• Visual disorders<br>• Paresis of extraocular muscles<br>• Nystagmus<br>• Headache<br>• Abnormal sella turcica region on computed tomography scan<br>• Affects cranial nerves III, IV, and VI<br>*Localized*<br>• III: ptosis, dilated pupils, inability to move eyes medially, superiorly, or inferiorly<br>• IV: inability to move eyes inferiorly or medially<br>• VI: diplopia<br>• Thalamus or hypothalamus: various endocrine changes (amenorrhea, infertility, loss of pubic hair, impotence, increased fatigue, sensitivity to cold) |
| **Schwannoma** (acoustic neurinoma, neurilemoma, cerebellopontile angle tumor)<br>• Accounts for about 10% of all intracranial tumors<br>• Onset of symptoms between ages 30 and 60; higher incidence in women than in men<br>• Affects the craniospinal nerve sheath, usually cranial nerves V and VII, and to a lesser extent, VI and X on the same side as the tumor<br>• Benign, but often classified as malignant because of its growth patterns; slow-growing—may be present for years before symptoms occur | *General*<br>• Unilateral hearing loss with or without tinnitus<br>• Stiff neck and suboccipital discomfort<br>• Secondary hydrocephalus<br>• Ataxia and uncoordinated movements of one or both arms because of pressure on brain stem and cerebellum<br>*Localized*<br>• V: early signs include facial hypoesthesia and paresthesia on the side of hearing loss; unilateral loss of corneal reflex<br>• VI: diplopia<br>• VII: paresis progressing to paralysis (Bell's palsy)<br>• X: weakness of palate, tongue, and nerve muscles on same side as tumor |

protective isolation to prevent further immuno-compromise.

Additional drugs used to treat brain tumors depend on the patient's specific needs. Most patients with brain tumors require an anticonvulsant. Most patients also benefit from the administration of steroids, which decrease cerebral edema. Steroids are given along with chemotherapy, during radiation treatment, and before and after surgery. Diuretics, such as mannitol or furosemide, may also be given for cerebral edema. Gastric irritation is managed with antacids and histamine$_2$-receptor antagonists (such as famotidine or cimetidine). Finally, codeine is effective for pain management.

### Surgery
Depending on the tumor's type, size, and location, surgery may be indicated to remove the tumor or a portion of it. Interventions include conventional dissection, laser surgery, and stereotaxic radiosurgery. A closed, bloodless procedure, stereotaxic radiosurgery uses a cobalt gamma knife and high-dose radiation to stop tumor growth and decrease tumor size.

## Nursing care
A patient with a brain tumor requires complex nursing care, including continuous monitoring to detect and treat increased ICP and to control cerebral edema. You'll also provide preoperative and postoperative care (if indicated), and therapeutic measures to overcome general deficits of cerebral function.

As you care for the patient, you must be keenly aware of any physiologic changes while also remaining responsive to the changing psychosocial needs of both the patient and his family. They'll require instruction about tumor management as well as considerable emotional support.

### Immediate care
As soon as the diagnosis is established, your primary responsibilities include monitoring the patient for signs of increased ICP and providing emotional support.
• Obtain baseline and serial assessments of the patient's vital signs and neurologic status.

Changes in his condition may signal cerebral edema and increasing ICP.
• Explain the purpose of any additional tests, and reinforce the doctor's explanation of treatment options. A positive, supportive approach can help the patient cope with the treatment, potential disabilities, and related life-style changes.

### Surgical care
Surgery may be performed to remove as much of the brain tumor as possible before radiation or chemotherapy.

*Preoperative care.* Prepare the patient for preoperative tests, such as routine laboratory studies, X-rays, a CT scan and, possibly, arteriography.
• Administer anticonvulsants and steroids as ordered.
• As needed, clarify what the doctor has told the patient about the type of surgery he'll be having. Answer any questions.
• Tell the patient what to expect after surgery, including his altered physical appearance and the course of treatment.

*Postoperative care.* After surgery, focus your care measures on monitoring the patient's clinical and neurologic status, easing his discomfort, and preventing complications.
• Closely monitor the patient's clinical status, including his vital signs and hemodynamic status. If an intracranial monitoring device has been inserted, monitor and interpret the ICP and cerebral perfusion pressure.
• Carefully manage the patient's temperature to minimize any additional cerebral metabolic demands.
• Assess the patient's neurologic status for signs of increased ICP. To minimize fluctuations in ICP, decrease external stimuli and keep the head of the patient's bed elevated 30 degrees. Place the patient's head and neck in a neutral position. Avoid having him perform Valsalva's maneuver and isometric exercises.
• Provide routine postoperative care, as for any craniotomy. Inspect the head dressing for signs of bleeding or CSF leakage. As ordered, admin-

ister analgesics to manage pain and antiemetics to control nausea and vomiting. Turn and reposition the patient frequently to prevent pulmonary compromise. Monitor fluid intake and output, and laboratory reports. To decrease the risk of complications related to immobility, use antiembolism stockings or compression boots, as indicated.

• Administer postoperative medications, including anticonvulsants, antacids, histamine blockers, steroids, and prophylactic antibiotics, as ordered.

### Continuing care

Tailor your interventions to fit the patient's treatment plan. For example, if radiation therapy and chemotherapy are indicated, focus on managing the adverse effects of these two treatments.

• Keep the patient's skin clean and dry. Avoid applying alcohol, powder, oils, or creams; these products may cause severe burning with the next treatment.

• Provide mouth care regularly to maintain oral mucosal integrity.

• Maintain adequate nutrition. You may need to provide small, frequent meals and snacks to avoid nausea. Administer antiemetics as needed.

### Patient teaching

• Teach the patient and his family about tumor management, treatment options, and medications. Help prepare them for necessary lifestyle changes.

• Review the possible adverse effects of all treatments. Help the patient and his family devise strategies to minimize these effects.

• For most patients with a brain tumor, the prognosis is no more than 2 years. Help the patient and his family develop effective coping strategies. Suggest ways to improve the patient's quality of life.

• As needed, refer the patient to a dietitian or a physical therapist. Inform the patient and his family about local social services agencies, community support groups, and home health care agencies that provide physical and rehabilitative services.

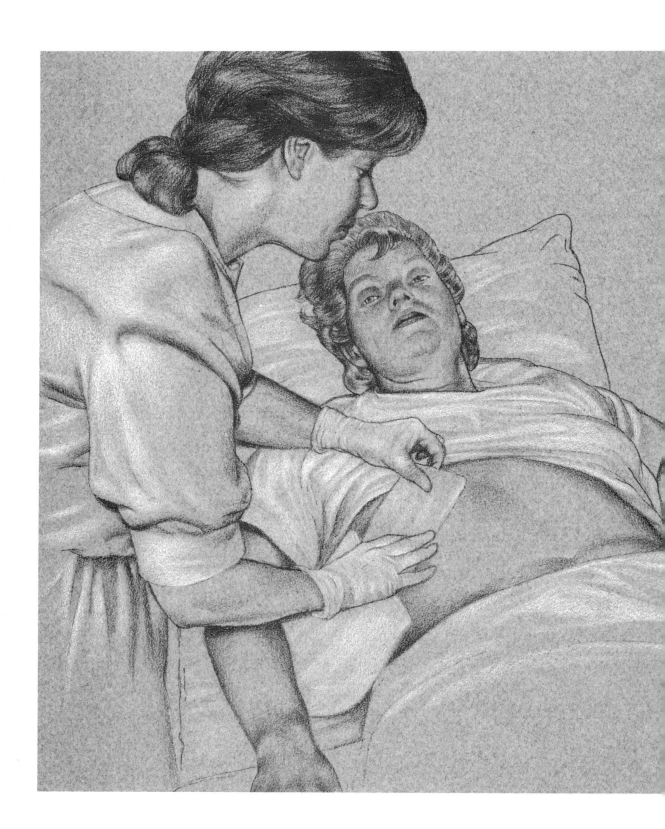

# CHAPTER 5

# Gastrointestinal disorders

The gastrointestinal (GI) system provides the essential nutrients to fuel the brain, heart, lungs, and other vital organs. So a GI malfunction can have far-reaching metabolic effects, severely affecting and, ultimately, jeopardizing a patient's life.

GI function is crucial in other respects too. Because of its impact on overall health, it profoundly affects the quality of life, including a person's mental health and stability. This makes psychological support mandatory for the patient with an acute GI disorder, who must cope with the possible need for major surgery and accompanying radical life-style changes.

An acute GI illness can result from a long-term disorder or from the sudden development of a condition requiring prompt management. Many patients with serious GI problems present with an acute abdomen—a condition for which immediate surgery must be considered. Some conditions causing an acute abdomen may not be life-threatening; others must be managed within a matter of hours to minimize the risk of serious consequences or death. The health care team must quickly determine the urgency of the patient's problem and decide whether he needs immediate surgery. This is where your careful history taking and physical examination come into play.

If the patient does require surgery, you'll need to carry out supportive measures and provide thorough preoperative preparation, then follow through with expert care during his postoperative recovery. Your care must include minimizing his anxiety before surgery and his discomfort after it. To carry out these responsibilities successfully, you must address both the emotional and physical needs of this patient.

This chapter describes how to provide high-quality care for acutely ill patients with selected GI disorders, including ulcerative colitis, cholelithiasis, peritonitis, pancreatitis, cirrhosis, and intestinal obstruction. Besides helping you become familiar with the causes, pathophysiology, and potential complications of these conditions, it describes assessment and intervention techniques that will build your confidence in managing patients with these problems.

# Ulcerative colitis

An inflammatory and often chronic disease, ulcerative colitis affects the mucosa of the colon, causing congestion, edema (leading to mucosal friability), and ulcerations. It usually starts in the rectum and sigmoid colon and may extend upward into the entire colon. Disease severity ranges from a mild, localized disorder to an acute, fulminant illness causing severe diarrhea and prostration, with many possible complications; it is also an illness of remissions and exacerbations, so careful patient teaching is essential.

Ulcerative colitis occurs primarily in young adults, especially women. It's most prevalent among Jews and higher socioeconomic groups. The exact incidence of the disease is unknown, but some studies indicate it affects as many as 1 in every 1,000 persons. Symptom onset

peaks between ages 15 and 20 and again between ages 55 and 60.

## Causes
The cause of ulcerative colitis is unknown. Proposed causes include a genetic predisposition, autoimmune disease, and allergy. Stress, once thought to cause the disease, is now believed to increase the severity of an acute exacerbation.

## Pathophysiology
Ulcerative colitis is characterized by acute, nonspecific inflammation of the colonic mucosa, especially the rectosigmoid area. The inflammatory process tends to extend gradually upward from the rectum and sigmoid colon. Multiple, irregular, superficial ulcerations develop in the involved areas. Unless the patient has coexisting Crohn's disease, the disease rarely affects the small intestine, except for the terminal ileum.

Repeated episodes cause thickening and scar tissue development in the intestinal wall. In severe disease, polypoid structures (pseudopolyps) form — probably from proliferative changes in the epithelium. Vascular congestion, edema, and ulceration impair absorption across the mucosa. Mucosal necrosis may lead to perforation with sepsis.

## Complications
General complications of ulcerative colitis include malnourishment, sepsis, and impaired growth and sexual development (in childhood onset). GI complications include abscesses, fissures, fistulas, toxic megacolon, colonic perforation, massive colonic hemorrhage, oral ulcers, and primary sclerosing cholangitis. (See *Managing toxic megacolon*.)

Except when confined to the rectum, ulcerative colitis increases the risk of colon cancer; this risk correlates directly to the extent, severity, and duration of ulcerative colitis. The cancer incidence is 0.2% after 1 year of ulcerative colitis but 13.5% after 30 years.

Other potential complications include:
• coagulation defects, if vitamin K is poorly absorbed
• pyoderma gangrenosum

• erythema nodosum polyarthritis
• ankylosing spondylitis
• ocular complications (such as iritis, uveitis, and other ocular lesions)
• anemia
• pleuropericarditis
• thrombophlebitis.

## Assessment

### Signs and symptoms

Check for a family history of inflammatory bowel disease. The patient may report blood and mucus in the stool or bloody, mucoid diarrhea up to 25 times daily. Diarrhea may be triggered by activity, stress, or meals. Other typical complaints include nausea and vomiting, lower abdominal cramps and pain, fecal incontinence, anorexia, weight loss, malaise, fatigue, and weakness. Find out about the patient's history of disease remissions and exacerbations.

Be sure to obtain a diet history; many patients with ulcerative colitis have an intolerance to dairy products.

On physical examination, check for hyperactive bowel sounds. You'll probably find the abdomen soft, with some tenderness and no signs of peritonitis (except if complications are present). Abdominal distention suggests severe disease, such as peritonitis or toxic megacolon. Other physical findings may include fever, perianal irritation, hemorrhoids, and dehydration.

### Diagnostic tests

The doctor must rule out Crohn's disease, another inflammatory bowel disease. (See *Managing Crohn's disease*, page 112.)

In ulcerative colitis, blood studies typically reveal hypochromic anemia from blood loss, polymorphonuclear leukocytosis, an elevated erythrocyte sedimentation rate, and hypoproteinemia. In patients with severe diarrhea, expect electrolyte imbalances (such as hypokalemia and hypomagnesemia). A stool specimen may show blood, pus, and mucus but is negative for pathogens when cultures are taken.

A barium enema identifies regional or generalized areas of involvement. Involvement may be mild, showing irritability; more severe involvement will be indicated by a shortened,

narrowed colon lumen, loss of physical landmarks (haustral markings), and pseudopolyps. (Barium enema is contraindicated if the patient has active signs and symptoms.)

Sigmoidoscopy usually reveals rectal involvement (95% of cases), mucosal hyperemia and friability, decreased mucosal detail, thick inflammatory exudate, petechiae, granulation, ulceration, and polypoid changes. Colonoscopy

---

COMPLICATIONS

# Managing toxic megacolon

A grave complication of ulcerative colitis, toxic megacolon is extreme colonic dilation characterized by loss of muscle tone in the colon. Eventually, the diameter of the transverse colon exceeds 2" (6 cm). This condition may lead to perforation of the colon, sepsis, and death. Mortality approaches 40%.

## Signs and symptoms

Signs and symptoms of toxic megacolon include a fever up to 104° F (40° C), leukocytosis, abdominal pain, rebound tenderness, diminished or absent bowel sounds, and increasing abdominal girth. Abdominal X-rays reveal intraluminal gas along a paralyzed segment of the colon.

## Interventions

• As ordered, discontinue antidiarrheals immediately and withhold all oral intake.
• Assist with insertion of an intestinal tube, if ordered, and connect the tube to intermittent suction. A large, soft rectal tube may be used to promote gas expulsion, but it must be inserted with extreme caution — preferably, by a doctor who's familiar with the condition of the patient's lower bowel mucosa — to avoid perforating the bowel.
• Begin aggressive I.V. fluid and electrolyte replacement, as ordered. Expect to administer I.V. hydrocortisone and antibiotics.
• Turn the patient every 2 hours to help redistribute gas and halt distention.
• Arrange for daily abdominal X-rays to detect free air and increasing distention.
• If supportive measures fail, prepare the patient for an emergency total colectomy, if ordered.

# Managing Crohn's disease

Like ulcerative colitis, Crohn's disease is a chronic inflammatory bowel disease. Because the two diseases require different treatment, proper diagnosis is essential.

Crohn's disease can affect both the large and small intestines. Most commonly, it involves the terminal ileum. Patchy bowel inflammation may extend through the layers of the bowel wall. As the disease progresses, the bowel wall thickens and the lumen narrows. Edema occurs and eventually the bowel becomes inflamed, ulcerated, and stenosed. Abscesses and fistulas form.

The exact cause of Crohn's disease is unknown. But research suggests that causes include allergies and other immune disorders, lymphatic obstruction, infection, and a genetic tendency. The disease is most common in Jews and least common in Blacks.

### Signs and symptoms

Initially, signs and symptoms may be mild and nonspecific. However, acute inflammatory findings mimic appendicitis and include abdominal pain in the right lower quadrant, cramping, tenderness, flatulence, nausea, fever, and diarrhea. Bleeding may occur; although usually mild, it may be massive. Bloody stools are possible as well.

Chronic symptoms are more persistent but milder. They may include diarrhea with abdominal pain in the right lower quadrant, steatorrhea, and marked weight loss. The patient may also report a general feeling of weakness and an inability to cope with stress.

### Diagnostic tests

Laboratory tests may show an increased white blood cell count and erythrocyte sedimentation rate, hypokalemia, hypocalcemia, hypomagnesemia, and a decreased hemoglobin level. A barium enema showing the string sign (segments of stricture separated by normal bowel) supports the diagnosis. Sigmoidoscopy and colonoscopy may reveal patchy areas of inflammation, helping to rule out ulcerative colitis. However, only a biopsy provides a definitive diagnosis.

### Interventions

• Provide treatment for Crohn's disease based on the patient's symptoms. If the patient is debilitated, provide total parenteral nutrition, as ordered, to maintain nutrition while resting the bowel.
• Administer anti-inflammatory corticosteroids, immunosuppressive agents, and metronidazole, as ordered. Opium tincture and diphenoxylate with atropine may help combat diarrhea, although they're contraindicated in patients with significant intestinal obstruction.
• Teach the patient about required life-style changes, which are central to effective treatment. Emphasize the importance of physical rest, a restricted fiber diet (no fruits or vegetables), and eliminating dairy products if the patient is lactose intolerant.
• If ordered, prepare the patient for surgery to correct bowel perforation, massive hemorrhage, fistulas, or acute intestinal obstruction. Surgery may involve resection of diseased bowel segments, total colectomy with ileostomy, or subtotal colectomy with temporary ileostomy or ileorectal anastomosis.

---

defines the extent of involvement, although this procedure is avoided during acute episodes. Colonoscopy with multiple biopsies can identify dysplasia and cancer; usually, it's recommended after the tenth year of the disease.

## Treatment

In fulminant disease, management focuses on restoring circulating blood volume to prevent shock. I.V. fluids, plasma, and blood are given, as indicated, and electrolyte imbalances are corrected. Total parenteral nutrition (TPN) is given if a prolonged exacerbation occurs. Nasogastric (NG) suction is indicated for colonic dilation.

## Drug therapy

In severe attacks, opiates and anticholinergics are withheld; if an infectious organism is present, the antiperistaltic action of these drugs may help the organism penetrate the impaired mucosa. Antidiarrheals may be withheld too, because they may slow intestinal motility, predisposing the patient to toxic megacolon.

I.V. antibiotics are used to treat or prevent sepsis. In severe cases, the doctor may order a corticosteroid, such as I.V. hydrocortisone or methylprednisolone or oral prednisone (20 to 60 mg/day). Corticosteroids have an anti-inflammatory effect, inhibiting prostaglandin synthesis. With clinical and sigmoidoscopic evidence of improvement, the prednisone dosage may be reduced by 5 mg/day each week.

To help prevent disease exacerbations, the doctor may prescribe oral sulfasalazine. The usual dosage is 3 to 4 g/day, with larger doses given during flare-ups. This drug is preferred over corticosteroids because it causes less serious adverse effects. Nausea, a common adverse effect, can be minimized by taking the drug with meals. Although largely nonabsorbable, sulfasalazine is metabolized in the intestines and its metabolite (sulfapyridine) is absorbed. Therefore, it may cause such systemic adverse effects as rashes, fever, arthralgia, anemia, and agranulocytosis.

For prolonged attacks, the doctor may prescribe mesalamine. This drug reduces inflammation and may decrease exacerbations in mild to moderate ulcerative colitis. Colonic response occurs in as little as 3 days, as shown by more fully formed stools. Mesalamine causes fewer adverse effects than sulfonamides and corticosteroids. To ensure direct contact with the colon, it's given as a rectal suspension via enema.

Anticholinergics, antidiarrheals (such as diphenoxylate and loperamide) and, less frequently, codeine may be prescribed to treat mild to moderate diarrhea. However, these drugs must be used with caution. Over time, most patients become adept at titrating the dosage of these and other medications in response to symptoms.

## Surgery
Refractory disease and life-threatening complications are indications for surgery. In a small number of cases, the surgeon may resect only involved areas of the colon. But the only really curative procedure is total colectomy (including the rectosigmoid stump) with ileostomy. The ileostomy may or may not have a continent pouch. (See *Ileostomies: Other choices*, page 114.)

Pouch ileostomy, in which a pouch is created from a small loop of the terminal ileum and a nipple valve, is formed from the distal ileum. The resulting stoma opens just above the pubic hairline; the pouch empties through a catheter inserted in the stoma several times a day. In ulcerative colitis, colectomy to prevent colon cancer is controversial because of its high mortality.

Ileoanal reservoir is a newer surgery that preserves the anal sphincter and provides the patient with a reservoir made from the ileum and attached to the anal opening. The procedure is performed in two steps. First, the rectal mucosa is excised. An abdominal colectomy is performed; then a reservoir is constructed and attached. Next, a temporary loop ileostomy is made to allow the new rectal reservoir to heal. Finally, the loop ileostomy is closed after a 3- or 4-month waiting period. Stools from the reservoir are similar to the stools from an ileostomy.

## Nursing care
### Surgical care
• Before and after surgery, provide emotional support to the patient. Colon removal causes a profound and permanent body image change.
• After surgery, care for the ileostomy or ileostomy pouch according to protocol. Initially after surgery, the pouch must be drained continuously until peristalsis returns. Thereafter, it's drained every 2 to 3 hours. The patient gradually becomes familiar with the procedure. (See *Draining a continent ileostomy,* page 115.)

Eventually, the small bowel segment will distend, allowing longer periods between emptying. The patient can expect to empty the pouch two to four times daily. (The pouch doesn't distend sufficiently to be emptied only once a day.) Teach the patient to recognize the sensation of pressure that means the pouch is full and needs to be drained.

### Continuing care
• Monitor the patient closely for complications.
• Obtain the patient's daily weight, and docu-

# Ileostomies: Other choices

The patient with ulcerative colitis may undergo a traditional ileostomy—the creation of an opening of the ileum onto the surface of the abdomen through which fecal matter empties. But the doctor may choose an alternative ileostomy: continent ileostomy or straight ileoanal anastomosis.

### Continent ileostomy

The surgeon constructs a nipple valve by intussuscepting several centimeters of terminal ileum into the surgically constructed pouch. He joins the valve's layers with sutures or staples, then sutures the valve to the abdominal wall, as shown below. Pouch evacuation occurs through the nipple valve.

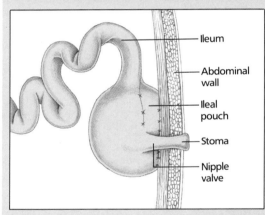

Ileum

Abdominal wall

Ileal pouch

Stoma

Nipple valve

### Straight ileoanal anastomosis

The surgeon sutures the distal ileum to the anal canal, as shown below, forming no pouch. Results compare favorably with ileoanal pouch procedures.

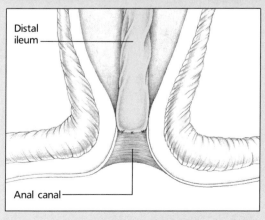

Distal ileum

Anal canal

ment fluid intake and output.
• Document the number and character of the patient's stools.
• Provide meticulous perianal skin care. Skin integrity is easily impaired when the patient has prolonged diarrhea because excreta will excoriate the area.
• Evaluate the patient's friends and family members as sources of support. As with most chronic illnesses, the patient must take charge of his own care.
• If the patient smokes, urge him to stop because smoking increases gastric secretions and intestinal motility.
• Verify that the patient understands the importance of communicating often with the doctor or clinic. Suggest he keep a diary between follow-up visits of his patterns of elimination, medication, stress, exercise, and other relevant life-style factors. This diary can be useful in helping him and the clinic evaluate and alter his therapy as needed.

*Diet and nutrition.* For the patient with ulcerative colitis, maintaining good nutrition is usually difficult, even during remission. He may associate mealtimes with pain, cramping, and diarrhea—and this can lead to anorexia. Gradual thickening of the colon causes malabsorption even during quiescent periods, when the patient's appetite may improve.
• Provide only foods the patient can tolerate. Teach him to avoid foods known to precipitate exacerbations. Many patients with ulcerative colitis can't tolerate dairy products; many are lactase deficient.
• Advise the patient to consume low-residue, high-protein foods and to avoid raw fruits and vegetables, nuts, caffeine, and cold fluids, which increase intestinal motility.
• Encourage the patient's family to bring foods from home that he knows he can tolerate; these preferences can then be incorporated into a more comprehensive plan of patient teaching.

*Medication.* Give medications as ordered.
• Give mesalamine by enema in divided doses of 800 mg to 2.4 g daily, as ordered, to main-

ain remission. For acute disease, give 1.6 to
.8 g daily, as ordered.
  If the patient is receiving sulfasalazine, inform
im that the drug may color his skin and urine
ellow.
  Make sure the patient who's receiving an an-
cholinergic, an antidiarrheal, or codeine knows
he warning signs of toxic megacolon and in-
ection.

*eostomy.* Have the patient demonstrate care
or the incision, ostomy, or pouch as indicated.
  Instruct the patient to increase his water and
alt intake because an ileostomy promotes
vater and salt loss.
  Sexuality is a concern for most ileostomy pa-
ients. Men with ostomies may experience im-
otence from damage to the pudendal nerves.
licit the patient's concerns and attempt frank
iscussion. As appropriate, arrange for visits by
stomates leading full lives. Refer the patient
or sexual therapy, if indicated.
  Arrange for other referrals, as appropriate —
or instance, the local chapter of the United
)stomy Association and the National Founda-
ion of Ileitis and Colitis.
  Arrange for the patient to see an enterosto-
nal therapy nurse for support and education.

**atient teaching**
  Be aware that patients with ulcerative colitis
ave been maligned for years. Many have been
old (even by health care professionals) that
he problem is "all in your head" and that
hey can control their symptoms. Yet often the
ack of control caused by sudden diarrhea and
he need to be near a bathroom at all times
ause significant stress.
  Inform the patient and his family members
hat the cause of ulcerative colitis is unknown,
lthough most evidence points to a genetic
redisposition or an immunologic cause. Inform
hem that no evidence suggests a behavioral
ause.
  Stress that there's no such thing as an "ul-
erative colitis personality." Each patient with
he disease has a unique personality.
  Emphasize that the patient isn't to blame for
he disease and that psychological factors are
nost likely an effect, not a cause, of ulcerative

# Draining a continent ileostomy

A continent ileostomy serves as an internal recep-
tacle for fecal discharge. Initially after surgery, the
pouch must be drained continuously until peristalsis
returns. Thereafter, it's drained every 2 to 3 hours.
Eventually, the patient will need to drain the pouch
unassisted, so encourage him to participate in the
procedure.

### Essential steps
• Gather equipment: tissues, water-soluble lubri-
cant, gauze squares, catheter, syringe, irrigating solution in a bowl, and emesis or receiving basin.
• Provide privacy. Explain the procedure to the patient, wash your hands, and put on gloves.
• Remove the stoma dressing.
• Lubricate the catheter and then gently insert it
into the stoma. When it reaches the nipple valve
(at about 2" [5 cm]), you'll feel resistance. Tell the
patient to take a deep breath, then exert gentle
pressure on the catheter to insert it through the
valve.
• If you still feel resistance, fill a syringe with 20 ml
of air or water and inject it through the catheter,
still exerting some pressure. The catheter should
then enter the pouch.
• Gently advance the catheter to the suture mark-
ing made by the surgeon.
• Place the other end of the catheter in a drainage
basin held below stoma level. Let the pouch drain
completely. Later, this procedure can be done at
the toilet, with drainage emptying into the toilet
bowl.
• After draining the pouch, remove the catheter
and gently wash the area around the stoma with
warm water. Pat the skin dry and apply a fresh
stoma dressing.
• Rinse the catheter with warm water.

colitis. For instance, although emotional stress
may alter blood supply to the intestinal mucosa and thus increase the number and severity of attacks, it's probably an effect of the
disease. However, urge the patient to avoid
stress as much as possible.
• Provide psychological support or refer the patient for counseling to help him deal with

# Helping a young patient cope with ulcerative colitis

The body-image and life-style changes imposed by ulcerative colitis can be difficult for anyone to cope with. They may be especially hard on a young adult, who sees his friends leading full, exciting lives while he struggles with an emotionally trying disease. A nurse who can't empathize with such a patient's plight may do him more harm than good.

Consider the case of Paul Gerace, age 20. Paul has a particularly severe case of ulcerative colitis. This is day 21 of his third hospitalization since his diagnosis just 1 year ago.

### Encountering an angry patient
Nurse Linda Maur enters Paul's room and places a bottle of total parenteral nutrition (TPN) on the overbed table. Paul angrily throws the tray on the floor.

Linda looks at Paul but doesn't reply. She picks up the TPN bottle and hangs it on an unused hook as she prepares the tubing for administration. This makes Paul even angrier, and he curses her.

### Reevaluating care
Linda is shaken. She thinks about the frenetic schedule she maintained at his age and finds she hasn't been considering Paul's feelings. She's been treating him as an anonymous patient, not as a previously healthy young man who has suddenly become a virtual invalid.

During the short lull of the evening shift, just before the night report, Linda enters Paul's room. She doesn't remonstrate him for his tantrum, but instead asks why he is so angry and encourages him to talk. Paul tells Linda that after his symptoms became unmanageable, he had to return home from his out-of-state college. He had enrolled in a local college and had just made some new friends when another exacerbation occurred. Now he's on his third admission, with three lost semesters and many lost relationships.

### Developing a better rapport
Later, on her now routine evening visit, Linda urges Paul to explore his strengths and supports. Paul says he has caring parents, two older sisters, and friends who still call.

Linda suspects that Paul's family members are so preoccupied with his possible need for surgery that they haven't thought about his socialization needs. She decides to speak to Paul's sisters about his feelings of loss. Soon, two of his old high school buddies pay him a visit.

### Dealing with a discouraged patient
The doctor and a round of consultants confer and agree that surgery is the most practical therapy for Paul. They present Paul and his family members with the surgical option of total colectomy. They believe he's been on TPN too long, explaining that it's not primary therapy and shouldn't be used simply to delay a decision about surgery.

That evening, Paul rails over his fate, emphasizing his extreme discomfort on being tied to an I.V. pole while everyone else his age is getting on with their lives. Even with the surgery, he says, life will be miserable, having to wear a colostomy pouch all the time.

Linda explains that Paul's quality of life will improve with surgery. She tells him about the experiences of other ostomy patients she's cared for. And she arranges for a visit by a 32-year-old former patient from the Ostomy Club.

Nevertheless, Paul decides against surgery, insisting he'll find alternative therapies. At the time of discharge, he can tolerate only liquids.

### Witnessing a change of heart
Two months later, however, Paul returns to the hospital, having opted for a continent ileostomy. His postoperative course is uneventful. A quick learner, he's adept at caring for his ileostomy by the time he's discharged.

A few months later, Paul comes back for a visit, timing it for the lull of evening. No longer is Paul angry, depressed, or cachectic, and he's gained 24 lb (10.9 kg). He appears to be in good spirits and thanks Linda for all her help.

He doesn't stay long — his girlfriend is waiting in the car. He tells Linda that his girlfriend knows and doesn't care in response to Linda's unasked question. A kiss good-bye, an elicited promise to visit again when he isn't too busy — and he's gone.

body-image and life-style changes. (See *Help-ng a young patient cope with ulcerative coli-is.*)

# Cholelithiasis

Cholelithiasis is the formation of calculi in the gallbladder. These calculi — basically a precipita-ion of bile salts, cholesterol, and calcium — de-velop during periods of sluggishness in the gallbladder due to conditions such as preg-nancy, diabetes mellitus, celiac disease, cirrhosis of the liver, pancreatitis, or inflammatory or obstructive lesions.

With treatment, the patient usually has a good prognosis. If infection occurs, the prog-nosis depends on its severity and the response to antibiotics.

### Causes
The precise cause of cholelithiasis is unknown. However, the following risk factors predispose a person to gallstone formation:
• a high-calorie, high-cholesterol diet
• elevated estrogen levels resulting from oral contraceptive use, postmenopausal hormone-replacement therapy, or pregnancy
• clofibrate therapy
• such diseases as diabetes mellitus, ileal dis-ease, hemolytic disorders, hepatic disease, and pancreatitis.

### Pathophysiology
Bile, made continuously by the liver, is concen-rated and stored in the gallbladder until needed by the duodenum to help digest fat. Conditions that cause changes in bile composi-ion or in the absorptive ability of the gallblad-der epithelium often encourage gallstone formation. (See *How gallstones form,* pages 118 and 119.)

### Complications
Cholelithiasis may lead to any of the disorders associated with gallstone formation. For in-tance, in *cholangitis,* the bile duct becomes in-ected; this disorder is commonly associated with choledocholithiasis and may follow percu-

taneous transhepatic cholangiography. Nonsup-purative cholangitis usually responds rapidly to antibiotic treatment. Suppurative cholangitis has a poor prognosis unless immediate surgery is done to correct the obstruction and drain the infected bile.

In *gallstone ileus,* a gallstone obstructs the small bowel. Typically, the stone travels through a fistula between the gallbladder and small bowel and then lodges at the ileocecal valve. Most common in older adults, this condition has a good prognosis after surgery.

In *cholecystitis,* the gallbladder is acutely or chronically inflamed — usually because a gall-stone becomes lodged in the cystic duct, caus-ing painful gallbladder distention. The acute form is most common during middle age; the chronic form, among older adults. The prog-nosis is good with treatment.

In *choledocholithiasis,* gallstones pass out of the gallbladder and lodge in the hepatic and common bile ducts, obstructing the flow of bile into the duodenum. The prognosis is good unless infection occurs.

## Assessment
### Signs and symptoms
Severity of symptoms depends on whether gallstones are stationary or mobile and whether they're obstructing the flow of bile. With small, nonobstructing calculi, the patient may be asymptomatic. With calculi lodged in the ducts or moving through the ducts, he may complain of spasms (biliary colic) and ex-cruciating abdominal pain in the right upper quadrant, which may radiate to the back, be-tween the shoulders, or to the front of the chest. The pain may be so severe that he seeks emergency care. Other clinical features include tachycardia, recurring fat intolerance, belching, flatulence, indigestion, diaphoresis, nausea, vomiting, chills, and low-grade fever. Typically, acute symptoms are precipitated by a high-fat meal (fat activates the gallbladder).

With total obstruction preventing bile drainage, the patient may appear jaundiced and report dark amber urine and clay-colored stools. Obstruction also causes poor absorption of fat-soluble vitamins and fat intolerance.

# How gallstones form

Bile is made continuously by the liver and stored in the gallbladder until needed by the duodenum to help digest fat. Calculi, or gallstones, are formed by the secretion of bile abnormally high in cholesterol, and can be complicated by fat entering the duodenum, biliary stasis, and ischemia.

## Bile secretion
Certain conditions—for example, age, obesity, and estrogen imbalance—cause the liver to secrete bile that's abnormally high in cholesterol or lacking the proper concentration of bile salts. Inflammation may occur when the gallbladder concentrates this bile. Excessive water and bile salts are reabsorbed, making the bile less soluble. Cholesterol, calcium, and bilirubin then precipitate into gallstones. This may cause nausea, belching, and abdominal pain.

## Fat entering the duodenum
Fat entering the duodenum causes the intestinal mucosa to secrete the hormone cholecystokinin, which stimulates the gallbladder to contract and

**Calculus in cystic duct**

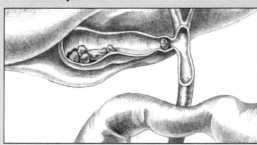

empty. If a calculus lodges in the cystic duct, as shown above, the gallbladder contracts but can't empty. This condition may lead to severe pain, nausea, and vomiting.

If a calculus lodges in the common bile duct, as shown at top right, the flow of bile into the duodenum becomes obstructed. Bilirubin is absorbed into the blood, causing jaundice. Other signs of obstruction include biliary colic, clay-colored stools, and fat intolerance.

### Diagnostic tests
Once the patient's pain is under control, he typically undergoes a battery of tests to rule out sources of other pain, such as from the heart. Consequently, the initial workup may include an electrocardiogram.

Ultrasonography can detect gallstones with great accuracy. Cholecystography visualizes gallstones and biliary duct obstruction, allowing the doctor to see the stones in their exact size and location.

Elevated total serum bilirubin, urine bilirubin, and alkaline phosphatase support the diagnosis of cholelithiasis. With obstruction, liver function studies are abnormal. With inflammation, the white blood cell (WBC) count is elevated.

## Treatment
Pain management is your main priority if the patient is in severe pain. Nausea and vomiting,

which may accompany pain, call for antiemetics. If the patient needs narcotics for pain relief, meperidine is the drug of choice because it's less likely to cause spasms in Oddi's sphincter. Anticholinergics or antispasmodics, such as atropine and papaverine, also may be used to relieve spasms.

If the patient is asymptomatic and has recovered from a first attack of biliary colic, the doctor may use conservative treatment, such as medication, diet, and life-style modifications. For instance, he may prescribe chenodiol to dissolve gallstones or prevent their formation, or vitamin supplements to replace fat-soluble vitamins (A, D, E, and K).

### Surgery
One of three procedures may be performed to remove calculi. In *traditional cholecystectomy*, the surgeon makes an incision on the right side of the diaphragm under the rib cage and in-

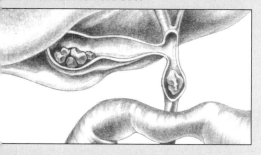

Calculus in common bile duct

## Biliary stasis and tissue ischemia
Biliary stasis and ischemia of the tissue surrounding the calculus also can cause irritation and inflammation of the common bile duct. When this occurs, clinical findings may include jaundice, high fever, chills, and an increased eosinophil count.

Inflammation may progress and lead to infection of any of the bile ducts. This causes scar tissue, edema, cirrhosis, portal hypertension, and variceal hemorrhage. The patient may exhibit fever, ascites, bleeding tendencies, confusion, and coma.

inserts a T tube. The T tube maintains patency in the hepatic duct system and is usually removed several days after the operation. This surgery typically requires a hospital stay of 5 to 7 days. *Endoscopic retrograde cholangiopancreatography* is a less invasive surgical procedure for which the surgeon inserts an endoscope to remove calculi.

With *laparoscopic cholecystectomy*, a newer procedure, the surgeon makes several small incisions of ³⁄₈″ to 1¹⁄₈″ (1 to 3 cm) on the abdomen — one at the umbilicus to insert the laparoscope (which is attached to a video camera) and others at the upper midline and the right midclavicular line to insert various grasping and dissecting forceps. Then he inflates the abdomen with carbon dioxide to allow visualization of the structures. The camera transmits images to a monitor, allowing the surgical team to view the procedure more closely. The surgeon clips and divides the cystic

duct and artery, and then uses a laser or cautery to excise the gallbladder from the liver. The gallbladder is removed through the incision at the umbilicus. The small wounds are closed with staples.

Laparoscopic cholecystectomy causes little postoperative pain and requires no dressings or tubes. The patient is discharged immediately and may eat a light meal the same evening. (See *Laparoscopic cholecystectomy,* page 120.)

## Nursing care
Monitor the cholelithiasis patient's vital signs and urine output closely, and check the abdominal dressing and any drains to ensure patency. Care for the patient focuses on preparing him for surgery; answering his questions about the procedure; and changing dressings, monitoring for complications, and relieving pain after surgery, if indicated.

### Surgical care
***For traditional cholecystectomy.*** Provide care as you would for any abdominal surgery.
• Before surgery, provide detailed preoperative teaching so the patient knows what to expect during the postoperative period. Mention that he may have an NG tube for gastric decompression, a Penrose drain, and a T tube postoperatively. The Penrose drain will drain serosanguineous fluid. The T tube, connected to a closed gravity system, will drain bile and help maintain duct patency. (See *Caring for the patient with a T tube,* page 121.)

Inform the patient that the incision will cause pain on inspiration. Teach him the coughing and deep-breathing methods he must use after surgery.
• After the surgery, change the dressing on the T tube or the Penrose drain frequently.
• Monitor the patient's serum potassium level closely; this electrolyte is lost via drainage of potassium-rich bile.

***For laparoscopic cholecystectomy.*** Focus on patient teaching and managing discomfort.
• Before surgery, teach the patient about the procedure and what to expect afterward.
• After surgery, control pain and manage other problems, as indicated. For instance, you may

## Laparoscopic cholecystectomy

In this procedure, the surgeon inserts a laparoscope through the incision at the umbilicus (below, left) and manipulates instruments through two other incisions guided by a video monitor. After dissecting and clipping the cystic duct and artery (below, right), he separates the gallbladder from the liver and pulls it up through the umbilical incision.

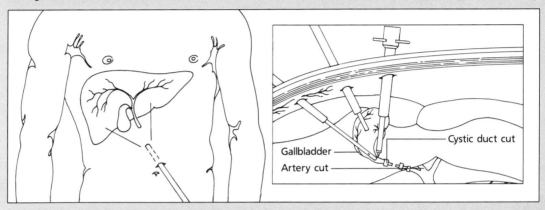

Cystic duct cut
Gallbladder
Artery cut

need to apply heat to the patient's shoulder to control pain due to general inflammation that has radiated to the shoulder.
• Keep him in semi-Fowler's position and promote early ambulation. Teach him to keep the small wounds clean and to avoid heavy lifting.

### Patient teaching
Diet is pivotal to continued nursing care. A proper diet can prevent future attacks and avoid the necessity of surgery. If the patient doesn't need surgery, he'll be discharged with dietary instructions, including the need to reduce his fat intake. Teach him about healthy dietary practices, referring him to a dietitian as needed.

# Peritonitis

Peritonitis is an acute or chronic inflammation of the peritoneum, which lines the abdominal cavity and covers the visceral organs. Inflammation may be generalized throughout the abdomen, extend to the pelvis, or remain local-

ized as an abscess. Typically, intestinal motility decreases, causing intestinal distention with gas. Mortality from peritonitis is 10%, with death usually a result of bowel obstruction.

### Causes
*Peritonitis* typically results from inflammation and perforation of the GI tract, allowing bacterial invasion. Common causes include appendicitis, diverticulitis, peptic ulcer, ulcerative colitis, volvulus (twisting of the bowel on itself), strangulated bowel obstruction, abdominal neoplasm, and stab wounds. *Chemical peritonitis* occurs when irritating substances (such as enzymes leaking from the pancreas in acute pancreatitis) come into contact with the peritoneum. Fallopian or ovarian tube rupture, bladder rupture, and a perforated gastric ulcer also may cause chemical peritonitis.

Spontaneous *bacterial peritonitis* may occur during late stages of cirrhosis. Neoplastic disease and certain drugs (for example, beta blockers and methysergide) can cause sclerosing peritonitis.

## Pathophysiology

Normally, the peritoneum is sterile. In peritonitis, however, it's invaded by bacteria or chemicals, causing infection of the peritoneal cavity. Accumulated fluids containing protein and electrolytes make the transparent peritoneum opaque, red, inflamed, and edematous. Because the peritoneal cavity is so resistant to contamination, such infection is commonly localized as an abscess instead of disseminated as a generalized infection.

## Complications

Pelvic abscess is the most common complication of peritonitis; abscess also can occur elsewhere in the abdomen. Intestinal obstruction, which may arise long after the inflammatory process resolves, can result from adhesions related to peritonitis. Septic shock may result from bacteria or toxins entering the bloodstream.

## Assessment

### Signs and symptoms

If you suspect peritonitis, inquire about recent abdominal surgery and find out if the patient has a history of ulcers or diverticulosis.

Cardinal signs of peritonitis include paralytic ileus, diminished to absent peristalsis, and progressive abdominal distention. The patient may report nausea, vomiting, and pain, which typically becomes increasingly severe and constant.

Ask the patient to describe the location of his pain. With localized inflammation, pain occurs in a specific abdominal area. With generalized inflammation, pain is diffuse and may be referred to the shoulder or thoracic area.

On physical examination, observe the patient's position — he may flex his knees to try to relieve pain. Also assess him for:
• fever
• abdominal distention and rigidity (a classic sign of generalized peritonitis)
• rebound tenderness referred to the area of peritonitis
• general or local abdominal tenderness to light percussion
• rectal or vaginal tenderness (suggesting pelvic peritonitis)
• prostration.

# Caring for the patient with a T tube

Your patient may return from a cholecystectomy with a T tube connected to a closed gravity system. The T tube maintains duct patency and drains bile. To ensure proper tube care and protect the patient's skin from bile, which is highly irritating, follow these guidelines.

### Monitor drainage
• Observe drainage for color and amount. Initially, expect bloody drainage, which turns greenish brown after several hours. After the first few days, drainage should measure 400 ml/day. Report amounts over 1,000 ml/day to the doctor. As bile starts to follow its normal route, drainage should decrease. If it starts to increase *after* first diminishing, suspect a ductal obstruction below the tube.
• Observe for drainage around the tube. You may need to use a sterile pouching system if there is any leakage.
• Don't aspirate, irrigate, or clamp the tube without a doctor's order. Irrigation isn't necessary, and free flow of bile is desirable.

### Promote drainage
• Keep the patient in low Fowler's position to promote bile drainage.
• Maintain the drainage bag at the correct level, as ordered, so bile will drain by gravity.
• Follow the doctor's orders for raising the level of the bag and clamping the T tube. Observe the patient for pain, chills, abdominal fullness, and nausea, which may indicate that the common bile duct isn't patent.

### Maintain tube patency
• To maintain the patency of the tube and prevent it from dislodging, help the patient turn and ambulate.
• To determine if bile is aiding digestion, clamp the tube for 1 to 2 hours before and after meals and assess the patient's response.
• Observe for signs that bile is flowing through normal channels: brown stools, reduced drainage from the tube, and no signs of jaundice. Initially, all or nearly all bile flows out of the T tube. As edema subsides, most bile flows into the duodenum. The T tube is removed when bile flows through normal channels (usually in 7 to 10 days).

### Diagnostic tests

Usually, the patient has leukocytosis; the WBC count may rise above 20,000/mm³. Abdominal X-rays may show gas and fluid collection, dilation, edema, and inflammation of the small and large intestines. With perforation, X-rays show free air in the abdominal cavity.

Paracentesis is done to collect and analyze ascitic fluid for amylase and protein measurement, culture and sensitivity, and cytology (the number of polymorphonuclear neutrophils). Cloudy fluid withdrawn during aspiration indicates peritonitis; high WBC and neutrophil counts are common in bacterial peritonitis.

## Treatment

Medical care is supportive and aims to control infection, restore fluid and electrolyte balance, and identify and correct the cause of peritonitis. Usually, massive antibiotic therapy is initiated.

Many patients require surgery to correct the underlying problem. Surgery may involve removal of an inflamed appendix or a gangrenous bowel, closure of a perforation, or abscess drainage.

## Nursing care

• Administer medications, such as analgesics and antibiotics, as ordered. Monitor the patient for desired and adverse effects.
• Maintain parenteral fluid and electrolyte administration as ordered.
• Monitor the patient's fluid status by assessing his skin turgor, mucous membranes, urine output, weight, and vital signs. Accurately record intake (including infused I.V. fluids) and output (including NG tube drainage).
• Suspect an abscess if fever, leukocytosis, or ileus fails to respond to treatment or if pain localizes or fails to improve daily. However, be aware that antibiotic therapy may mask some of these signs.
• Maintain bed rest. Keep the patient in semi-Fowler's position to help him breathe deeply with less pain and thus prevent pulmonary complications.
• Perform frequent oral hygiene and provide lubrication to combat mouth and nose dryness

(caused by fever, dehydration, and NG intubation).
• Provide psychological support and encouragement.

### Surgical care

*Preoperative care.* If time allows before surgery, reinforce the doctor's explanation of the procedure.
• Teach the patient how to cough and deep breathe, which he'll need to do during postoperative recovery.
• Tell the patient what to expect during the postoperative period.

*Postoperative care.* Immediately after surgery, monitor the patient's pain, vital signs, level of consciousness (LOC), respiratory status, bowel signs, abdominal distention, incisional drainage, urine output, NG tube drainage, and I.V. fluid intake at least once every hour, or as ordered.
• Place the patient in Fowler's position to promote gravity drainage through the drainage tube.
• Allow the patient nothing by mouth until NG tube suction is discontinued. Administer parenteral feedings as ordered.
• Administer blood transfusions, if necessary and ordered.
• Frequently assess for peristaltic activity by listening for bowel sounds and checking for flatus, bowel movements, and a soft abdomen. When peristalsis resumes and the patient's temperature and pulse rate become normal, gradually increase parenteral fluids and increase oral fluids, as ordered. If an NG tube is in place, clamp it for short intervals. If the patient tolerates this without nausea or vomiting, begin oral fluids, as ordered and tolerated.
• Watch for signs of dehiscence (such as a patient complaint that "something gave way") and abscess formation (continued abdominal tenderness and fever).
• Encourage and assist ambulation, as ordered—usually on the first postoperative day.
• If necessary, refer the patient to the social service department or a home health care agency to help him obtain needed services during convalescence.

Depending on the surgical procedure, the patient may have specific dietary limitations. Provide appropriate dietary instructions.

**Patient teaching**

Explain what peritonitis is and identify the underlying condition that caused it.

Because the wound usually is open at the time of discharge, you'll need to teach the patient how to clean and irrigate it (usually with 0.9% sodium chloride solution) and how to change the dressing. Request a demonstration in return from the patient.

Instruct the patient on what drainage changes to expect; for instance, drainage usually appears green and diminishes in quantity each day. Instruct him to report any swelling, increasing drainage, bleeding, redness, pain, tenderness, warmth, or odor from the incision.

Discuss the proper use of prescribed medications; review the administration regimen and both the desired and adverse effects.

Have the patient demonstrate that he can take his temperature accurately using his home thermometer and interpret the results correctly.

Instruct the patient to perform as much activity as he can tolerate. Caution him to avoid heavy lifting for 6 weeks, however.

Make sure the patient knows when to return for a follow-up medical visit.

# Pancreatitis

Pancreatitis is an acute or chronic inflammation of the pancreas. Usually a severe intra-abdominal disease, it affects more males than females. Recovery may be complete, but some patients have recurring attacks and about 10% develop chronic pancreatitis.

The prognosis is good when pancreatitis follows biliary tract disease but poor when associated with alcoholism. When accompanied by necrosis or hemorrhage, the disease has a mortality of up to 60%.

**Causes**

Pancreatitis results primarily from biliary tract disease (gallstones) or alcohol abuse. In biliary tract disease, bile flows backward into pancreatic ducts and directly injures acinar cells.

Alcohol abuse is the most common cause of chronic pancreatitis. Alcohol stimulates hydrochloric acid and secretin production, which in turn stimulates pancreatic secretions. It also causes pylorospasm and regurgitation of duodenal contents into the pancreatic ducts, resulting in inflammation.

Other causes of pancreatitis include abnormal organ structure, metabolic or endocrine disorders (such as hyperlipidemia and hyperparathyroidism), and certain drugs. Pancreatitis sometimes occurs as a complication of renal failure, kidney transplantation, or endoscopic retrograde cholangiopancreatography (ERCP).

**Pathophysiology**

Acute pancreatitis involves autodigestion of enzymes normally excreted by the pancreas. Fluid, serum, plasma, albumin, and blood are lost into the retroperitoneal space. With severe episodes, necrosis of the acinar cells and hemorrhage from necrotic blood vessels may occur.

**Complications**

Leakage of fluid into the pancreatic bed and ileum may cause severe intravascular fluid volume deficit, leading to hemodynamic instability and shock. Fluid leakage also may cause pleural effusion.

Because the inflammation is so close to the bowel, paralytic ileus may occur. Damage to the islets of Langerhans may lead to diabetes mellitus; diabetes and exocrine pancreatic insufficiency may outlast the acute episode. Prerenal azotemia may arise in the first 24 hours, requiring temporary supportive dialysis.

Pseudocysts — sacs filled with fluid rich in pancreatic enzymes — are common complications of pancreatitis. They may arise in the mediastinal and retrorectal areas as well as the pancreas. Smaller pseudocysts may resolve spontaneously but infected pseudocysts may require incision and drainage. Erosion of a blood vessel may cause hemorrhage into the cyst, a dangerous complication.

Pancreatic abscesses also may occur. These suppurative lesions, usually infected by bacteria, require incision and drainage, followed by antibiotic therapy.

Internal or external fistulas may form from enzyme leakage or draining of pseudocysts or abscesses. Most fistulas resolve spontaneously over several months.

During initial treatment of pancreatitis, infusion of a large volume of fluid increases the risk of adult respiratory distress syndrome and cardiac dysfunction.

## Assessment
### Signs and symptoms
Expect the patient's history to reveal a risk factor, such as a previous pancreatitis episode, alcohol abuse, biliary tract disease, hyperlipidemia, or use of certain drugs (such as glucocorticoids, sulfonamides, thiazides, and oral contraceptives). He may complain of nausea, vomiting, and weakness. Epigastric pain may be severe and steady, radiating to the back; it may abate when the patient leans forward in a sitting position.

On inspection, the patient may seem anxious, diaphoretic, pale, and mildly jaundiced. Obtain his vital signs, noting any fever, tachycardia, or hypotension. You may detect a tender upper abdomen (usually without guarding or rigidity) and abdominal distention.

### Diagnostic tests
The doctor will make a presumptive diagnosis based on clinical and laboratory findings. Blood tests typically reveal an elevated serum amylase level (above 200 Somogyi units/dl) within 24 hours of onset. Most reliable within 48 hours of onset, an elevated serum amylase level is highly indicative of pancreatic cell injury. The serum lipase level also rises within 24 hours; the degree of elevation and time of return to normal vary with disease severity (usually, the serum lipase level remains elevated longer than the serum amylase level).

Other findings include an increased WBC count (10,000 to 30,000/mm$^3$) and elevated serum glucose, bilirubin, blood urea nitrogen (BUN), and alkaline phosphatase levels. Urinalysis may reveal proteinuria and glycosuria.

A computed tomography (CT) scan may show an enlarged pancreas, a gas-distended small intestine, or pseudocysts. ERCP may identify pancreatic cysts, abscesses, and gallstones. A chest X-ray may reveal left-sided elevation of the diaphragm and pleural effusion.

## Treatment
Treatment of acute pancreatitis is entirely supportive and focuses on resting the pancreas. Bed rest and temperature control are used to reduce the metabolic rate and thus decrease pancreatic secretions. Continuous NG suction is used to keep the stomach decompressed and reduce duodenal activity to prevent secretion of enzymes. All oral intake is withheld; because peritonitis causes considerable volume depletion, maintaining the patient's fluid and electrolyte balance is crucial.

### Drug therapy
Antibiotic therapy depends on the involved organism. To restore hemodynamic stability, expect to administer 0.9% sodium chloride solution, colloids, fresh frozen plasma, and serum albumin or other blood products. Most patients require TPN to maintain weight and achieve a positive nitrogen balance.

To manage pain, the usual choice is meperidine, administered as needed by the I.M. route. The patient with impaired renal or hepatic function requires smaller, more frequent meperidine doses. Hydromorphone is sometimes used instead of meperidine. But opiates are avoided whenever possible because they may cause smooth-muscle contractions, triggering spasms of the ampulla of Vater.

Other drug therapy may include:
• antispasmodics to decrease pancreatic outflow
• anticholinergics to reduce pancreatic secretions
• antacids to neutralize gastric secretions

• histamine$_2$-receptor blockers (such as famotidine, cimetidine, and ranitidine) to reduce gastric pH
• pancreatic replacement therapy to supplement pancreatic enzymes (if the patient has extensive permanent damage to pancreatic cells).

## Surgery

Surgery is reserved for patients at risk for multisystem organ failure from severe autodigestion of pancreatic enzymes and for those with unmanageable edema, hemorrhage, necrosis, or biochemical abnormalities. The surgeon debrides and resects necrotic areas; then he flushes and drains accumulated toxins from the abdominal cavity. Drains remain in place for several weeks.

External drainage is established with surgical placement of a three-way irrigation catheter and Penrose drain. One port of the three-way catheter is used as an air vent, the second for irrigating fluids, and the third for suction drainage. To drain toxins produced by necrotic pancreatic tissue, irrigation with 0.9% sodium chloride solution continues, sometimes for several weeks after surgery.

An abscess or unresolving pseudocyst must be surgically incised and drained. Internal drainage of a pseudocyst may involve anastomosis between the pancreatic ducts and the jejunum. External sump drains requiring irrigation may be placed.

# Nursing care

• If your patient is an alcoholic, be sure you know the risks and complications of alcohol withdrawal during pancreatitis treatment. (See *When your alcoholic patient has pancreatitis,* page 126.)
• Monitor for complications by checking the patient's vital signs, breath sounds, urine output, and arterial blood gas (ABG) levels. Monitor blood glucose levels to detect any islet cell involvement.
• Assess for abdominal signs—Cullen's (bluish skin around the umbilicus), indicative of pancreatitis; Grey Turner's (bluish brown skin in the flank), indicative of intraperitoneal bleed-

ing; rigid abdomen and increasing abdominal girth, both indicative of paralytic ileus or obstruction.
• Stay alert for fever, increasing pain, and leukocytosis, which signal a pseudocyst or abscess. To prevent or manage these problems, expect to give I.V. antibiotics.
• To maintain intact skin after surgery, carry out special skin care using stomal bags and products. External fistulas drain pancreatic enzymes and impair skin integrity. Apply skin barriers and ostomy drainage bags carefully to maintain the skin until the fistula heals, which may take weeks to months. The patient may require TPN for the duration.
• Closely monitor complete blood count and serum calcium and creatinine levels. Calcium binds with free lipids, possibly causing hypocalcemia and placing the patient at risk for seizures.

## Continuing care

• If the doctor prescribes pancreatic enzymes, instruct the patient to take the medication with meals and snacks to help digest food and promote fat and protein absorption.
• Advise him to report abdominal distention, cramping, and fatty, frothy stools, which are formed in chronic pancreatitis. Acinar cells, which secrete enzymes, are progressively destroyed; eventually, lipase and protease secretions are so reduced that fat absorption is severely impaired, resulting in fatty stools.

*Diet and nutrition.* Introduce oral feedings gradually, as ordered.
• Progress from clear fluids to a high-carbohydrate, low-fat diet. Carbohydrates are less stimulating to the pancreas; fats, in contrast, trigger secretion of pancreozymin, which in turn stimulates the pancreas.
• Restrict caffeine and other stimulants because they increase peristalsis, which stimulates the pancreas.

## Patient teaching

• Abstinence from alcohol is essential to prevent chronic pancreatitis or recurrence of acute

# When your alcoholic patient has pancreatitis

Biliary tract damage induced by alcohol is a leading cause of pancreatitis. Make sure you're familiar with the special problems posed by alcoholism in a patient with pancreatitis.

Alcohol withdrawal and detoxification complicate the care of a patient with pancreatitis and necessitate the utmost caution. The intensity of withdrawal varies with the degree and duration of alcohol abuse. Alcohol inactivation depends entirely on the patient's metabolism. If he already has liver disease, for instance, metabolism of alcohol can be greatly impaired.

## Pathophysiology

Alcohol abuse causes precipitation of protein and atrophy of the acini in the pancreas. Consequently, the small ducts become obstructed, blocking proper drainage of the pancreas. These chronic and irreversible changes occur well before acute pancreatitis develops.

The exact mechanism leading to an acute pancreatitis attack is unknown. Alcohol absorbed in the stomach stimulates hydrochloric acid and secretin production, which may trigger pylorospasm. Most alcohol is absorbed in the duodenum, however. Alcohol may trigger acute attacks by causing regurgitation of duodenal contents into the pancreatic ducts.

## Risks

Detoxification can lead to sudden death caused by cardiogenic shock, cardiac standstill, ventricular fibrillation, and abrupt left ventricular failure. A falling blood alcohol level has an antidiuretic effect, which increases fluid retention. Because this patient is predisposed to overhydration, fluid administration is challenging. Many withdrawal protocols advise against forcing fluids unless other factors, such as severe malnutrition, vomiting, or diarrhea, are present. Administering fluids to an overhydrated patient in alcohol withdrawal may thus be extremely counterproductive and induce life-threatening congestive heart failure.

The electrolyte imbalances that accompany pancreatitis are also aggravated by alcohol withdrawal. Hypokalemia and hypomagnesemia together account for 5% to 25% of deaths occurring during withdrawal.

Most detoxification protocols involve substituting alcohol with drugs that depress the central nervous system (CNS) and then tapering these drugs slowly to soften the withdrawal effects. Benzodiazepines (such as chlordiazepoxide and diazepam) are commonly used. However, the alcoholic needs larger-than-normal doses because of his greater tolerance for CNS depressants. Benzodiazepines are best given orally because they're poorly absorbed parenterally. However, the patient with pancreatitis can't have any oral intake because this might stimulate his pancreas. For this reason, diazepam may be given I.V.

## Interventions

• Replacing fluid lost into the peritoneal cavity and via nasogastric suctioning is the primary goal of caring for the patient with pancreatitis. Administer fluids with caution and only in proportion to losses, based on the patient's hourly urine output and central venous or pulmonary artery pressure monitoring.

• Be aware that the antidiuretic effect of withdrawal makes the patient's response to fluid infusion unpredictable. With the large amounts of fluids given in acute pancreatitis—up to 8 liters/day—he can quickly become overhydrated. You'll need to monitor his fluid status closely.

---

pancreatitis. Refer the alcohol-dependent patient for counseling.

• Smoking increases gastric acid secretion. If your patient smokes, urge him to stop. Refer him to a smoking cessation program, as appropriate.

# Cirrhosis

Cirrhosis is a chronic degenerative disease of the liver in which the lobes are covered with fibrous tissue, the parenchyma degenerates, and the lobules are infiltrated with fat. Diffuse destruction and fibrotic regeneration of hepatic cells occur.

Major forms of cirrhosis include Laënnec's, postnecrotic, biliary, and cardiac cirrhosis. Laënnec's cirrhosis is most prevalent among malnourished, alcoholic men and accounts for more than half of the cirrhosis cases in the United States.

Cirrhosis can occur at any age. Among Americans ages 35 to 55, it's the fourth leading cause of death.

## Causes

Laënnec's cirrhosis is closely linked with frequent and excessive intake of alcohol, a hepatotoxin. This cirrhosis form may have a genetic basis; some people have a familial tendency toward cirrhosis or a sensitivity to alcohol. However, many alcoholics don't develop cirrhosis, whereas others develop it despite an adequate nutritional status.

Postnecrotic cirrhosis follows subacute hepatic necrosis from toxic or viral hepatitis. The most common form of cirrhosis worldwide, it affects more women than men.

Primary biliary cirrhosis is caused by interlobular bile duct destruction resulting from an autoimmune response. Secondary biliary cirrhosis results from obstruction of the hepatic or common bile duct by stones, tumors, or conditions causing edema. Stasis and backflow of bile eventually lead to the physiologic changes associated with liver disease. Liver cells become severely damaged and are replaced by scar tissue.

## Pathophysiology

Regardless of the cause or form of cirrhosis, the pathophysiology is the same. The liver parenchyma is destroyed, lobules are separated by fibrous scar tissue, and structurally abnormal nodules form. These changes prevent the smooth flow of blood through the liver. As necrotic tissue yields to fibrosis, alterations in liver structure and vasculature impair blood and lymph, ultimately causing hepatic insufficiency.

## Complications

Depending on the extent of liver damage, cirrhosis may lead to portal hypertension, bleeding esophageal varices, hepatic encephalopathy, and hepatorenal syndrome. Acutely bleeding esophageal varices can prove fatal. (See *What happens in portal hypertension,* page 128.)

## Assessment
### Signs and symptoms

In the early stage of cirrhosis, clinical findings may be vague. Typical complaints include abdominal pain, diarrhea, nausea, and vomiting. As the disease progresses, the patient may report chronic dyspepsia, constipation, pruritus, and weight loss as well as signs of easy bleeding (such as frequent nosebleeds), easy bruising, and bleeding gums.

Because the liver has such wide-ranging functions (including detoxification of all ingested substances, formation of blood clotting factors and vitamins, and other metabolic activities), liver damage causes signs and symptoms in every body system. Thus, a body-systems approach provides a useful framework for physical examination.

*Integumentary findings,* which reflect the liver's inability to break down and excrete estrogen metabolites, may include palmar erythema (redness of the palms) and spider angiomas of the nose, cheeks, and upper trunk. Also look for petechiae and purpura, which result from impaired coagulation. Observe the sclerae and skin for jaundice, which results from abnormal metabolism or flow of bilirubin from the liver into the blood as it fails to be metabolized.

*Metabolic findings* include fluid and electrolyte imbalances. Excessive fluid accumulates in the peritoneal cavity, causing ascites. Ascites typically manifests as weight gain and an enlarged, fluid-filled abdominal cavity; you also may detect striae and distended abdominal veins. Keep in mind that ascites doesn't always indicate fluid overload because the intravascular space may be dehydrated. (See *How ascites develops,* page 129.)

COMPLICATIONS

# What happens in portal hypertension

Portal hypertension—elevated pressure in the portal vein—occurs when blood flow meets increased resistance. A complication of cirrhosis, the disorder also may stem from mechanical obstruction and occlusion of the hepatic veins (Budd-Chiari syndrome).

## Blood bypasses the liver

As pressure in the portal vein rises, blood backs up into the spleen and flows through collateral channels to the venous system, bypassing the liver. Consequently, portal hypertension causes splenomegaly with thrombocytopenia, dilated collateral veins (esophageal varices, hemorrhoids, or prominent abdominal veins), and ascites.

## Esophageal varices begin to bleed

In many patients, the first sign of portal hypertension is bleeding from esophageal varices—dilated, tortuous veins in the submucosa of the lower esophagus. Rupture of these varices typically causes massive hematemesis, requiring emergency care to control hemorrhage and prevent hypovolemic shock.

Care for the patient who has portal hypertension with ruptured esophageal varices focuses on careful monitoring for signs and symptoms of hemorrhage and subsequent hypotension, compromised oxygen supply, and altered level of consciousness.

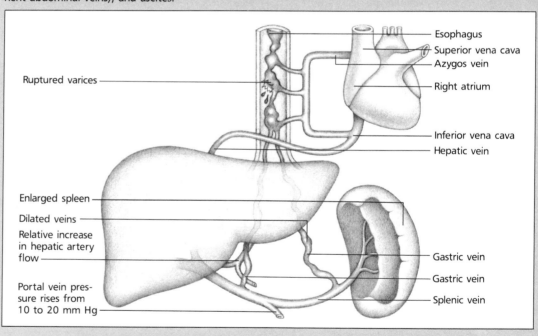

*Endocrine findings* reflect ineffective hormonal breakdown and elimination by the liver. In cirrhosis, serum levels of certain hormones become markedly elevated. For instance, in males, excess estrogen causes gynecomastia, testicular atrophy, and impotence. Females may experience amenorrhea or dysfunctional uterine bleeding.

*Hematologic findings* include bleeding problems stemming from the liver's inability to synthesize prothrombin and other blood clotting factors. In an acute situation, coagulopathy puts the patient at risk for bleeding from puncture wounds, ulcers, and esophageal varices. Also expect leukopenia, anemia, and thrombocytopenia because the enlarged spleen removes excess amounts of red blood cells (RBCs).

GI findings are obvious in both early and late stages of cirrhosis. These may include anorexia, dyspepsia, nausea, vomiting, diarrhea, hematemesis, and hemorrhoidal or esophageal varices.

Central nervous system (CNS) findings reflect an elevated serum ammonia level. During normal protein metabolism, ammonia is produced and converted to urea, which is then excreted by the kidneys. In cirrhosis, the liver doesn't metabolize protein properly, so ammonia accumulates in the serum and acts as a cerebral toxin. The higher the ammonia level, the more severe the CNS symptoms. Ammonia accumulation and intoxication cause hepatic failure and peripheral encephalopathy. (See Causes of hepatic encephalopathy, page 130.)

Symptoms of ammonia intoxication range from lethargy, fatigue, and memory loss to coma. Asterixis (liver flap) also indicates an increased serum ammonia level. To elicit this sign, ask the patient to extend his arms with hands outstretched; typically, he can't hold this position and makes a series of rapid flapping motions.

In an alcoholic with cirrhosis, you may detect CNS signs of vitamin $B_{12}$ deficiency, such as ataxia, poor muscle coordination, and fatigue.

Cardiovascular findings include peripheral edema, which results from the same conditions that cause ascites.

## Diagnostic tests
Blood tests may reveal elevated liver enzymes (alanine aminotransferase [formerly SGPT] and aspartate aminotransferase [formerly SGOT]), total serum bilirubin, and indirect bilirubin levels; decreased total serum albumin and protein levels; prolonged prothrombin time; reduced hemoglobin, hematocrit, and serum electrolyte levels; and deficiencies of vitamins A, C, and K. Suggestive urine findings include increased lev-

## How ascites develops

In ascites, fluid containing large amounts of protein and electrolytes accumulates in the peritoneal space. In patients with cirrhosis, ascites can develop in three ways.

In the first, the liver vasculature becomes stiff and noncompliant, causing increased portal vein pressure (portal hypertension). Plasma proteins are transported from hepatic vessels via the larger sinuses into the lymph space. When lymph channels become overloaded, water in the proteins leaks into the peritoneal cavity. Excess protein builds up in the peritoneal space, drawing water into that space and causing ascites.

The second cause of ascites, hypoalbuminemia, occurs as a result of the liver's inability to synthesize albumin. Hypoalbuminemia reduces colloid osmotic pressure, allowing fluid to leak from the intravascular space into the peritoneal space.

A third cause of ascites is the liver's inability to metabolize aldosterone. Excessive aldosterone causes accelerated sodium reabsorption by the proximal tubules, in turn causing water retention. Sodium retention causes potassium excretion, resulting in hypokalemia.

els of urobilinogen. Typically, the fecal urobilinogen level is reduced.

Liver biopsy provides a definitive diagnosis, showing hepatic tissue destruction and fibrosis. Abdominal X-rays reveal liver size and cysts or gas in the biliary tract or liver. They also may show liver calcification and massive ascites.

CT and liver scans may determine liver size, identify liver masses, and visualize hepatic blood flow and obstruction more accurately than X-rays. Esophagogastroduodenoscopy may show bleeding esophageal varices, stomach irritation or ulceration, or duodenal bleeding and irritation.

## Treatment
Cirrhosis can't be cured, so treatment is based on the patient's symptoms. Drugs are given to combat symptoms and the patient's diet is modified. Repeated hemorrhagic episodes may require sclerotherapy (injection of a sclerosing

# Causes of hepatic encephalopathy

The following chart lists the causes of hepatic encephalopathy along with their corresponding effects.

| CAUSE | EFFECT |
|---|---|
| Central nervous system (CNS) depressants (such as narcotics) | • Increase CNS depression from inability of liver to detoxify these drugs, causing serum drug level to rise |
| Constipation | • Increases ammonia from bacterial action on fecal matter |
| Dehydration | • Potentiates ammonia toxicity |
| Diuretics | • Increase renal formation of ammonia. May eventually cause azotemia, which increases endogenous ammonia production; also may cause hypokalemia |
| GI hemorrhage | • Increases ammonia in GI tract |
| Hypokalemia | • Increases renal production of ammonia, which then enters the systemic circulation; the brain needs potassium to metabolize ammonia |
| Hypovolemia | • Increases blood ammonia level by causing hepatic hypoxia; reduced blood flow impairs CNS, hepatic, and renal function |
| Increased metabolism | • Increases work load of liver |
| Infection | • Increases catabolism; enhances CNS sensitivity to toxins |
| Metabolic alkalosis | • Promotes ammonia transport across blood-brain barrier; increases renal production of ammonia |
| Paracentesis | • Causes loss of sodium and potassium and decreases blood volume |
| Uremia (renal failure) | • Causes retention of nitrogenous metabolites |

the systemic circulation.) A typical diet includes daily intake of 1.5 g protein/kg of body weight to maintain plasma osmotic balance and promote liver cell regeneration. As cirrhosis progresses, protein intake may be reduced to prevent encephalopathy. Sodium intake is usually restricted to limit edema and reduce ascites.

Drug therapy requires special precautions because the cirrhotic liver can't detoxify harmful substances efficiently. The doctor may order vasopressin to reduce acute bleeding, propranolol to decrease portal hypertension and prevent GI bleeding, and neomycin and lactulose to decrease the serum ammonia level and thus lower the risk of encephalopathy. Neomycin reduces bacteria in the bowel, decreasing ammonia formation; lactulose traps ammonia so it's excreted in the stools.

Other medications used to relieve symptoms of cirrhosis include antacids to reduce gastric distress and prevent GI bleeding and potassium-sparing diuretics, such as spironolactone, to inhibit the effect of excessive aldosterone on the tubules, preventing sodium and water absorption and averting potassium elimination. Fresh frozen plasma, vitamin K injections, and blood transfusions may be needed to prevent bleeding.

### For ascites
In a patient with ascites, the doctor may perform paracentesis to remove ascitic fluid from the abdomen and relieve abdominal pressure. Pressure valves located along the tube open and close, causing fluid to drain with changes in intra-abdominal and intrathoracic pressure during inspiration and expiration.

Paracentesis may cause intraoperative and postoperative complications, including life-threatening bleeding. To control bleeding, the doctor may order transfusions of packed RBCs and fresh frozen plasma, along with vitamin K injections. The threat of infection necessitates meticulous care and aseptic technique.

### For esophageal varices
The patient with esophageal varices receives vasopressin and undergoes esophageal tamponade to combat bleeding. In tamponade, the

agent directly into the vessels using endoscopy).

Dietary modification is crucial for the cirrhosis patient. Unless he has complications, he should consume a high-calorie diet (3,000 calories/day) with a high carbohydrate content, moderate protein content, and low fat content. Optimal protein intake varies with the extent of liver damage. (In cirrhosis, protein breakdown leads to direct entry of ammonia into

doctor inserts a Sengstaken-Blakemore tube through the nose, preferably in an intubated patient because of the high risk of airway obstruction. The tube has esophageal and gastric balloons that compress bleeding vessels. As with any other NG tube connected to suction, the gastric lumen drains the stomach of blood, fluid, and air. Alternatively, a Minnesota tube may be used. Its esophageal aspiration lumen suctions esophageal secretions that accumulate on top of the balloon.

### Surgery

Surgery may be attempted if medical management no longer relieves the severe symptoms of hepatic failure. The doctor may perform surgery to divert ascites into the venous circulation, using a peritovenous shunt. Shunt insertion causes weight loss, decreased abdominal girth, greater sodium excretion from the kidneys, and improved urine output. Reinfusion of ascitic fluid into the vascular space alleviates ascites and improves comfort.

## Nursing care

Caring for the patient with cirrhosis focuses on careful monitoring of his diet, sodium, and fluid intake (especially if he's taking diuretics), and his LOC, and teaching him to avoid or reduce substances that increase his risk of bleeding. Emphasize that he must completely abstain from alcohol.
• Administer diuretics, potassium, and protein and vitamin supplements, as ordered. If your patient is receiving a potassium-sparing diuretic, monitor for hyperkalemia.
• Find out which foods the patient prefers and provide these within prescribed dietary limitations. Offer frequent, small meals.
• If the patient is at risk for or already has hepatic encephalopathy, make sure his diet contains little or no protein.
• Restrict sodium and fluid intake, as ordered.

### Supportive care

• Monitor vital signs, intake and output, and electrolyte levels to determine the patient's fluid volume status.
• To assess for fluid retention, measure and record the patient's abdominal girth every shift.

Weigh him daily and document his weight.
• If your patient has a Sengstaken-Blakemore tube, be sure to protect his airway. Assess the balloon regularly for proper pressure. Too much pressure may cause the esophagus to rupture. To check pressure, connect the esophageal balloon to a sphygmomanometer and use a Y-connector on the other side to attach the bulb. Close off the port leading to the tube; then pump the mercury column to about 25 mm Hg. Turn the stopcock off to the bulb. When the mercury stops vacillating, read the pressure; it should never exceed 22 mm Hg.
• Document the degree of scleral and skin jaundice.
• Check for bleeding gums, ecchymoses, epistaxis, and petechiae. Stay with the patient during hemorrhagic episodes.
• Inspect stools for amount, color, and consistency. Test stools and vomitus for occult blood.
• Provide frequent skin care. Bathe the patient without soap and massage him with emollient lotions. Keep his fingernails short. Handle him gently. Turn and reposition him often to keep his skin intact.
• Increase the patient's exercise tolerance by providing rest periods before exercise.
• Address the patient by name and tell him your name to orient him. Mention the time, place, and date frequently throughout the day. Place a clock and a calendar where he can easily see them.
• Use appropriate safety measures to protect the patient from injury. Avoid physical restraints if possible, since they often provoke anxiety.
• Watch for signs of anxiety, epigastric fullness, restlessness, and weakness.
• Observe the patient closely for behavioral and personality changes. Report increasing stupor, lethargy, hallucinations, or neuromuscular dysfunction. Arouse the patient periodically to assess his LOC. Watch for asterixis, a sign of developing hepatic encephalopathy.
• Provide or assist with oral hygiene before and after meals.
• Encourage the patient to express his thoughts and feelings about having cirrhosis. Provide emotional support. Also, don't hesitate to offer him and his family members a realistic evaluation of his present health status while commu-

# Causes of intestinal obstruction

These illustrations show various conditions that can cause intestinal obstruction.

### Scar tissue

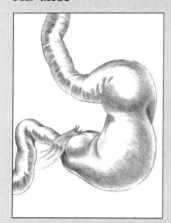

Development of scar tissue constricts the lumen of the bowel, blocking the intestinal flow.

### Mesenteric occlusion

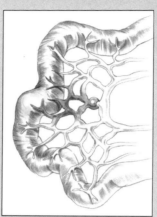

Occlusion in the area of the mesenteric artery, which serves parts of the intestine, blocks blood flow.

### Intussusception caused by polyps

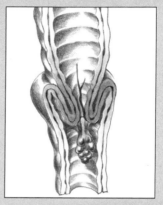

A polyp on the intestinal wall causes prolapse of one segment of the bowel into the lumen of another segment.

### Neoplasm

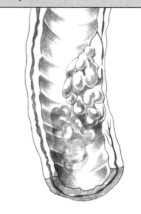

Abnormal new tissue growth obstructs the bowel.

nicating hope for the immediate future.

**Patient teaching**
• To minimize the risk of bleeding, teach the patient to avoid nonsteroidal anti-inflammatory drugs, straining to defecate, and blowing his nose or sneezing too vigorously. Suggest he use an electric razor and a soft toothbrush.
• Inform the patient that rest and good nutrition conserve energy and decrease metabolic demands on the liver. Urge him to eat frequent, small meals. Teach him to alternate periods of rest and activity to reduce oxygen demand and prevent fatigue.
• Teach the patient to conserve energy while performing activities of daily living. For example, suggest he sit on a bench while bathing or dressing.
• If the patient has esophageal varices, tell him to help prevent bleeding and hemorrhage by avoiding alcohol, aspirin, and foods that irritate the esophagus. Tell him to avoid actions that provoke coughing and vomiting because they may also provoke bleeding.
• Stress the need to avoid infections and abstain from alcohol. Refer him to Alcoholics Anonymous, if appropriate.

# Intestinal obstruction

Intestinal obstruction is the complete or partial blockage of the lumen of the small or large intestine, preventing intestinal contents from passing through the lumen. Intestinal obstruction may be simple, strangulated, or close-looped; these types may be acute or chronic.

In a simple obstruction, blockage prevents the passage of bowel contents, with no other complications. A strangulated obstruction closes off the lumen and impedes blood supply to part or all of the obstructed section. In a close-looped obstruction, both ends of the af-

### Ileocecal intussusception

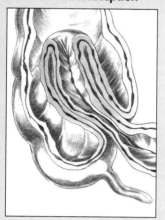

Prolapse of the valve between the small intestine and the cecum of the large intestine causes an obstruction.

### Strangulated inguinal hernia

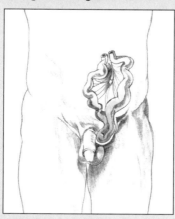

A hernia in the inguinal area causes an obstruction in the blood flow.

### Volvulus involving the sigmoid colon

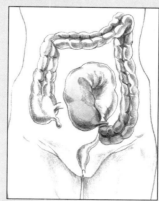

Twisting of the sigmoid colon causes an obstruction.

fected bowel section are occluded, isolating it from the rest of the intestine.

Mortality from intestinal obstruction is 10% to 20%. With strangulated obstruction, mortality may be as high as 75%.

### Causes

Intestinal obstruction results from mechanical or nonmechanical (neurogenic) blockage of the intestinal lumen. Causes of mechanical obstruction include hernia, adhesions, neoplasms, stenosis, intussusception, volvulus, and foreign bodies. (See *Causes of intestinal obstruction.*)

Nonmechanical obstruction may result from paralytic ileus, spinal cord lesion, or peritoneal irritation (for example, from hemorrhage, peritonitis, surgery, wound dehiscence, infection, or pancreatitis). Vascular problems, such as thrombosis of mesenteric vessels, emboli, and atherosclerosis, and cardiopulmonary resuscitation can cause intestinal obstruction.

### Pathophysiology

In all forms of intestinal obstruction, physiologic effects are similar. Fluid, air, gas, and increased bacterial growth accumulate. Peristalsis increases as the intestine attempts to move its contents through the obstruction. Forceful peristaltic movement may injure the intestinal mucosa, causing distention at and above the obstruction site. Distention increases venous pressure, blocking blood flow and interrupting normal absorptive processes. The bowel starts to secrete water, sodium, and potassium into the fluid pooled in the lumen, further decreasing absorptive ability. Anoxia and compression of the mesenteric blood supply may cause necrosis.

### Complications

Upper intestinal obstruction may lead to metabolic alkalosis secondary to dehydration and loss of hydrogen ions in gastric contents.

Lower intestinal obstruction may cause metabolic acidosis secondary to loss of intestinal alkaline fluids.

Peritonitis occurs as bacteria and toxins pass across the intestinal membranes into the abdominal cavity. Hypovolemic shock may arise as 6 to 8 liters/day of fluid enter the small bowel. Retention of large amounts of fluid in the intestine and peritoneal cavity causes intravascular volume depletion. Unrelieved intestinal obstruction leads to ischemia, necrosis (gangrene) of the bowel, and ultimately death.

## Assessment

### Signs and symptoms

Review the patient's history for a precipitating factor, such as recent abdominal surgery, spinal cord injury, radiation therapy, gallstones, colon cancer, Crohn's disease, diverticular disease, or ulcerative colitis. The family history may reveal colorectal cancer in one or more relatives.

Typically, the patient complains of abdominal pain, which may be severe, persistent, and colicky. He may describe obstipation and recent nausea and vomiting. Projectile vomiting suggests an obstruction high in the small intestine; typically, this vomitus contains bile. Vomitus caused by an obstructed large intestine may be orange-brown and foul-smelling, perhaps containing fecal material.

You may assess fever and signs of dehydration and shock. Abdominal examination may reveal distention. With strangulation or peritonitis, you may detect tenderness and rigidity.

Auscultation may reveal loud, high-pitched borborygmi. Sometimes, bowel sounds are hyperactive above and hypoactive below the obstruction site. Document any hiccups, which suggest a mechanical obstruction.

### Diagnostic tests

Upright and lateral decubitus abdominal X-rays may show dilated, air-filled loops of bowel, with trapped gas and fluid. Free air indicates bowel perforation.

ABG analysis may reveal metabolic acidosis or, less commonly, metabolic alkalosis. Blood tests may show increased hematocrit and hemoglobin levels (from hemoconcentration secondary to fluid loss into the bowel lumen), leukocytosis, and electrolyte imbalances. The BUN level may rise from dehydration.

GI studies, such as sigmoidoscopy, colonoscopy, or barium enema, may help determine the cause of obstruction. Before these tests are done, perforation must be ruled out.

## Treatment

Although surgery is usually mandatory, medical interventions are attempted in some patients — for instance, those with paralytic ileus or partial obstruction (especially if obstruction is recurrent or followed surgery or a recent episode of diffuse peritonitis). Medical interventions typically include measures to correct fluid and electrolyte imbalances, broad-spectrum antibiotics, nonopiate analgesics or sedatives, decompression with an NG or nasointestinal tube connected to low suction, and rectal tube insertion (in paralytic ileus).

A nasointestinal tube provides continuous bowel decompression. However, some doctors avoid this tube, believing the simpler, more widely available NG tube effectively decompresses the stomach and reduces intestinal lumen distention with less discomfort to the patient. Nonetheless, a nasointestinal tube has an important benefit — the mercury-filled balloon at its tip acts as a bolus, stimulating peristalsis as it advances down the intestinal lumen.

Occasionally, colonoscopy is done to remove an obstruction and sigmoidoscopy is done to reduce volvulus.

### Surgery

Intestinal obstruction is a surgical emergency. The type of surgery chosen depends on the cause of the obstruction. Commonly, surgery involves resection of the obstructed segment and anastomosis of the healthy bowel. Some patients require a colostomy, ileostomy, or total colectomy.

Preoperatively, the patient must be stabilized and usually undergoes bowel decompression, broad-spectrum antibiotic therapy, and measures to treat shock, peritonitis, and fluid and electrolyte imbalances.

# Nursing care
• Establish I.V. access for fluid replacement.
• As ordered, assist with NG tube (Salem sump) or nasointestinal tube placement to relieve vomiting, prevent aspiration, and reduce distention.
• Administer TPN, as ordered, if prolonged decompression is necessary.
• Administer medications, as prescribed, to manage pain and nausea.
• Correct fluid and electrolyte imbalances, as ordered.
• Monitor intake and output carefully. Measure all vomitus and tube drainage and document the character and odor.
• Stay alert for signs and symptoms of shock caused by fluid loss into the intestinal lumen.
• Closely monitor serum electrolyte levels, abdominal girth, and weight.
• Carefully evaluate the patient's therapeutic response. Signs and symptoms of increasing obstruction sometimes are masked by the obstruction.
• Provide surgical care as you would for any patient undergoing major abdominal surgery. Be aware that emergency surgery may leave the patient psychologically unprepared for a surgically created ostomy. Postoperatively, he'll need special psychological and emotional support.
• If cancer was found, treatment options and the prognosis will vary greatly. For other causes of obstruction, such as strangulated hernia, surgical repair is the definitive treatment.

## Patient teaching
• Base patient teaching on the underlying cause of the obstruction.
• Instruct the patient to consume a high-fiber, high-fluid diet after discharge (unless contraindicated).

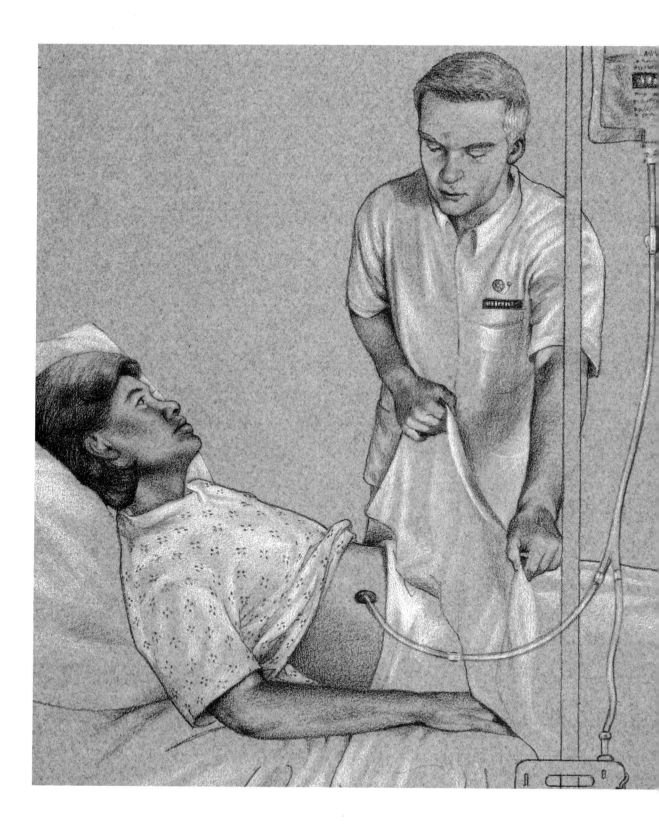

# CHAPTER 6

# Renal disorders

Kidney-related diseases affect more than 8 million Americans each year, so you're likely to encounter such patients often. Renal diseases and disorders can impair fluid, electrolyte, and acid-base balances. And without prompt intervention, they can progress to renal failure.

This chapter will familiarize you with the most common renal problems seen in the acute-care setting: acute renal failure, acute pyelonephritis, and renal calculi. First, the chapter presents the causes, pathophysiology, and complications of each of these disorders. Then it explains how to assess your patient, which diagnostic tests will be performed, and which treatment options the doctor may choose. Finally, the chapter discusses nursing care — the immediate interventions to take during the acute stage of illness, how to care for your patient before and after surgery, and the expert continuing care your patient will need.

# Acute renal failure

Acute renal failure is the sudden cessation of renal function due to obstruction, reduced circulation, or intrarenal (parenchymal) disease. When the kidneys suddenly stop functioning, the glomerular filtration rate (GFR) falls abruptly. When urine output falls below 500 ml/24 hours, acute renal failure is accompanied by oliguria; below 100 ml/24 hours, anuria. Waste products — mainly blood urea nitrogen (BUN) and creatinine — are retained.

If the original renal insult or decreased perfusion is not corrected, permanent damage will occur to the nephrons, and acute renal failure will progress to chronic renal failure. The rapid onset and potential reversibility of acute renal failure distinguish it from chronic renal failure. Acute renal failure is usually reversible with medical treatment. Chronic renal failure progresses through three stages which, untreated, may progress to end-stage renal disease and death.

In the initial stage of chronic renal failure, renal function is reduced, but no metabolic wastes accumulate because the healthier kidney compensates for the diseased one.

In the second stage, unaffected nephrons can no longer compensate, and metabolic wastes start to accumulate in the blood. The GFR decreases, determining the degree of insufficiency. Renal insufficiency is classified as mild, moderate, or severe.

Finally, excessive metabolic wastes accumulate in the blood. The kidneys can no longer maintain homeostasis and the patient requires dialysis.

## Causes
Depending on the cause, acute renal failure is classified as prerenal, intrarenal, or postrenal. *Acute prerenal failure* is characterized by diminished blood flow to the kidneys, as from hypovolemia, shock, embolism, excessive blood loss, sepsis, pooling of fluid due to ascites or burns, and cardiovascular disorders, such as heart disease, congestive heart failure, arrhythmias, and tamponade. Dehydration lowers intravascular volume and thus reduces blood supply to the kidneys. This reduction can cause oliguria or even anuria if dehydration is sufficiently severe.

*In acute intrarenal failure,* the kidney tissue itself is damaged secondary to inflammatory or immunologic processes. Acute tubular necrosis (ATN) is the most common cause of acute intrarenal failure. This problem may develop in a critically ill patient following an ischemic or nephrotoxic injury. ATN injures tubular segments of the nephron, causing lesions and necrosis. Depending on the type and extent of cell damage, ATN may be reversible. (See *Acute tubular necrosis.*)

Other causes of acute intrarenal failure include systemic lupus erythematosus, malignant hypertension, periarteritis nodosa, vasculitis, sickle cell anemia, nephrotoxins, ischemia, renal myeloma, acute pyelonephritis, intrarenal precipitation, disseminated intravascular coagulation, and hepatorenal syndrome (commonly associated with cirrhosis).

*Acute postrenal failure* results from bilateral obstruction of urine outflow anywhere from the calyces to the urinary meatus. Underlying causes include renal calculi, thrombi, papillary necrosis, tumors, benign prostatic hyperplasia, strictures, and urethral edema from catheterization.

## Pathophysiology
In acute renal failure of tubular or vascular etiology, oliguria occurs during early stages. Impaired renal function leads to progressive azotemia (uremia, or retention in the blood of excessive amounts of nitrogenous compounds). With a tubular abnormality, oliguria presumably results from tubular leakage or obstruction (such as from debris, casts, or interstitial edema). Typically, the GFR decreases.

When the glomeruli aren't structurally damaged, oliguria may stem from vascular changes, particularly renal artery constriction. In the early stages of acute renal failure, vasoconstriction in the renal cortex leads to ischemia, reduced GFR and, ultimately, oliguria. (See *Comparing types of acute renal failure,* page 140.)

*Phases of acute renal failure.* In most patients, acute renal failure progresses through three phases. During the *oliguric phase,* which may last 10 to 20 days, urine output ranges from 50 to 400 ml/24 hours. Protein typically spills into the urine. Renal blood flow drops to about 30% of normal, and the GFR falls to less than 1% of normal, causing such fluid and electrolyte imbalances as hyponatremia, hyperkalemia, and metabolic acidosis.

However, about 30% of patients have increasing azotemia without oliguria. Nonoliguric acute renal failure is rarely fatal. Typically, urine output measures 1 liter/24 hours or more. Azotemia peaks in 10 to 12 days, and laboratory values gradually return to normal over another 10 to 12 days.

The *diuretic phase* starts when urine output increases above 500 ml/24 hours. Accumulated substances, such as serum urea and creatinine, serve as osmotic diuretics. Diuresis may start as early as 24 hours after onset of acute renal failure. Increased urine output doesn't signal a total return of renal function, however. Tubular function remains altered, as reflected by significant potassium and sodium loss in the urine. Fluid and electrolyte balances fluctuate widely during the diuretic phase, and the inability to conserve water may cause dehydration.

The *recovery phase* may last for several months after the initial episode of acute renal failure. Although renal function may be adequate, residual impairment may decrease the patient's renal reserve. Eventually, the GFR, renal blood flow, and tubular function return to normal, and the kidneys resume proper urine concentration. During the recovery phase, modifying protein intake and preventing fluid overload can improve the patient's fluid and electrolyte balances.

## Complications

Acute renal failure may progress to end-stage renal disease, uremic syndrome and, ultimately, death. Uremic syndrome is characterized by increasing serum concentrations of urea, creatinine, uric acid, potassium, phosphate, phenols, sulfates, and guanidine bases. This condition leads to generalized edema (from water and sodium retention) and acidosis (from failure to eliminate normal acidic products). Complica-

# Acute tubular necrosis

Acute tubular necrosis (ATN) accounts for about 75% of all cases of acute renal failure. Mortality can be as high as 70%, depending on the severity of complications.

## Causes and complications

ATN is caused by ischemic or nephrotoxic injury, as from extensive surgery or critical illness. Causes of ischemic injury, which disrupts blood flow to the kidneys, include circulatory collapse, severe hypotension, trauma, hemorrhage, dehydration, and transfusion reaction. Nephrotoxic injury may follow ingestion or inhalation of certain drugs or chemicals (such as aminoglycosides or nonsteroidal anti-inflammatory drugs, and X-ray contrast dyes) or an allergic reaction. Nephrotoxic ATN is potentially reversible because it doesn't damage the basement membrane of the nephrons.

Infections, which complicate about two-thirds of ATN cases, are the leading cause of death in patients with ATN. Other potential complications of ATN include GI hemorrhage, fluid and electrolyte imbalances, cardiovascular disorders, and neurologic problems.

## Pathophysiology

In ATN, muscle damage leads to rhabdomyolysis. Myoglobin, a substance contained in striated muscle tissue, is released into the bloodstream and obstructs the tubular portion of the nephrons with cellular debris or tissue swelling. Casts also may plug the tubules. If damage is confined to the tubular epithelium, the cells may regenerate. However, damage extending to the basement membrane is permanent because this layer can't regenerate.

## Signs and symptoms

Clinical findings may include oliguria (urine output below 500 ml/24 hours), petechiae, ecchymoses, hematemesis, dry and pruritic skin, dry mucous membranes, uremic breath odor, muscle weakness, lethargy, somnolence, confusion, disorientation, agitation, muscle twitching, and seizures. The heart rate may be irregular and increased (tachycardia). You may auscultate bibasilar crackles and detect peripheral edema.

PATHOPHYSIOLOGY

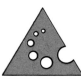

# Comparing types of acute renal failure

Different types of renal failure—prerenal, intrarenal, and postrenal—have different pathophysiologies. *Prerenal failure* due to reduced perfusion causes fluid retention and increased water reabsorption. *Intrarenal failure* caused by acute tubular necrosis may culminate in pyelonephritis and vasoconstriction, triggering oliguria. *Postrenal failure* results from urine flow obstruction and causes kidney ischemia and tissue atrophy. Features of all three types are listed below.

| TYPE AND DESCRIPTION | PATHOPHYSIOLOGY |
|---|---|
| **Prerenal failure**<br>• Reduced glomerular filtration rate (GFR) and increased proximal tubular reabsorption of sodium and water<br>• Most common form of acute renal failure<br>• Reversible if detected and treated within 24 hours | • Reduced perfusion causes fluid retention, reexpanding the extracellular space.<br>• Reduced glomerular blood flow rate decreases postglomerular plasma flow, altering pressure within tubular and intratubular spaces and increasing proximal tubular sodium and water reabsorption.<br>• Increased water reabsorption raises urea concentration in filtrate.<br>• Reduced blood pressure in kidney stimulates juxtaglomerular apparatus receptors, enhancing renin production. |
| **Intrarenal failure**<br>• Destruction of glomeruli or tubulointerstitial structures<br>• May lead to obstruction or ischemia | • Immunologic injury may affect nephron's interstitial tissue or vascular bed.<br>• Inflammatory changes precipitate tissue injury, with scarring and glomerular function loss. Acute proximal tubular necrosis may occur with renal poisoning. (Pyelonephritis usually involves suppurative necrosis, abscess formation, or both; eventually, such changes destroy glomeruli.)<br>• Crystalline deposits in tubules obstruct urine flow.<br>• Vasoconstriction reduces renal blood flow, decreases GFR and tubular fluid flow, and triggers oliguria. |
| **Postrenal failure**<br>• Results from mechanical or functional urine flow obstruction anywhere along urinary tract<br>• Increases back pressure on kidney's filtration system, impairing glomerular filtration | • Increased pressure leads to dilation and enlargement of kidney, pelvis, calyces, and tubules.<br>• GFR decreases, disrupting tubular cell function.<br>• Leakage of solutes from blood prevents sodium reabsorption and potassium and hydrogen secretion in distal tubules.<br>• Vasodilation of renal cortex and medulla blocks vasopressin action, inhibiting sodium transport.<br>• Renin release and prostaglandin production raise blood pressure.<br>• Progressively decreased blood flow through glomeruli causes kidney ischemia.<br>• Prolonged pressure causes tissue atrophy.<br>• Nephrons stop functioning or have reduced filtration rate. |

tions of these effects involve virtually every body system and may cause multisystem failure. (See *Multisystem effects of renal failure,* pages 142 and 143.)

## Assessment
### Signs and symptoms
Clinical findings in acute renal failure may vary with the form of the disorder. In acute prerenal failure, signs and symptoms may resemble those of congestive heart failure (CHF) or dehydration. Expect hypotension, tachycardia,

and reductions in urine output, cardiac output, and central venous pressure (CVP). The patient may be lethargic, with a lowered level of consciousness.

If the patient also has CHF, symptoms can include increased interstitial pressure in the lungs and pulmonary edema. (See *Congestive heart failure in a patient with acute renal failure,* page 144.)

In acute intrarenal failure, glomerular or tubular damage causes decreased urine output, hypotension, elevated CVP, and tachycardia. In acute postrenal failure, signs and symptoms such as oliguria or intermittent anuria, severe uremia, lethargy, and difficulty urinating reflect obstruction of the lower urinary tract.

Any form of acute renal failure may cause nausea, vomiting, headache, weight gain, and tremor. If acute renal failure progresses untreated, you may detect cardiac changes, including friction rub, cardiac irritability, and peaked T waves on an electrocardiogram (ECG).

Assess jugular vein pulses as the patient lies supine. Flat veins may indicate blood volume depletion, a possible cause of renal ischemia. Measure blood pressure in both arms in three different positions — with the patient lying, standing, and sitting. Then measure his heart rate. Suspect volume depletion if you note orthostatic hypotension and a significant rise in the heart rate when the patient stands.

Inspect for periorbital, peripheral, sacral, or dependent edema. Check for signs of dehydration, such as recent weight loss, poor skin turgor, and dry mucous membranes. Palpate for bladder distention, kidney enlargement, and tenderness at the costovertebral angle (the angle formed at each side of the body by the bottom rib and the vertebral column).

When examining a patient with suspected acute renal failure, remember that lethargy or confusion may be the first sign of this disorder. At the first sign of confusion or lethargy in any patient, obtain serum electrolyte levels.

## Diagnostic tests

As nitrogenous wastes accumulate in the blood, the BUN and serum creatinine levels rise progressively. The normal BUN-creatinine ratio is approximately 20:1. If the BUN level rises more rapidly than the creatinine level, suspect altered protein catabolism or volume depletion, not renal failure. If both BUN and creatinine levels rise but remain in a 20:1 ratio, suspect renal failure.

Creatinine clearance assesses GFR and helps estimate the number of functioning nephrons. The patient with acute renal failure may also have subnormal hemoglobin and hematocrit levels; altered electrolyte levels; below-normal blood pH, serum calcium, and serum albumin levels; and an elevated serum phosphorus level.

Urinalysis, essential in evaluating renal function, measures urine specific gravity, detects hematuria or proteinuria, and permits microscopic examination of casts and other particles. Specific gravity reflects urine osmolality and the kidneys' urine concentrating ability. Excessive secretion of cell casts and other particles in the urine (which may accompany proteinuria and hematuria) indicates renal disease. Other microscopic urine findings may include red blood cells (RBCs), white blood cells (WBCs), bacteria, and tubular epithelial cells.

Urine sodium and creatinine levels help classify renal failure. In acute prerenal failure, for instance, urine osmolality and creatinine concentration are below normal and the urine sodium level is high because the kidneys can't conserve water and sodium.

Kidney-ureter-bladder (KUB) X-rays identify kidney shape and size and reveal any calculi in the urinary tract. The kidneys appear normal or enlarged in ATN; smaller in most cases of chronic renal failure; and asymmetrical in unilateral renal artery disease, ureteral obstruction, and chronic pyelonephritis. Computed tomography may provide better visualization of an obstruction.

Renal ultrasonography safely and accurately reveals kidney size and any dilation of the renal pelvis or calyces. A radionuclide renal scan detects bilateral differences in renal perfusion (suggesting major renal disease) and differences in dye excretion (suggesting parenchymal disease or obstruction as a cause of acute renal failure). In ATN, this scan may show slow, diffuse and, eventually, dense radionuclide uptake.

Renal angiography, which may reveal obstruction or dysplasia of the renal artery, exacerbates renal failure and is ordered only for select patients. Digital subtraction angiography, a variation of this test, uses little dye and thus poses less risk for the patient with acute renal failure.

If all other tests are inconclusive, renal biopsy may be done to determine the cause of acute renal failure.

COMPLICATIONS

# Multisystem effects of renal failure

Renal failure causes functional changes that can affect all body systems, leading to the clinical findings listed here.

| Cardiovascular system | GI system | Genitourinary system | Hematologic system |
|---|---|---|---|
| • Accelerated progression of atherosclerosis | • Anorexia | • Amenorrhea (women) | • Anemia |
| • Cardiac tamponade | • Bleeding | • Impotence (men) | • Bleeding tendencies |
| • Congestive heart failure | • Nausea and vomiting | • Loss of libido | |
| • Hypertension | • Pancreatitis | | |
| • Pulmonary edema | • Peritonitis | | |
| • Uremic pericarditis | • Stomatitis | | |
| | • Uremic breath odor | | |

## Treatment

Goals of treatment are to correct the primary cause of acute renal failure, prevent further renal damage and complications, and maintain fluid and electrolyte balances, to decrease the work of the kidneys and permit tissue regeneration. Treatment varies with the phase of acute renal failure.

*Oliguric phase.* Serum electrolyte levels and the ECG must be monitored closely to detect fluid and electrolyte imbalances, such as potentially lethal hyperkalemia. To reduce serum potassium, the doctor may order ion exchange resins (sodium polystyrene sulfonate) by mouth or retention enema. Because the drug's action depends on its ability to move through the GI tract, it may be given with sorbitol, which induces GI water loss.

As a temporary emergency measure to treat hyperkalemia, the patient may receive I.V. glucose and insulin or calcium gluconate. Sodium bicarbonate reduces serum potassium by causing potassium to move into the cell, raising the plasma pH. To reduce an elevated serum phosphate level, the doctor may order aluminum hydroxide, a phosphate-binding agent.

A patient with a high and rising serum potassium level needs immediate peritoneal dialysis, hemodialysis, or continuous renal replacement via hemofiltration. Dialysis can keep a patient alive until the cause of renal failure is corrected. In some cases, it's used as a long-term treatment.

Both peritoneal dialysis and hemodialysis involve the movement or diffusion of particles through a semipermeable membrane from an area of high concentration to an area of low concentration. Pores in the membrane allow passage of electrolytes, BUN, and creatinine while preventing larger particles, such as blood cells and proteins, from passing through. Osmosis governs water movement through the membrane: Water moves from areas of lower osmolality to areas of higher osmolality.

In *peritoneal dialysis,* the patient's own peritoneal membrane acts as the semipermeable membrane, replacing the damaged kidney by way of a closed drainage system. Dialysate instilled into the peritoneal cavity at regular intervals draws wastes as well as excess fluid and electrolytes across the peritoneal membrane by osmosis and diffusion. The waste-laden dialysate is periodically drained into a collection bag and discarded.

| Integumentary system | Metabolic system | Musculoskeletal system | Neurologic system |
|---|---|---|---|
| • Dry skin and mucous membranes<br>• Ecchymoses and sub-cutaneous bruises<br>• Pale, sallow complexion<br>• Pruritus<br>• Uremic frost (pale, frostlike deposit of white crystals on skin) | • Fixed urine specific gravity<br>• Hyperkalemia<br>• Polyuria, nocturia<br>• Hyperphosphatemia<br>• Hypocalcemia, increased parathyroid hormone level<br>• Metabolic acidosis<br>• Sodium retention | • Bone pain and tenderness<br>• Metastatic calcifications<br>• Muscle weakness<br>• Osteomalacia<br>• Osteoporosis<br>• Spontaneous fractures | • Headache<br>• Neuropathy (muscle weakness, paresthesia, paralysis)<br>• Uremic encephalopathy (lethargy, coma, seizures, asterixis, and muscle twitching) |

In *hemodialysis,* a thin porous plate of cellophane acts as the semipermeable membrane. Blood and dialysate circulate on opposite sides of the membrane, permitting solute and fluid removal from the blood. Hemodialysis avoids many of the problems associated with peritoneal dialysis. However, it requires access to an artery or a vein, expensive and sophisticated equipment, and a specially trained staff member.

Each patient is assessed individually to determine if peritoneal dialysis or hemodialysis is the more appropriate treatment. (See *Comparing hemodialysis and peritoneal dialysis,* page 145.)

*Hemofiltration* has become a popular alternative to dialysis in patients with acute renal failure. To treat hypercatabolism, hyperkalemia, acidosis, or fluid overload, the doctor may order slow continuous ultrafiltration or continuous arteriovenous (AV) hemofiltration. In these procedures, the patient's blood pressure controls the rate of blood flow. Typically, the femoral artery and vein provide access.

Slow continuous ultrafiltration and continuous AV hemofiltration share the advantage of maintaining minimal extracorporeal volume (less than 100 ml). However, they may clear urine poorly. To enhance clearance, the doctor may opt for continuous AV hemodialysis, in which dialysate solution is infused in countercurrent flow to the blood flow circuit. (See *Continuous renal replacement therapy,* page 146.)

Other measures used to combat acute renal failure may include I.V. fluids and medications to restore adequate renal blood flow, along with mannitol, furosemide, or ethacrynic acid to initiate diuresis and minimize renal failure. If acute renal failure is caused by hypovolemia secondary to hypoproteinemia, albumin may be infused to correct the deficit.

During the oliguric phase, dietary protein intake must be limited to roughly 1 g/kg of body weight to minimize protein breakdown and prevent accumulation of waste products that result from protein metabolism, including creatinine and BUN.

***Diuretic phase.*** Blood chemistry evaluations continue to guide fluid and electrolyte replacement.

# Congestive heart failure in a patient with acute renal failure

Maintaining proper fluid and electrolyte balance poses a challenge in this patient. His fluid balance needs to be sufficient to perfuse the kidneys, yet restricted enough not to overload the pulmonary circulation and compromise the effective pumping of the cardiac muscle.

### Pathophysiology

The patient with congestive heart failure (CHF) can't maintain a cardiac output sufficient to meet his body's needs. Because of previous damage to the left ventricle, blood returning to the lungs can't be pumped into the systemic circulation. This leads to increased pressure in the lungs; if the pressure exceeds pulmonary capillary oncotic pressure, fluid leaks into the pulmonary interstitial spaces, causing pulmonary edema.

Right ventricular pressure rises from backflow of pressure in the pulmonary vasculature. Consequently, the right ventricle can't pump blood into the pulmonary system, and venous return to the right side of the heart decreases. As pressure continues to back up in the systemic circulation, the kidneys and other organs become congested with venous blood.

Decreased perfusion and congestion in the renal arteries damage the nephrons, resulting in acute tubular necrosis or cell death. Because the nephrons aren't functioning adequately, metabolic wastes and water accumulate in the serum and urine output drops dramatically.

### Risks

Treating the patient for CHF may worsen acute renal failure. Damage to the kidneys may result from further fluid overload and accumulation of waste products, or dehydration secondary to diuretic therapy. Acute renal failure may also progress to chronic renal failure, in which case the patient will require dialysis.

### Drug therapy

Morphine may be used to induce vasodilation and to decrease venous return, preload, myocardial oxygen consumption, and pain.

The doctor may prescribe diuretics to reduce blood volume and preload and increase urine output; digoxin to strengthen cardiac contractions; dopamine, dobutamine, or amrinone to support blood pressure and perfuse the kidneys; and nitrates to dilate the veins, reduce preload, and decrease cardiac and pulmonary congestion.

Captopril or hydralazine may be used to dilate arterial or resistant vessels and reduce afterload, thus increasing forward flow. Phosphate binders, sodium bicarbonate, or sodium polystyrene sulfonate help correct electrolyte imbalances.

### Interventions

- Administer medications as ordered.
- Restrict dietary sodium and potassium to relieve fluid retention.
- Closely monitor the patient's fluid intake and output, blood pressure, and heart rate. As ordered and indicated, limit fluids to 1,500 ml/day or less.
- Weigh the patient daily. A net gain of 2¼ lb (1 kg) may signal a fluid gain of 1 liter.
- Assess for peripheral edema, lung crackles, jugular vein distention, $S_3$, new murmurs or arrhythmias, bounding pulses, and ascites.
- Regularly check serum creatinine, blood urea nitrogen, and electrolyte levels.

*Recovery phase.* Treatment includes a high-calorie, high-protein diet and gradual return to normal activities.

## Nursing care
### Oliguric phase

- To meet daily calorie needs, provide high-carbohydrate feedings, which have a protein-sparing effect. Restrict fluids and foods rich in sodium, phosphorus, and potassium (such as bananas, citrus fruits and juices, and coffee). Limit potassium intake to 40 to 60 mEq/day and sodium to 2 g/day.
- If necessary, administer total parenteral nutrition to meet daily nutrient requirements and maintain fluid balance.
- When administering stored whole blood and certain I.V. medications (such as penicillin G),

# Comparing hemodialysis and peritoneal dialysis

| HEMODIALYSIS | PERITONEAL DIALYSIS |
|---|---|
| **Indications** | |
| • Hypercatabolism<br>• Hyperkalemia<br>• Severe respiratory insufficiency<br>• Large, draining abdominal wound<br>• Intra-abdominal adhesions<br>• Diffusely infected abdominal wall<br>• Critical volume excess | • Severe blood-clotting disorders<br>• Cardiovascular disease<br>• Exhausted veins<br>• Atherosclerosis |
| **Advantages** | |
| • Takes only 3 to 8 hours, making it useful in emergencies<br>• Effective; most patients need fewer than three treatments per week<br>• Removes low-molecular-weight substances from the patient's blood more efficiently than peritoneal dialysis<br>• Can be performed at home (after completion of a training program) | • Can be performed right away in most patients<br>• Low risk, with few life-threatening complications<br>• Less stressful to the cardiovascular system, causing no blood loss<br>• Less risky for patients with bleeding problems because they receive little or no heparin<br>• Rarely causes dialysis disequilibrium syndrome (caused by rapid fluid and electrolyte shifts) because it leads to more gradual shifts<br>• Removes middle-molecular-weight substances more efficiently than hemodialysis<br>• Simpler, requiring less complex equipment and little training<br>• Performed via peritoneal catheter instead of through the veins<br>• Costs less than hemodialysis<br>• Can be performed by the patient anywhere without assistance |
| **Disadvantages** | |
| • Requires expensive equipment and a specially trained nurse<br>• Requires venous access<br>• Necessitates larger heparin doses<br>• Confines patient to special treatment unit<br>• Can't be used for patients with shock or hypotension and must be used cautiously in infants, small children, and patients with cardiovascular disease<br>• May cause such complications as internal or external hemorrhage, septicemia, anemia, hepatitis, cardiovascular problems, air emboli, dialysis disequilibrium syndrome, muscle cramps, itching, pain, intracranial bleeding from excess heparin, nausea, vomiting, headache, and shunt or fistula problems | • Can take 10 to 72 hours to complete<br>• May need to be done more than three times per week<br>• Carries a high peritonitis risk<br>• May cause protein depletion and respiratory distress<br>• Can't be used for patients who've had recent abdominal surgery or extensive abdominal trauma<br>• May cause such complications as arrhythmias, hyperglycemia, pain, and constipation, as well as catheter site infection, inflammation, or leakage |
| **Procedure** | |
| • The doctor creates arteriovenous (AV) access—for example, with an AV shunt or a fistula.<br>• The patient requires heparin to prevent clotting.<br>• Blood moves from the patient's artery through the arterial lines and into the dialyzer, where diffusion, osmosis, and ultrafiltration occur. The dialysate draws wastes, excess fluid, and electrolytes across the semipermeable membrane.<br>• A synthetic semipermeable membrane separates the blood and dialysate compartments in the dialyzer and permits water and solutes to move to and from the blood.<br>• Dialyzer pressure adjustments increase or decrease the ultrafiltration rate as needed.<br>• Detoxified blood leaves the dialyzer, is filtered and monitored for bubbles, and returns to the patient through the venous lines. | • The doctor inserts a peritoneal catheter for access to the peritoneal cavity.<br>• Instilled into the peritoneal cavity, the dialysate draws wastes, excess fluids, and electrolytes across the peritoneal membrane by osmosis and diffusion at periodic intervals. The waste-laden dialysate drains into a collection bag.<br>• The patient's peritoneal membrane acts as the semipermeable membrane and transmits body wastes to the dialysate from the peritoneal fluid.<br>• Medications, such as antibiotics, potassium, or heparin, may be added to the dialysate as needed.<br>• The instill-dwell-drain cycle continues until waste and excess fluid removal is completed and the patient's acid-base and electrolyte balances become normal. |

# Continuous renal replacement therapy

Continuous renal replacement therapy (CRRT) is a safer alternative than hemodialysis or peritoneal dialysis in unstable patients with acute renal failure.

### What types of CRRT are available?

CRRT may involve continuous arteriovenous (AV) hemofiltration, slow continuous ultrafiltration, or continuous AV hemodialysis.

Continuous AV hemofiltration requires only arterial and venous vascular access, a hemofilter, and a fluid collection device. Replacement fluids are given to compensate for extracorporeal volume collected each hour. Continuous AV hemofiltration is the treatment of choice when moderate fluid and solute removal is indicated.

Replacement fluids aren't required in slow continuous ultrafiltration because of the slower filtration rate. Slow continuous ultrafiltration is the treatment of choice in patients with mild renal insufficiency.

Continuous AV hemodialysis is the preferred method for fluid overload and when the patient requires aggressive management of uremia.

### How is CRRT done?

CRRT is a continuous rather than intermittent process and may take 8 to 24 hours or more. It uses an extracorporeal system in which blood moves from the patient's arterial circulation through a filter and then is returned to the venous circulation. The hydrostatic pressure of the patient's blood pressure drives blood through the system and drives the filtrate across the membrane and out of the circulation.

The CRRT membrane is highly permeable, so more fluid can be removed with a smaller pressure gradient. The amount of fluid that can be removed depends on the degree of volume overload and the patient's blood pressure. The higher the arterial pressure, the higher the pressure gradient across the filter and the more rapid the filtration.

### When is CRRT used?

• To treat patients in unstable condition (gradual fluid removal is safer than the rapid removal of dialysis).
• To reduce the risk of dialysis disequilibrium syndrome (for example, in patients with congestive heart failure or cardiovascular compromise).
• To allow more liberal nutrient administration with a lower risk of azotemia and fluid overload

remember that they contain a high concentration of potassium. Monitor the patient receiving I.V. medications and whole blood carefully for signs of hyperkalemia, such as nausea, vomiting, and diarrhea. ECG changes include bradycardia and prolonged QRS intervals.
• Monitor arterial blood gas values for severe acidosis. If acidosis develops, the patient may require mechanical ventilation, sodium bicarbonate therapy, or dialysis.
• Regularly monitor the patient's pulse, blood pressure, temperature, respirations, and fluid intake and output. Record daily weight, CVP readings, and serum and urine electrolyte levels to help determine fluid replacement needs. Be sure to include parenteral and oral intake as well as output from perspiration, urine, wound drainage, gastric drainage, and stools.
• Expect to replace fluids at about 10 ml/kg of body weight/24 hours (using dextrose 5% to 50% in water) to compensate for insensible fluid losses. If the patient has a fever, add fluid at 1 ml/kg of body weight over the basic amount for each degree Celsius of fever, as ordered.
• To help detect hyperkalemia, monitor the ECG for peaked T waves.
• Monitor the patient closely for signs of altered fluid volume by assessing intake and output and daily weight. Stay alert for edema, jugular vein distention, and abnormal heart and breath sounds.
• If needed, enforce bed rest to conserve the patient's energy and lower his metabolic rate

uring the most severe stage of acute renal ilure. Assist with activities of daily living as eeded.

**ialysis.** If your patient needs dialysis, continue ɔ assess his fluid and electrolyte status osely.
 Consult the doctor and dietitian regarding et and use of nutritional supplements. If the atient is undergoing hemodialysis, encourage m to eat high-calorie foods, such as butter, ɔney, and hard candy.
 If the patient is undergoing peritoneal dialysis, ᴉake sure his intake consists mainly of high- rotein foods (meats, fish, fowl, and eggs). his patient will absorb extra calories from glu- ɔse in the peritoneal dialysate, and thus won't eed an increased caloric intake.
 Assess the patient's dialysis or hemofiltration te regularly for adequate perfusion and signs f infection. At a hemodialysis site, expect a alpable thrill, a bruit on auscultation, and ᴧarmth of the shunt tubing or AV fistula site. Never take a blood pressure reading on the de of the body with an AV shunt.
 Continue to assess the patient's level of con- ɔiousness frequently. Stay alert for signs of di- ɣsis disequilibrium syndrome (headache, ausea, vomiting, restlessness, stupor, or ɔma), caused by rapid fluid and electrolyte ᴉifts.

**iuretic phase**
 To evaluate the patient's fluid status, monitor is daily weight, intake and output, and heart ιte. Check orthostatic blood pressure. Report ᴧassive diuresis (over 3,000 ml/day), which an lead to severe electrolyte imbalances.
 Expect to replace three-fourths of the pre- ᴉous day's fluids and electrolytes lost through rination, vomiting, or hemorrhage.
 Be aware that the patient is at risk for fluid nd electrolyte imbalances, infection, GI bleed- ιg, and respiratory failure during diuresis. ᴧonitor his clinical status and laboratory results ᴇgularly.

# Acute pyelonephritis

Also called acute infective tubulointerstitial ne- phritis, acute pyelonephritis is a sudden inflam- mation of one or both kidneys caused by bacterial invasion. It primarily affects the inter- stitial area and the renal pelvis and, less often, the renal tubules. With treatment and contin- ued follow-up care, the prognosis is good and extensive permanent damage is unlikely.

Pyelonephritis affects more women than men — probably because a woman's shorter urethra and the proximity of the urinary me- atus to the vagina and rectum allow bacteria to reach the bladder more easily. Women also lack the antibacterial prostatic secretions that men produce. Sexual activity in women in- creases the risk of bacterial contamination of the urinary system.

### Causes
Acute pyelonephritis results from bacterial con- tamination via the urethra, from catheteriza- tion, or from cystoscopy. The infecting bacteria are usually the normal intestinal and fecal flora that grow readily in urine — *Escherichia coli*, *Proteus*, *Pseudomonas*, *Staphylococcus aureus*, and *Streptococcus faecalis* (enterococcus).

Pregnancy, diabetes mellitus, and chronic renal calculi predispose a person to acute py- elonephritis. About 5% of pregnant women develop asymptomatic bacteriuria; if untreated, about 40% of these women develop pyelone- phritis.

For patients with diabetes mellitus, auto- nomic neuropathy and subsequent bladder atony promote urinary stasis and increase the risk for acute pyelonephritis. Similarly, in pa- tients with spinal cord injury, multiple sclerosis, and tabes dorsalis, neurogenic bladder causes incomplete emptying and urinary stasis. The risk of acute pyelonephritis also rises with com- promised renal function and glycosuria, both of which may support bacterial growth in the urine.

Other causes of acute pyelonephritis in- clude urinary obstruction from tumors, stric- tures, or benign prostatic hyperplasia; urologic surgery; and hematogenic infection (such as septicemia and endocarditis).

### Pathophysiology
The infection spreads from the bladder to the ureters and then to the kidneys — typically from urine reflux at the junction of the ureter and bladder (vesicoureteral reflux). An inflammatory process begins with mobilization of WBCs, leading to local edema. Scar tissue then forms, reducing tubular reabsorption and secretion, which in turn alters renal function. Bacteria refluxed to intrarenal tissues may create colonies of infection within 24 to 48 hours.

### Complications
Acute pyelonephritis may lead to arteriosclerosis, calculus formation, further renal damage, renal abscess with possible metastasis to other organs, and septic shock. In some patients, pyelonephritis becomes chronic.

Emphysematous pyelonephritis also may occur. In this condition, common in patients with diabetes mellitus and ureteral obstruction, gas forms in the collecting system. The gas originates from gas-producing bacteria, such as *E. coli* or *Pseudomonas.*

## Assessment
### Signs and symptoms
Symptoms may develop rapidly over a few hours or perhaps over a few days. The patient with acute pyelonephritis appears acutely ill and typically complains of intense and constant pain over one or both kidneys that increases on palpation.

Urinary symptoms include urgency, frequency, burning or pain on urination, nocturia, and hematuria (usually microscopic but possibly gross). Urine may appear cloudy and smell like fish or ammonia.

Other signs and symptoms include a temperature of 102° F (38.9° C) or higher, shaking chills, anorexia, and general fatigue. Although symptoms may disappear within days even without treatment, residual bacterial infection is likely and may cause recurring symptoms.

### Diagnostic tests
Diagnosis requires urinalysis as well as culture and sensitivity tests. Typical findings include:
• pyuria; urine sediment reveals leukocytes singly, in clumps, and in casts, possibly with a few RBCs.
• significant bacteriuria; urine culture shows more than 100,000 organisms/mm³. A Gram stain may be done to identify gram-positive or gram-negative organisms.
• low specific gravity and osmolality, from a transient decrease in urine concentrating ability
• proteinuria, glycosuria, and ketonuria (rare).

Blood tests also help diagnose acute pyelonephritis. A complete blood count usually shows an elevated WBC count (up to 40,000/mm³) and an increased neutrophil count. The erythrocyte sedimentation rate is elevated. Blood cultures may be drawn to determine if the causative organism has reached the bloodstream.

KUB X-rays and excretory urography may reveal calculi, tumors, or cysts in the kidneys or urinary outlets. For some patients, a cystourethrogram may be indicated, at least for the first pyelonephritis episode. A gallium scan may help identify active pyelonephritis or abscesses in the perinephric region of the kidneys.

## Treatment
### Drug therapy
Treatment centers on antibiotic therapy appropriate to the specific infecting organism, as identified by urine culture and sensitivity tests. For example, an enterococcal infection calls for ampicillin, penicillin G, or vancomycin. *Staphylococcus* requires penicillin G or, if the bacterium is resistant, a semisynthetic penicillin (such as nafcillin) or a cephalosporin. Infection by *E. coli* may be treated with sulfisoxazole, nalidixic acid, or nitrofurantoin; *Proteus,* with ampicillin, sulfisoxazole, nalidixic acid, or a cephalosporin; and *Pseudomonas,* with gentamicin, tobramycin, or carbenicillin.

If the infecting organism can't be identified, therapy usually consists of a broad-spectrum antibiotic, such as ampicillin or cephalexin. Antibiotics must be used cautiously in elderly patients because of the combined effects of aging and pyelonephritis on renal function. Pregnant patients also require cautious antibiotic therapy; in these patients, urinary analgesics, such as phenazopyridine, can help relieve pain.

Symptoms usually dissipate after several days of antibiotic therapy. Although the patient's urine typically becomes sterile within 48 to 72 hours, the course of therapy ranges from 10 to 14 days. Follow-up measures include reculturing urine 1 week after drug therapy ends and then periodically for the next year to detect residual or recurring infections.

A patient with an uncomplicated infection usually responds well to therapy and avoids reinfection. Extensive follow-up care is indicated for the patient at risk for recurring urinary tract and kidney infection — for example, one with a long-term indwelling urinary catheter or one on maintenance antibiotic therapy.

### Surgery

If infection results from obstruction or vesicoureteral reflux, antibiotics may be less effective and surgery may be necessary to relieve the obstruction or correct the anomaly. Surgery may involve pyelolithotomy, nephrectomy, ureteroplasty, or ureteral reimplantation.

In *pyelolithotomy,* the surgeon removes large calculi in the renal pelvis that are contributing to blocked urine flow and subsequent infection. However, two noninvasive techniques that crush calculi — extracorporeal shock wave lithotripsy (ESWL) and percutaneous ultrasonic pyelolithotomy — have decreased the frequency of surgical calculus removal.

*Nephrectomy,* removal of the entire kidney, is reserved for patients whose infections fail to respond to all other treatments. *Ureteroplasty* is repair of the ureter.

In *ureteral reimplantation,* the ureter is reimplanted through another site in the posterior bladder wall. This procedure may be done in an effort to preserve renal function and eliminate infection in patients with incompetent ureterovesical valve closure.

### Nursing care

• Promptly collect the necessary specimens for urinalysis and culture and sensitivity tests.

• Begin antibiotic therapy as soon as it's ordered. Monitor peak and trough levels of nephrotoxic agents such as gentamicin, vancomycin, tobramycin, and tetracycline.
• Administer analgesics and other medications as needed and ordered; for example, give narcotics to relieve severe pain, antispasmodics to help prevent pain, or phenazopyridine to anesthetize the urinary tract.
• Use strict sterile technique when inserting a urethral catheter. Make sure you keep the catheter bag and tubing below bladder level. Clean the catheter with soap, water, or povidone-iodine at least twice daily.
• Monitor the patient's vital signs, and carefully record his intake and output.
• To evaluate renal function, monitor laboratory results, such as BUN, creatinine, and serum electrolyte levels.

### Surgical care

• If ordered, start an I.V. line before surgery, administer antibiotics, and give a preoperative sedative.
• Manage the patient's pain and monitor for postoperative complications such as decreased mobility and anesthetic effects.
• Confirm that catheters, drains, and dressings are secure and correctly in place. Assess the amount and color of any drainage.
• Monitor vital signs and document intake and output very closely during the first 8 to 12 hours after surgery.

### Continuing care

• Encourage fluid intake of up to 3,500 ml/day (unless contraindicated by the patient's renal or cardiovascular status).
• Acidify the patient's urine by providing an acid-ash diet — for example, one that includes meats, fish, fowl, whole grains, cranberries, plums, and prunes.
• Assist the patient with activities of daily living as needed. Encourage self-care when she's ready, and encourage her to ambulate as tolerated and ordered.

### Patient teaching

• Instruct the patient to complete the prescribed antibiotic regimen (usually 10 to 14 days).

• Tell her to avoid large doses of potentially nephrotoxic agents, such as aminoglycosides, cephalosporins, vancomycin, and nonsteroidal anti-inflammatory drugs (such as aspirin and ibuprofen); radiographic testing using contrast dyes; and exposure to heavy metals and organic solvents.

• Make sure the patient knows the signs and symptoms of urinary tract infection (UTI), such as urinary burning, urgency, frequency, and hematuria. Emphasize the need to seek prompt treatment if these occur.

# Renal calculi

Renal calculi are stones in the urinary tract — in particular, those that form in the bladder or pass through the lower urinary tract. Stones that form in the renal parenchyma cause a condition called *nephrolithiasis;* those that form in the ureter cause *ureterolithiasis.*

Calculi formation follows precipitation of substances normally soluble in urine, such as calcium oxalate, calcium phosphate, magnesium ammonium phosphate, urate, and cystine. Renal calculi vary in size and number. (See *Comparing types of renal calculi,* opposite, and *Removing renal and ureteral calculi,* pages 152 and 153.)

Approximately 500,000 Americans suffer from episodes of renal calculi formation yearly, and up to 12 million will develop renal calculi in their lifetimes. The risk of calculus formation peaks between ages 30 and 50. Calculi rarely form in children. However, in cystinuria, they begin to form shortly after puberty.

## Causes
Renal specialists disagree about why calculi form but concur on the following causative factors:

• *Fluid intake.* The lower the fluid intake, the greater the concentration of calculus-forming substances in the urine.

• *Infection.* By changing the urine pH, infection creates an environment that promotes calculi formation. Blood clots, clumps of dead tissue, and bacteria in infected urine may serve as nu-

clei for the formation of magnesium ammonium phosphate or calcium calculi.

• *Diet.* A diet high in purines (uric acid), oxalate, calcium, phosphate, and other substances that can be excreted into the urine may promote calculus formation.

• *Immobility and inactivity.* By promoting urinary stasis, immobility and inactivity allow calculus-forming substances to collect.

• *Obstruction.* This condition causes urinary stasis, allowing calculus-forming substances to aggregate. Obstruction also promotes inflammation and infection, compounding the problem.

• *Foreign body.* Calculi can grow on a foreign body, such as an indwelling urinary catheter.

• *Metabolic factors.* Hyperparathyroidism, renal tubular acidosis, elevated uric acid levels (usually with gout), defective oxalate metabolism, genetically defective cystine metabolism, excessive vitamin D or calcium intake, sarcoidosis, milk-alkali syndrome, Cushing's disease, and cancer can also create an environment conducive to calculus formation.

## Pathophysiology
Theories about renal calculi formation abound. According to one theory, urine supersaturation with a crystallizing salt triggers precipitation and calculus formation; crystals continue to form as long as supersaturation lasts.

However, some people with supersaturated urine never develop calculi. This leads some experts to speculate that calculus inhibitors in the urine — citrate, peptides, pyrophosphate, magnesium, and zinc — normally guard against calculus formation. Presumably, susceptible people lack these inhibitors.

## Complications
Sudden and complete obstruction by a calculus impairs renal function. Intermittent or partial obstruction dilates the calyces and renal pelvis. Ureteral obstruction causes hypertrophy of the ureteral muscle; if the obstruction remains, ureteral scarring decreases the muscle's peristaltic activity.

By causing urinary stasis, obstructive calculi allow infections to persist. Struvite calculi, the aftermath of UTIs, harbor bacteria. Antibiotics may clear the infection but don't effectively

# Comparing types of renal calculi

| TYPE | DESCRIPTION | POSSIBLE CAUSES | INTERVENTIONS |
|---|---|---|---|
| Calcium (oxalate, phosphate, or mixture) | • Account for two-thirds of calculi<br>• Small, rough, and hard<br>• Shaped like needles or a staghorn<br>• Color varies from gray to white | • Hypercalciuria<br>• Hyperuricosuria<br>• Hyperoxaluria<br>• Hyperparathyroidism | • Force fluids.<br>• Restrict calcium and oxalate intake.<br>• Give hydrochlorothiazide, as ordered.<br>• Prepare patient for parathyroid gland removal. |
| Struvite (magnesium ammonium phosphate) | • Second most common calculus type<br>• Crumble easily<br>• Shaped like a staghorn<br>• Yellow | • Infection by microbes that split urea | • Force fluids.<br>• Decrease urine pH.<br>• Give antibiotics as ordered. |
| Uric acid | • Small and hard<br>• Dye enhancement needed for X-ray visualization<br>• Color varies from yellow to red | • Gout<br>• High uric acid levels caused by chronic diarrhea or low fluid intake | • Force fluids.<br>• Restrict purines.<br>• Give sodium citrate or sodium and potassium bicarbonate, as ordered, to alkalinize urine.<br>• Give allopurinol, as ordered, to reduce urine uric acid level. |
| Cystine | • Small calculi may clump into staghorn shape<br>• Smooth and waxy | • Cystine-containing crystals in urine | • Force fluids.<br>• Give penicillamine and pyridoxine, as ordered.<br>• Give sodium bicarbonate, as ordered, to increase urine pH. |
| Triamterene | • A recently recognized calculus type | • Triamterene ingestion | • Withhold triamterene from patients at risk for developing calculi. |

penetrate the calculi. As a result, struvite calculi allow UTIs to become chronic.

A calculus also can cause local tissue irritation and inflammation. Tissue that contacts the calculus may become ulcerated or fibrotic. A calculus that erodes through the kidney or causes a kidney abscess to rupture may result in perirenal abscess. Finally, renal calculi may contribute to the development of renal pelvic cancer.

## Assessment
### Signs and symptoms
A thorough patient history may provide the first clue to urinary calculi. Although findings vary with the size, location, and cause of the calculi, severe pain in the lower back is a key symptom.

If the patient reports such pain, ask for a detailed description of its pattern and quality. His reply may provide telling evidence of his condition. For example, violent hyperperistalsis, spasms, and colic pain suggest sudden distention of the renal pelvis or ureter caused by calculus obstruction. Typically, colic begins suddenly, progresses rapidly, and peaks over a 30-minute period. At its peak, it's sharp, stabbing, intense, and unaffected by position changes. Pain may persist until the calculus stops moving or an analgesic takes effect. In contrast, dull renal pain suggests pressure on the renal parenchyma and capsule from urine retention.

Pain at the costovertebral angle or flank pain between the last rib and iliac crest suggests renal or upper ureteral calculi. Other signs and symptoms of renal calculi include:
• nausea and vomiting (from a reflex response

(Text continues on page 154.)

# Removing renal and ureteral calculi

Renal or ureteral calculi can be removed through endoscopy, surgery, and extracorporeal shock wave lithotripsy (ESWL).

### Endoscopy
*Percutaneous nephrolithotomy* removes renal or upper ureteral calculi. Using fluoroscopy, the doctor inserts a nephroscope through the renal parenchyma. Then he removes the calculi with a basket catheter.

*Endoscopic stone manipulation,* shown in the illustration below, removes small calculi (less than 1 cm in diameter) located in the lower third of the ureter. Using a cystoscope, the doctor inserts a special loop or basket catheter up the ureter to capture and remove the calculus.

*Ureteroscopy* using a ureteroscope may allow visualization and removal of a calculus in the middle third of the ureter. *Ureteral probes* or *electrohydraulic shock waves* fragment and remove large calculi. If the doctor can't remove a calculus, he may leave a loop or ureteral catheter in place to dilate the ureter and permit later calculus manipulation. He may also leave a ureteral catheter in place after the procedure to prevent obstruction from edema.

Also called percutaneous nephrolithotripsy, *percutaneous ultrasonic lithotripsy,* shown below, removes renal or upper ureteral calculi. In this procedure, the doctor uses an electrohydraulic or ultrasonic probe to fragment a larger calculus with electrical or ultrasonic energy. He first locates the calculus with a fiber-optic light and a magnifying lens, then removes larger fragments with a basket catheter and smaller pieces with suction created by a continuous irrigation flow through the sheath. Afterward, he places a catheter in the tract to drain the kidney and control bleeding—a major complication.

### Surgery
*Pyelolithotomy* involves incising the renal pelvis to remove calculi confined to the renal pelvis or ureteropelvic junction. With *extended pyelolithotomy,* the surgeon makes a longer incision to expose more of the collecting system, which may be necessary if the calculus is trapped or extends into the calyx. With *coagulum pyelolithotomy,* the surgeon injects calcium chloride, cryoprecipitate, and thrombin into the collecting system. These substances clot and trap calculi, which the surgeon then removes along with the clots.

### Endoscopic stone manipulation

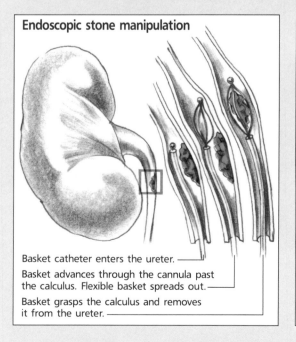

Basket catheter enters the ureter.
Basket advances through the cannula past the calculus. Flexible basket spreads out.
Basket grasps the calculus and removes it from the ureter.

### Percutaneous ultrasonic lithotripsy

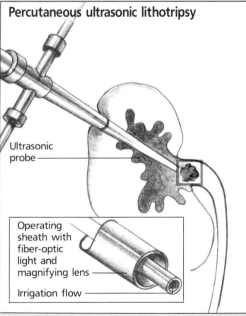

Ultrasonic probe
Operating sheath with fiber-optic light and magnifying lens
Irrigation flow

*Nephrolithotomy,* shown below, involves incising the renal parenchyma to reach staghorn calculi and calculi too tightly embedded to be removed by pyelolithotomy. A ureteral catheter is placed into the ureter to make sure no other stones have migrated down the ureter. A nephrostomy tube may be placed to drain urine temporarily while the kidney tissue damaged by calculi heals. A drain may be placed at the level of the incision.

In *ureterolithotomy,* the surgeon makes an incision in the ureter to reach calculi larger than 1 cm embedded in the ureter. He also may use this procedure to remove calculi not removable by ureteroscopy. Most ureteral calculi require a flank incision, but distal ureteral calculi may call for an oblique incision in the lower abdominal quadrant.

*Nephrectomy* (kidney removal) may be performed when one kidney is severely damaged or nonfunctional but the other kidney is functioning. In *partial nephrectomy,* the doctor removes part of the kidney (usually the lower pole) in a patient with severe obstruction and permanent kidney damage. Unless removed, the damaged region may produce more calculi.

## ESWL

*ESWL,* shown below, uses spark-induced shock waves to shatter renal or upper ureteral calculi identified by fluoroscopy. During this procedure, the patient lies in a tank of water. Electrodes on the bottom of the tank emit 500 to 1,500 shock waves directed at the calculi over 30 to 60 minutes. An X-ray image intensifier with two monitors is used to visualize the calculus at the focal point of the shock wave. To prevent arrhythmias, the shock waves are synchronized with the patient's R waves, as monitored by an electrocardiogram.

The pulverized calculi should pass in the patient's urine within a few days.

ESWL can't be used for patients with calculi that can't be visualized by fluoroscopy, for example, those located below the pelvic brim. For calculi resting below the pelvic brim, the doctor may use endoscopy to push them back into a region accessible by ESWL. ESWL is also not recommended for patients with obstruction or infection.

## Nephrolithotomy

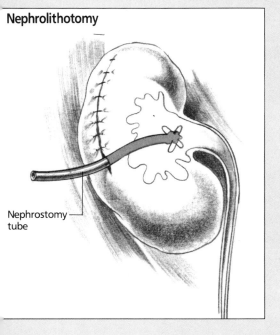

Nephrostomy tube

## ESWL

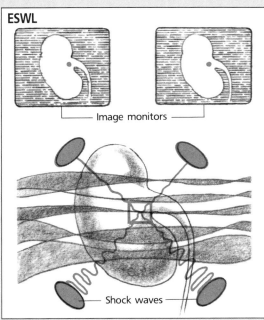

Image monitors

Shock waves

between the autonomic and sensory nerve pathways of the urinary and GI systems)
• abdominal distention (from peritoneal inflammation)
• persistent or intermittent hematuria (from local irritation)
• bladder discomfort or burning on urination (from calculi near the ureterovesical junction, which cause inflammation of the bladder wall around the ureteral orifice)
• urinary frequency or urgency (from bladder inflammation)
• anuria (rare, from bilateral obstruction or, in a patient with one kidney, from unilateral obstruction).

### Diagnostic tests

Various tests help confirm and locate suspected calculi. Urinalysis may reveal either gross or microscopic hematuria, suggesting calculus abrasion of the urinary tract mucosa. A significant number of WBCs indicates infection, suggesting struvite calculi. During active calculus formation, crystals in the urine may reveal which type of calculus is present. Urine pH also may indicate the calculus type or may help evaluate the therapeutic effectiveness of urine acidification or alkalinization. Urine culture and sensitivity tests can provide further evidence of an active infection.

The doctor may order a 24-hour urine study for creatinine clearance. In impaired renal function, serum creatinine and BUN levels are elevated.

KUB and oblique-angle abdominal X-rays help identify calculi in the urinary tract. Excretory urography evaluates the structure and excretory function of the kidneys, ureter, and bladder; failure of the contrast medium to become promptly visible in the collection system indicates an obstruction. If the patient is allergic to the contrast medium used in this test, retrograde pyelography or tomography may be used to locate the calculi.

Ultrasonography may help identify obstructive changes, such as hydronephrosis, and detect larger calculi. Noninvasive and nontoxic, ultrasonography is useful for pregnant women and patients with anuria or chronic renal failure.

## Treatment

Approximately 90% of renal calculi measure less than 5 mm in diameter. Thus, treatment usually involves encouraging natural calculi passage, such as through vigorous hydration. Other measures include antimicrobial agents to combat infection, and I.V. analgesics (such as morphine or meperidine) and antispasmodic agents (such as oxybutynin and propantheline) to relieve pain.

Diuretics may be given to prevent stasis and thus avoid further calculus formation (thiazides promote calcium excretion into the urine). Sodium bicarbonate may be administered orally, I.V., or in combination to dissolve uric acid calculi. A combination of sodium bicarbonate and oral penicillamine may be used to dissolve cystine calculi.

Irrigation of the urinary system may be a primary treatment or it may be done postoperatively to dissolve residual stone fragments or prevent calculi recurrence. Alkalinizing solutions may be given via a ureteral catheter or nephrostomy tube. A patient with calcium phosphate or struvite calculi may undergo renal pelvis irrigation with hemiacidrin.

### Surgery

Calculi too large for natural passage may require surgical removal. About half of patients with renal calculi must have surgery to remove the calculi and relieve pain, prevent infection, or restore renal function.

Common surgical procedures include manipulation with catheters or retrieval instruments inserted via cystoscope (for ureteral calculi) and ultrasonic fragmentation and endoscopic removal (for ureteral or renal pelvis calculi).

Recent advances have dramatically altered surgical options. New procedures incorporate nephroscopy, ureteroscopy, or ESWL to extract or crush and remove calculi. While not without risks, these treatments have many advantages over traditional surgery. For instance, they usually shorten healing time and hospital stays and cause less tissue damage, thus minimizing scarring. Potential complications include infection, bleeding, kidney and ureteral perforation,

ureteral tearing or fistula, and bowel or peritoneal injury.

## Nursing care

During calculi passage, assess the patient's
pain and administer analgesics generously, as
ordered.

Encourage the patient to walk, if possible, to
promote spontaneous calculi passage.

Administer I.V. fluids, as ordered, and encourage abundant oral fluid intake.

Maintain total urine output at 3 to 4 liters/
day of dilute, colorless urine. Provide fruit
juices, such as cranberry juice, if needed, to
help acidify the urine.

Strain all urine, and carefully measure and record fluid intake and output.

### Surgical care

If ordered, establish I.V. access, administer antibiotics, and give the preoperative sedative.

After surgery, the patient will probably have
an indwelling urinary catheter or a nephrostomy tube.

Be sure to identify the catheter origin site
(nephrostomy, ureteral, suprapubic, or urethral).
Some patients may have more than one catheter, so be sure to determine which portion of
the urinary tract each appliance drains. Monitor
closely for catheter patency, and inspect the
catheter drainage system for kinks and leaks.

Notify the doctor if you suspect catheter obstruction.

Anticipate drain care if the patient underwent
ureterolithotomy, pyelolithotomy, or nephrolithotomy. After nephrectomy, he probably won't
have a drain unless an infection develops.

During the early postoperative period, urine
leakage may increase wound drainage. Be sure
to change the dressing frequently and check
for skin changes. Excessive drainage may call
for placing an ostomy appliance over the drain
to contain leaking fluid.

Keep accurate fluid intake and output records.
Expect urine output to exceed 50 ml/hour; for
adults, the minimum acceptable rate is 30 ml/
hour. Check and document urine color, describing any clots.

Explain all care procedures to the patient, including the reason for the catheter. Advise him
that his urine may be bloody at first.

• Assess the patient frequently for pain. If he
has an indwelling or urethral catheter, he may
report bladder spasms. The patient with a nephrostomy tube may have renal pain on tube
manipulation. Manage pain with oral, I.M., or
I.V. analgesics, as ordered.

• If your patient underwent ESWL, encourage
him to walk because movement promotes passage of calculi fragments. Some patients have
pain when passing calculi fragments after this
procedure. Suspect colic from ureteral obstruction if an oral analgesic (such as acetaminophen or codeine) doesn't relieve the pain, or if
the patient reports nausea and vomiting beyond the immediate postanesthesia phase.

• Monitor vital signs regularly, and stay alert for
signs and symptoms of infection, such as a rising fever or chills. Administer antibiotics, as
needed and ordered.

### Continuing care

Because calculi tend to recur and can impair
renal function, most patients must make permanent changes in life-style and habits.

• Advise the patient with a hyperuricemic condition to reduce meat consumption. Meat is
rich in purine and contributes to uric acid production.

• If your patient has hypercalciuria, instruct him
to limit his dietary calcium intake.

• Advise the patient to increase his fluid intake
and to exercise regularly to help keep urine
and tiny calculi moving.

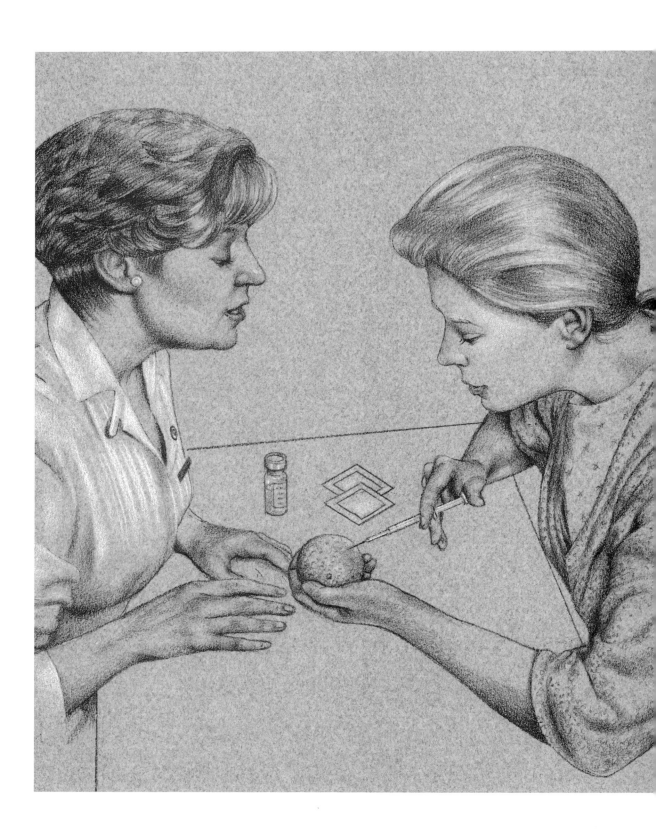

# Endocrine and metabolic disorders

The endocrine system consists of three major components: glands, hormones, and receptors. Cell metabolism, another key bodily component, determines the final use of nutrients by the body. Since hormones directly or indirectly affect every cell in the human body, and metabolism helps the body maintain life functions, an endocrine or metabolic disorder will likely affect all of your patient's body systems.

Initial assessment of an endocrine or metabolic disorder poses a particular challenge: Your patient won't have an obvious traumatic injury, and he's unlikely to exhibit clear-cut manifestations of cardiovascular, respiratory, neurologic, GI, or other body system disorders. Instead, his signs and symptoms may suggest a systemic illness or may appear in seemingly paradoxical combinations. And once you begin to assess an endocrine problem, you're faced with another dilemma—various endocrine emergencies share many of the same characteristics.

To provide competent care, you must be

able to recognize subtle clues indicating an endocrine or metabolic disorder. Otherwise, the disorder may elude detection until it's well advanced, complicating treatment, and seriously compromising or delaying your patient's recovery.

This chapter provides the essential information you'll need to accurately and swiftly assess, treat, and care for your patient. It discusses two of the most common endocrine and metabolic disorders you'll encounter when caring for the acutely ill patient — diabetes mellitus and potassium imbalances.

First, the chapter defines both of these disorders, describes their causes and underlying pathophysiology, and reviews potential complications. Then it discusses assessment findings obtained from the health history, the physical examination, and diagnostic studies. After describing current medical treatment, including implantable, computer-regulated insulin pumps, sulfonylurea drugs, and surgery, the chapter presents all aspects of the nursing care your patient will need — the immediate measures you must take as well as the continuing care you must provide to ensure his well-being, such as intrasite rotation of insulin injections, exercising the diabetic patient, and recognizing signs and symptoms of hypokalemia and hyperkalemia.

# Diabetes mellitus

A chronic disease of absolute or relative insulin deficiency or resistance, diabetes mellitus is characterized by disturbances in carbohydrate, protein, and fat metabolism.

The National Diabetes Data Group classifies diabetes mellitus as:
• Type I, or insulin-dependent diabetes mellitus
• Type II, or non-insulin-dependent diabetes mellitus (further subdivided into obese and nonobese diabetes)
• other types of diabetes mellitus (associated with certain conditions or syndromes).

## Causes
Type I diabetes is caused by destruction of pancreatic beta cells. By the time the disease becomes apparent, 80% of beta cells have been destroyed. Destruction probably represents an autoimmune process, although details remain obscure. The disease is strongly linked to human leukocyte antigens (HLAs) DR3 and DR4 as well as to more specific HLA loci, such as DQ3.2. It may be also be linked to certain viral infections.

Type II diabetes, the most common diabetes form, presumably arises from abnormal insulin secretion secondary to beta cell dysfunction, coupled with hepatic and peripheral resistance to insulin action. However, as with Type I diabetes, its precise cause hasn't been fully explained. Hereditary factors probably play a major role in its development. In the obese form of Type II diabetes (which accounts for approximately 75% of Type II diabetes cases), obesity may help a genetic predisposition express itself.

Causes of other types of diabetes include pancreatic disease, particularly chronic pancreatitis in alcoholics; hormonal abnormalities, such as pheochromocytoma, acromegaly, and Cushing's syndrome; genetic syndromes, such as lipodystrophies, myotonic dystrophy, and ataxia-telangiectasia; certain drugs, including thiazide diuretics, adrenal corticosteroids, and oral contraceptives; and severe physiologic stress, for example, from severe burns, acute myocardial infarction, and other life-threatening conditions (such as stress hyperglycemia). Some types of diabetes may disappear when the underlying cause is corrected.

## Pathophysiology
In Type I diabetes, experts believe genetic susceptibility is followed by an environmental stimulus — for example, a virus or other foreign antigen. This antigen provokes a normal immune response in the body, but if it's similar in chemistry and configuration to the beta cell, it also stimulates an autoimmune attack against these cells. The attack causes insulitis, an inflammatory response in the pancreas.

In insulitis, the islets of Langerhans are infiltrated with activated T lymphocytes and the immune system mistakes beta cells for foreign substances. Cytotoxic antibodies develop and act in concert with cell-mediated immune mechanisms to destroy beta cells. When more than 90% of the beta cells have been destroyed, hyperglycemia becomes manifest.

Researchers are less certain about the pathophysiology of Type II diabetes. It's unknown how the two physiologic defects linked with Type II diabetes — abnormal insulin secretion and insulin resistance at the hepatic and peripheral (primarily fat and muscle) levels — develop. One theory holds that genetic susceptibility may be the underlying cause of the beta cell dysfunction responsible for abnormal insulin secretion, whereas both genetic susceptibility and obesity may cause insulin resistance.

The pathophysiology of other types of diabetes varies. Pancreatic disease causes beta cell destruction. Hormonal abnormalities may increase levels of hormones that raise blood glucose levels, such as cortisol, epinephrine, glucagon, and human growth hormone. Impaired glucose tolerance typically is linked to genetic syndromes. Many drugs are known to antagonize the effects of insulin or to increase the glucose level directly. In stress hyperglycemia, endogenous glucagon and epinephrine are released.

***Disease progression.*** All forms of diabetes progress the same way regardless of the underlying cause. Insulin transports glucose into cells for use as energy and for storage as glycogen. It also stimulates protein synthesis and free fatty acid (FFA) storage in adipose tissue. Insulin deficiency compromises body tissues' access to essential nutrients for fuel and storage.

Glucose, the body's major energy source, enters the bloodstream via digestion of dietary carbohydrates or through gluconeogenesis and glycogenolysis. It is then actively transported to cells that need energy. However, most cells can't use glucose without insulin, which causes glucose transport through cell membranes to increase. If insulin isn't available, glucose remains trapped in the blood; eventually, some spills into the urine. The resulting hyperglyce-

mia causes osmotic diuresis, leading to polyuria, dehydration, and subsequent polydipsia, and electrolyte imbalances. Bicarbonate excretion also increases. If osmotic diuresis becomes severe (as from absolute insulin deficiency in Type I diabetes), cardiac output drops, causing hypotension and circulatory collapse.

Meanwhile, glucose-starved cells lack the energy to function. The body tries to compensate by using protein as an alternate fuel, breaking it down into amino acids from which the liver can form new glucose. In an effort to boost the amount of glucose available to cells, storage glycogen is converted to glucose. (The body can't differentiate a glucose shortage from an insulin insufficiency.) However, these processes prove ineffective and only worsen hyperglycemia.

The body also uses fat as an alternate fuel source, leading to weight loss. Unlike protein, fat can be used directly by most cells. However, it's an inefficient cellular fuel and breaks down into FFAs and glycerol (a glucose substance that exacerbates hyperglycemia). The liver further breaks down FFAs into ketone bodies.

In Type I diabetes, fat is broken down so rapidly that the liver can't handle the excessive ketone bodies. Ketone bodies then spill into the bloodstream, causing ketoacidosis. In Type II diabetes, enough insulin is present to prevent a rapid breakdown of fat, allowing cells to function — even if only sluggishly — and ketoacidosis rarely occurs.

## Complications

Complications of diabetes mellitus can be acute or long-term. Acute complications include hypoglycemia and hyperglycemia. Severe hyperglycemia can lead to two acute metabolic complications — diabetic ketoacidosis (DKA) and hyperosmolar nonketotic syndrome (HNKS). These life-threatening conditions require immediate medical intervention.

Long-term diabetes complications include various chronic illnesses affecting virtually all body systems. The most common are cardiovascular disease, peripheral vascular disease, retinopathy, nephropathy, diabetes-related foot problems, and peripheral and autonomic neu-

COMPLICATIONS

# Understanding the effects of diabetes mellitus

Diabetes mellitus can have widespread effects. This table presents the potential complications of diabetes mellitus, according to the affected body system.

| Cardiovascular | Neurologic | Musculoskeletal | Gastrointestinal |
|---|---|---|---|
| • Arrhythmias | • Autonomic neuropathy | • Bunions | • Constipation |
| • Atherosclerosis | • Blunted hypoglycemia awareness | • Calluses | • Diarrhea |
| • Congestive heart failure | • Carpal tunnel syndrome | • Claw toes | • Fecal incontinence |
| • Coronary artery disease (such as myocardial infarction and angina) | • Cerebrovascular accident | • Hammer toes | • Gastroparesis |
| • Fulminating vascular infections | • Distal symmetrical polyneuropathy (such as small- or large-fiber neuropathy) | • Neuroarthropathy (Charcot's joint) | • Increased salivation |
| • Gangrene | • Focal neuropathy (such as cranial neuropathy, truncal neuropathy, mononeuropathy, radiculopathy, and plexopathy) | • Neuropathic foot ulcers | • Periodontal disease |
| • Hyperlipidemia | | | |
| • Hypertension | | | |
| • Intermittent claudication | | | |
| • Orthostatic hypotension | | | |
| • Vascular ulcers | | | |

ropathy. (See *Understanding the effects of diabetes mellitus.*)

Diabetes also may cause fetal and neonatal complications. For instance, the fetus of a diabetic mother is two to three times more likely to suffer fetal distress or congenital malformations.

## Assessment
### Signs and symptoms
The patient with Type I diabetes usually has pronounced symptoms of rapid onset. With Type II diabetes, symptoms typically are vague, long-standing, and of gradual onset. Diagnosis comes from tests that reveal hyperglycemia or glycosuria or from diabetes-related abnormalities detected on routine examination, such as eye changes noted on ophthalmologic examination. With other types of diabetes, symptom onset may be either rapid or gradual.

Regardless of the form of diabetes, expect a chief complaint that reflects hyperglycemia, such as polyuria, polydipsia, polyphagia, weight loss, or fatigue. Some patients complain of weakness, vision changes, frequent skin infections (such as boils, carbuncles, or furuncles), dry and itchy skin, impotence, and vaginal discomfort.

The patient with Type I diabetes may report a history of viral infections or autoimmune disease. The patient with Type II diabetes may have a family history of diabetes or gestational diabetes or may have delivered a neonate weighing more than 9 lb (4 kg). With other types of diabetes, explore the family history for endocrine disease, genetic syndromes, pancreatic disease, recent stress or trauma, or use of drugs that raise the blood glucose level.

Physical examination may reveal signs of hyperglycemia and its accompanying complica-

| Renal | Genitourinary | Integumentary | Metabolic | Eye |
|---|---|---|---|---|
| • Diabetic nephropathy<br>• End-stage renal disease<br>• Kidney infections<br>• Progressive renal insufficiency | • Decreased vaginal lubrication<br>• Dyspareunia<br>• Impotence<br>• Urinary tract infection<br>• Vesical atony or neurogenic bladder | • Anhidrosis<br>• Diabetic dermopathy<br>• Dry skin<br>• Hypertrophied skin<br>• Necrobiosis lipoidica diabeticorum<br>• Skin infections<br>• Skin lesions | • Diabetic ketoacidosis<br>• Hyperglycemia<br>• Hyperkalemia<br>• Hyperosmolar nonke-totic syndrome<br>• Hypoglycemia<br>• Hypokalemia<br>• Infections<br>• Lactic acidosis | • Blindness<br>• Cataracts<br>• Diabetic macular edema<br>• Neovascular glaucoma<br>• Nonproliferative diabetic retinopathy<br>• Open-angle glaucoma<br>• Proliferative diabetic retinopathy<br>• Retinal detachment<br>• Vitreous hemorrhage |

tions. Signs of hyperglycemia include dehydration and neurologic dysfunction, such as confusion. In a patient with Type I diabetes who's experiencing DKA, you may detect fruity breath odor, Kussmaul's respirations, facial flushing from fever, dehydration, or superficial vasodilation (secondary to carbonic acid increase). In a patient with Type II diabetes who's experiencing HNKS, you may assess rapid respirations; GI disturbances, such as vomiting, ileus, or gastric stasis; and neurologic disturbances, such as changes in the patient's level of consciousness, seizures, or paralysis.

*Other body system findings.* Because diabetes has such widespread effects, expect abnormal findings in many body systems — especially the eyes, cardiovascular system, renal system, nervous system, and skin (particularly the feet).

Ophthalmologic examination may reveal cataracts or typical early changes suggesting diabetic retinopathy, such as retinal microaneurysm (often followed by microinfarction and exudate formation). These changes may progress to proliferative retinopathy, a serious condition that is characterized by retinal neovascularization (new blood vessel formation) and that may lead to retinal detachment, vitreous hemorrhage and, eventually, vision loss.

Cardiovascular abnormalities may include elevated blood pressure (suggesting hypertension, commonly associated with diabetes) and decreased peripheral pulses (suggesting peripheral vascular disease). Other potential indicators of heart disease include abnormal heart or breath sounds (which may mean heart failure) and an abnormal pulse rate or rhythm (which suggests arrhythmias).

Although kidney function is assessed mainly

from renal function studies, you should stay alert for oliguria despite adequate fluid intake and for signs of fluid retention, such as ankle edema and distended neck veins. Puffy eyelids and fingers may reflect diabetic nephropathy. Neurologic assessment may reveal diminished sensory or motor responses and decreased reflexes.

Skin inspection, especially of the legs and feet, may reveal various abnormalities that suggest peripheral vascular disease and diabetic neuropathy. The skin may appear dry and flaky, with lesions and signs of infection anywhere on the body. Lesions visible on inspection include ulcers (such as neurotrophic ulcers that don't elicit pain when pressure is applied) and the erythematous papules or nodules associated with necrobiosis lipoidica diabeticorum. You may detect reddish brown papular spots (diabetic dermopathy), which may progress to crusts and scar tissue. Other skin abnormalities linked to diabetes include hypertrophy, ingrown toenails, corns, and calluses. You also may detect abnormalities in skin color and temperature, especially in the lower extremities.

### Diagnostic tests
In nonpregnant adults, any of the following findings confirms the diagnosis of diabetes mellitus:
• a random blood glucose level equal to or above 200 mg/dl
• a fasting blood glucose level equal to or greater than 140 mg/dl on at least two occasions
• with a normal fasting blood glucose level, a blood glucose level above 200 mg/dl at 2 hours and on at least one other occasion during the glucose tolerance test.

Other diagnostic and monitoring tests include urinalysis to detect acetone and blood testing for glycosylated hemoglobin (hemoglobin $A_{1C}$ or $A_1$), which reflects the patient's average blood glucose level in the past 2 to 3 months.

## Treatment
Treatment of diabetes aims to normalize carbohydrate, fat, and protein metabolism; prevent or minimize long-term complications; and avoid hypoglycemia and other treatment complications. To achieve these goals, the doctor may prescribe dietary modifications, exercise, and drugs (insulin or oral antidiabetic agents) as necessary.

### Nutritional therapy and exercise
With all forms of diabetes, the patient must adhere to a strict diet that's carefully planned to meet his nutritional needs, control his blood glucose level, and reach and maintain his appropriate weight. The doctor or dietitian will estimate total daily energy needs based on the patient's ideal weight, then formulate a diet with appropriate carbohydrate, fat, and protein content. The American Diabetes Association (ADA) recommends a diet consisting of 55% to 60% carbohydrates, no more than 30% fat, and the remaining daily calories from protein. The diet should include 40 g of fiber and no more than 3,000 mg of sodium; concentrated sweets may be prohibited or limited. The patient must follow the diet consistently and eat proper meals at regular intervals.

The type of exercise prescribed varies. Most exercise regimens include an aerobic exercise, such as walking, running, cycling, or swimming, which the patient should perform at least three times a week for 45 to 60 minutes per session.

### Drug therapy
Insulin therapy aims to correct hyperglycemia while avoiding hypoglycemia. The patient with Type I diabetes needs daily insulin administration because of his absolute insulin deficiency. The patient with Type II diabetes may need insulin to control blood glucose levels unresponsive to proper diet and oral antidiabetic agents or during periods of acute stress (for example, acute illness or surgery). Patients with other types of diabetes usually require daily insulin therapy to maintain blood glucose control.

Single-agent or combination insulin therapy may be prescribed. The insulin type or types used depend on the patient's hyperglycemia pattern. (See *Comparing insulin types.*)

For instance, the doctor may prescribe daily intermediate-acting insulin for one patient and a mixture of rapid-acting insulin (to control morning hyperglycemia) and intermediate-acting insulin (to control later hyperglycemia) for another patient. Or, instead of one daily injection, he may prescribe a split (or mixed) insulin schedule, or continuous administration via an insulin pump. (See *Insulin pumps,* page 164.) To meet the patient's specific needs, effective insulin therapy must be determined by trial and error.

When developing the patient's insulin regimen, the doctor will consider insulin purity. The purer the insulin, the less marked its antigenic effect. Pure pork and human insulins, for example, cause less antigenicity than pure beef or combination beef and pork insulins and are therefore less likely to cause insulin allergy, insulin resistance, and lipodystrophy.

*Oral antidiabetics.* Sulfonylureas initially regulate blood glucose levels by increasing beta cell insulin secretion. This effect diminishes after a few months, but the drugs have a second, more important effect — they decrease cellular insulin resistance, enhancing blood glucose regulation. Some doctors prescribe sulfonylureas for Type I diabetic patients with severe insulin resistance caused by acquired insulin antigenicity, although this use remains controversial.

Several sulfonylurea agents are available in the United States to treat Type II diabetes unresponsive to diet alone. Traditional sulfonylureas (first-generation antidiabetic agents) include tolbutamide, tolazamide, acetohexamide, and chlorpropamide. Newer sulfonylureas (second-generation antidiabetic agents) include glipizide and glyburide.

Besides the sulfonylureas currently in use, two other types of oral antidiabetic drugs, biguanides and alpha-glucosidase inhibitors (starch blockers), are being investigated for potential use in Type II diabetes. Biguanides, such as metformin and phenformin, differ from sulfonylureas in structure and action.

Metformin doesn't stimulate insulin secretion or cause hypoglycemia. Other details about its action are poorly understood. The drug may work by enhancing the sensitivity of insulin receptors. Used only after a reasonable

## Comparing insulin types

| PRODUCT | FORM |
|---|---|
| **Rapid acting (30 minutes to 4 hours)** | |
| Humulin R (Regular) | Human |
| Novolin R (Regular) | Human |
| Novolin R Penfill (Regular) | Human |
| Velosulin Human (Regular, buffered) | Human |
| Iletin II (Regular) | Pork |
| Purified Pork R (Regular) | Pork |
| Velosulin (Regular) | Pork |
| Iletin I (Regular) | Beef and pork |
| Regular | Pork |
| Semilente | Beef |
| **Intermediate acting (2 to 4 hours)** | |
| Humulin L (Lente) | Human |
| Humulin N (NPH) | Human |
| Insulatard Human (NPH) | Human |
| Novolin L (Lente) | Human |
| Novolin N (NPH) | Human |
| Novolin N Penfill (NPH) | Human |
| Iletin II (Lente) | Pork |
| Iletin II (NPH) | Pork |
| Insulatard (NPH) | Pork |
| Purified Pork (Lente) | Pork |
| Purified Pork N (NPH) | Pork |
| Iletin I (Lente) | Beef and pork |
| Iletin I (NPH) | Beef and pork |
| Lente | Beef |
| NPH | Beef |
| **Long acting (4 to 6 hours)** | |
| Humulin U (Ultralente) | Human |
| Ultralente | Beef |
| **Mixtures** | |
| Humulin 70/30 (70% NPH, 30% regular) | Human |
| Humulin 50/50 (50% NPH, 50% regular) | Human |
| Mixtard (70% NPH, 30% regular) | Pork |
| Mixtard Human 70/30 (70% NPH, 30% regular) | Human |
| Novolin 70/30 (70% NPH, 30% regular) | Human |
| Novolin 70/30 Penfill (70% NPH, 30% regular) | Human |

# Insulin pumps

For the patient who needs long-term insulin therapy, an insulin pump offers advantages over conventional insulin delivery methods, such as standard injection and jet injection. Insulin pumps work on either a closed-loop or open-loop system.

## Closed-loop systems
The self-contained closed-loop system both detects and responds to changing blood glucose levels. Most closed-loop systems include a glucose sensor, a programmable computer, a power supply, a pump, and an insulin reservoir. The computer triggers continuous insulin delivery from the reservoir. The closed-loop system does have a drawback — it's used only in hospitals because of its large size and because it withdraws blood and infuses insulin I.V. A smaller version now under development would be implanted under the patient's skin.

## Open-loop systems
The open-loop pump infuses insulin but can't respond to changing blood glucose levels. Also called a continuous subcutaneous insulin infuser, the pump delivers insulin in small (basal) doses every few minutes and in large (bolus) doses that the patient releases manually. The system consists of a reservoir containing regular insulin, a small pump, an infusion rate selector allowing insulin release adjustments, a battery, and a plastic catheter with an attached needle leading from the syringe to the subcutaneous injection site. The patient can fasten the pump to his belt or waist-level clothing.

The infusion rate selector automatically releases half of the total daily insulin requirement. The patient releases the remainder in bolus amounts before meals and snacks. He must change the syringe daily and the needle, catheter, and injection site every other day.

## Who benefits from insulin pumps
• Patients with widely fluctuating blood glucose levels despite optimal insulin and dietary regimens
• Patients who don't or can't eat regular meals
• Pregnant women

## Who shouldn't use an insulin pump
• Patients who can't or won't comply with standard dietary, insulin, and self-monitoring regimens
• Patients who miss scheduled medical appointments
• Patients who can't recognize hypoglycemia
• Patients with diabetes complications, such as advanced renal disease, proliferative retinopathy, or severe autonomic neuropathy

## Possible disadvantages
Despite recent advances that have made insulin pumps smaller and more programmable, the pumps do have potential disadvantages, such as infection at injection sites, catheter clogging, and insulin loss from a loose connection between the reservoir and the catheter.

---

trial of diet therapy, it's particularly effective in treating obese patients.

Phenformin (formerly DBI-TD) was removed from the U.S. market in 1977 after researchers linked it to a high risk of lactic acidosis. However, some patients still need this drug. The Food and Drug Administration makes it available to nonketotic diabetic patients who meet these conditions:
• elevated blood glucose levels
• signs and symptoms of hyperglycemia
• signs and symptoms that persist despite dietary measures or sulfonylurea therapy, or sulfonylurea hypersensitivity

• responsiveness to phenformin
• no underlying risk factors that could complicate phenformin use
• risk of insulin-induced hypoglycemia that jeopardizes the patient's job or poses a threat to him or others
• disability that bars insulin self-administration.

Alpha-glucosidase inhibitors such as acarbose decrease postprandial blood glucose peaks by changing the way the body handles glucose. These drugs delay absorption of sucrose and complex carbohydrates from the GI tract by blocking alpha-glucosidase enzymes in the small intestine. Carbohydrates that enter the large intestine are converted to short-chain fatty acids by bacteria and are then absorbed.

### Surgery
Pancreas and islet cell transplantation is only occasionally used in Type I diabetic patients because of the high risk of rejection and complications, the low availability of donor organs, and the successful long-term manageability of diabetes. (See *Pancreas and islet cell transplantation,* page 166.)

## Nursing care
### Immediate care
Take immediate measures to bring the patient's blood glucose level to within an acceptable range (usually less than 180 mg/dl) and to correct or prevent DKA and HNKS.

• For the diabetic patient who's *not* experiencing DKA or HNKS, measure the blood glucose level several times a day, as ordered, until it stabilizes. Keep the doctor informed of blood glucose results. In Type I diabetes, also monitor urine for ketone bodies.

• Administer regular insulin as prescribed until blood glucose is under control. Then expect to start insulin therapy, which may involve other insulin types. In patients with confirmed Type II diabetes, expect to switch the patient to an oral antidiabetic agent as prescribed or, in a patient with newly diagnosed Type II diabetes, to begin a trial period of diet therapy only. Check all meal trays and snacks to make sure the patient is receiving the prescribed diet, and verify that meals and snacks are delivered on time.

• Monitor the patient closely for signs and symptoms of DKA, HNKS, and hypoglycemia (caused by a too-rapid drop in blood glucose levels).

*For DKA.* Suspect DKA if a patient with diabetes exhibits Kussmaul's respirations, a fruity breath odor, and signs and symptoms of severe dehydration. Notify the doctor immediately, and expect him to order fluid replacement, increased insulin therapy, electrolyte replacement, and possibly antiacidosis therapy.

• Administer I.V. fluids rapidly at the prescribed rate. Expect to give 1,000 to 2,000 ml over the first 2 hours. Typically, you'll administer a hypotonic or 0.9% sodium chloride solution, depending on the patient's condition. When the glucose level is slightly above normal, the doctor may switch to a glucose solution, which helps prevent hypoglycemia and reduces the risk of cerebral edema.

• Administer small regular doses of insulin I.V., I.M., or by a combination of routes, as prescribed. Usually, you'll give an initial I.V. bolus followed by a continuous infusion. Monitor the patient's blood glucose level frequently during insulin infusion. Alert the doctor when it reaches 250 to 300 mg/dl; he may wish to decrease the insulin dosage to prevent hypoglycemia. Typically, insulin reduces the blood glucose level by 75 to 100 mg/dl each hour.

Once the patient emerges from this crisis, expect to resume his usual insulin regimen, unless he's newly diagnosed.

• Monitor electrolyte levels closely, and expect to administer potassium replacement as indicated. A patient with an extremely low pH may require antiacidosis therapy with bicarbonate. For most patients, however, fluid and insulin replacement alone will correct metabolic acidosis.

*For HNKS.* If you suspect your diabetic patient is developing HNKS, notify the doctor immediately and prepare to give fluid and electrolyte replacements and insulin therapy.

• Administer I.V. fluids rapidly at the prescribed rate. You may need to administer a hypertonic saline solution or, if the patient is in hypovolemic shock, an isotonic solution. If the patient is an older adult, monitor him closely for fluid overload.

• As ordered, give low insulin doses (usually by continuous I.V. infusion) to gradually decrease the blood glucose level. The patient with HNKS has a greater insulin sensitivity than one with DKA, so expect to give less insulin. Monitor the blood glucose level closely to avoid hypoglycemia. When it approaches 250 to 300 mg/dl, notify the doctor; expect to give I.V. glucose and discontinue the continuous insulin infusion. You may need to give further insulin subcutaneously if ordered.

• Monitor the patient's electrolyte levels closely.

# Pancreas and islet cell transplantation

Many experts believe that controlling blood glucose levels can help stave off certain complications of diabetes. For some Type I diabetic patients, pancreas and islet cell transplantation may be the best way to gain that control. Just as important to many Type I diabetic patients is the prospect of living free from the demands and limitations of self-administered insulin.

Recognizing the potential benefits of pancreas transplantation, doctors attempted the first one in the mid-1960s. That and later attempts throughout the 1970s failed. But more recently, new surgical techniques and improved immunosuppressant drugs have increased the success rate (further enhanced when performed with kidney transplantation).

## Choosing a candidate
Which diabetic patients are most likely to undergo pancreas transplantation? Here are some questions doctors consider before suggesting this surgery.
• Does the patient have diabetes complications?
• Are the complications getting worse?
• Does the patient have life-threatening glucose control problems?
• Does he have renal problems that could warrant a kidney transplant at the same time?
• Is his quality of life poor or unacceptable to him?

Because pancreas transplantation is less successful than other organ transplantations, most patients don't undergo the procedure until other options are exhausted. Most have end-stage diabetic glomerulopathy and receive a combined kidney-pancreas transplant to prevent or relieve vascular complications.

## Surgery
Whether the patient receives only a pancreas or both a pancreas and a kidney, the original organs remain in his body. The new organs, which may come from either a cadaver or a living donor, are transplanted nearby (see illustration). Although transplantation of a living-donor organ has a better success rate than that of a cadaver organ, living-donor organ transplantation is done in only one center nationwide. Alternatively, the surgeon may transplant fetal or adult islet cell tissue into such sites as the portal vein, muscle, or spleen.

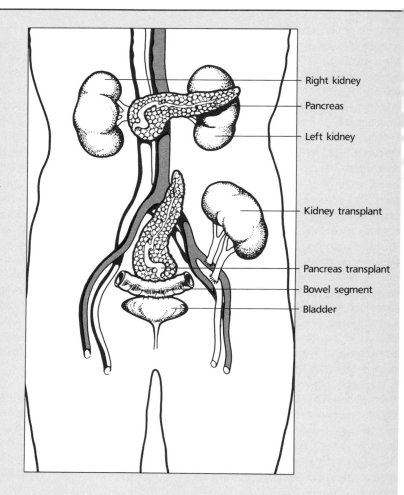

Right kidney
Pancreas
Left kidney
Kidney transplant
Pancreas transplant
Bowel segment
Bladder

## Postoperative care
After surgery, the patient requires immunosuppressant therapy, most commonly with cyclosporine, to prevent organ rejection. To relieve the drug's toxic effects on the liver and kidneys, the doctor may prescribe cyclosporine in combination with more conventional therapy, such as prednisone or azathioprine.

To control pancreatic secretions, the doctor may choose a drainage or suppression technique—for example, deliberate cutaneous fistula, duct ligation, ductoureterostomy, free peritoneal drainage, or pancreatic duct occlusion by synthetic polymers (such as prolamine or neoprene).

Potassium replacement therapy (potassium chloride or potassium phosphate added to the I.V. solution) may be necessary after fluid replacement, which shifts potassium back to cells and lowers the serum potassium level.

When DKA or HNKS resolves, investigate the reason for the crisis and incorporate measures into the plan of continuing care to prevent a recurrence.

### Continuing care
Focus on maintaining the patient's blood glucose level within an acceptable range and preventing or minimizing long-term complications.

*Diet and nutrition.* Doctors regard diet as the cornerstone of diabetes care because it directly controls the body's major glucose source.
• Carefully control your patient's food intake to prevent wide fluctuations in blood glucose levels. If he's receiving insulin or a sulfonylurea, he'll have to adhere to his prescribed diet even more carefully to avoid hypoglycemia.
• Arrange for a dietitian to teach your patient how to plan his meals. Reinforce the teaching as necessary, and make sure the patient who's receiving insulin understands that meal timing is as important as food types and amounts. He must space his meals (including snacks, if ordered) evenly throughout the day.

The dietitian may recommend the *food exchange system.* Based on the carbohydrate, fat, and protein content of six basic food groups, this widely used method promotes more flexible meal planning. Exchange groups include milk products, vegetables, fruits, breads, meats, and fats.

*Exercise.* Exercise is an important part of diabetes management. Besides improving the patient's physical and psychological fitness, an exercise program enhances glucose control by providing an outlet for stress (which can lead to hyperglycemia if left unchecked). Exercise also increases insulin sensitivity, which may help reduce insulin or oral antidiabetic requirements. Also, it lowers the risk of atherosclerosis associated with diabetes and may promote weight loss when used in conjunction with dietary measures for the overweight patient

with Type II diabetes.
• The doctor will tailor the exercise plan to the patient's physical condition, medical status, and risk of complications. If necessary, suggest a consultation with a physical therapist, who can help plan an appropriate program.
• Help the patient choose an aerobic exercise, such as walking, cycling, running, or swimming. Aerobic exercise uses glucose as fuel, decreasing the blood glucose level. It also improves cardiovascular fitness; this is important because the diabetic patient is at increased risk for cardiovascular disease.
• Teach the patient to avoid anaerobic exercises such as weight lifting and push-ups. These exercises *don't* use glucose as fuel and may raise the blood glucose level as the body reacts to exercise-induced stress. Anaerobic exercises also cause rapid rises in heart rate and blood pressure, which are potentially dangerous for any patient prone to cardiovascular disease.
• Inform the patient that exercise is effective only when performed consistently. Instruct him to exercise at least three times a week on alternate days, with each session lasting 45 to 60 minutes. Advise him to start each session with a warm-up phase consisting of 5 to 10 minutes of slow exercise. The conditioning phase, the main component of the exercise program, is next, lasting 25 to 30 minutes. Instruct him to end the session with a 15-minute cool-down phase consisting of exercise that gradually reduces the heart rate to normal.
• Teach the patient to test his blood glucose level before starting each exercise session. Make sure he understands the safety guidelines he must follow to prevent hypoglycemia or increased hyperglycemia during and after exercise.

*Insulin therapy.* Administer insulin as prescribed.
• Most likely, you'll administer subcutaneous injections using a standard insulin syringe. However, you may need to give insulin in other ways. For example, insulin may be injected subcutaneously using an insulin injector device such as the NovoPen, which uses a disposable needle and replaceable insulin cartridges. This

method eliminates the need to draw insulin into a syringe.

• You may also deliver insulin with jet-injection devices, which don't use a needle. These devices, such as the Medi-Jector, Mitajet, and Preci-Jet, draw up insulin from standard bottles and deliver it into subcutaneous tissue with a pressure jet. They allow the patient to mix insulins if needed, although they require a special procedure to draw up the insulin. Studies suggest that jet-injected insulin disperses and is absorbed more rapidly because it avoids the pooling of injectate in tissue that commonly occurs with needle injection. However, jet-injection devices are expensive and require special cleaning procedures.

• A third alternative is multiple-dose insulin regimens delivering insulin into subcutaneous tissue with an insulin pump. A small needle is inserted into subcutaneous tissue (usually in the abdomen) and taped into place. The needle is then connected to a syringe filled with insulin (located inside the insulin pump). The infusion rate selector automatically releases about half the total daily insulin requirement evenly over 24 hours. The patient releases the remainder in bolus amounts before meals and snacks. He must change the syringe daily and must change the needle, catheter, and injection site every other day.

• When administering insulin subcutaneously, rotate injection sites. Because the absorption rate differs at each site, most doctors recommend rotating insulin injections within a specific area, such as the abdomen. (See *Administering insulin by intrasite rotation.*)

• During severe hyperglycemic episodes, you may administer regular insulin I.M. or I.V. Never administer any other types of insulin by these routes because they contain substances that could be harmful.

• Monitor the patient for complications of insulin therapy, such as hypoglycemia, insulin lipodystrophy (subcutaneous tissue hypertrophy or atrophy, usually caused by using the same injection site continuously), insulin allergy, insulin resistance, the dawn phenomenon (an early morning rise in blood glucose levels requiring increased amounts of insulin to maintain blood glucose control), and the Somogyi phenome-

non. (See *Recognizing the Somogyi phenomenon,* page 170.)

• Two newer methods of insulin administration are intranasal delivery and use of an infusion pump called the programmable implantable medication system. These experimental methods may someday offer an alternative to the diabetic patient.

Intranasal administration involves a nasal spray consisting of aerosolized insulin and a surfactant. Currently only regular insulin can be administered by this method. Because nasal solutions are less potent than subcutaneous insulin, the patient must inhale more than he'd need to inject. Before this method becomes commercially available, further studies are needed to determine the surfactant's effects during long-term intranasal administration, the impact of nasal congestion on absorption rates, and the related incidence of severe hyperglycemia and hypoglycemia.

The programmable implantable medication system consists of a disk-shaped implantable pump unit that holds and delivers insulin and a delivery catheter that feeds insulin directly into the peritoneal cavity. The pump, encased in a titanium shell, contains a tiny computer that regulates the insulin dosage. It runs on a battery that lasts about 5 years. The patient uses a small, hand-held, external radio transmitter to control insulin release from the pump. Because the system has no built-in blood glucose sensor, the patient must measure his glucose level several times a day to track his insulin requirements. This technique, now undergoing clinical trials, requires more extensive studies before it can become readily available.

• Ophthalmic insulin delivery using an eyedropper may soon be available. Researchers are using genetic engineering to produce insulin in ophthalmic buffer solutions.

Benefits of ophthalmic delivery include rapid systemic absorption and less pain than with standard insulin injection. Potential drawbacks include limited volume capacity in the eye, patient resistance to eyedrops, and less precise dosing than with standard injection. However, ophthalmic insulin delivery seems to be more precise than intranasal delivery.

# Administering insulin by intrasite rotation

Rather than rotating insulin injection sites around the body, which diabetic patients have been taught to do for years, experts now recommend a technique called intrasite rotation. For example, if the patient receives a morning injection in his thigh, he should receive subsequent morning injections in his thigh. If he receives a before-dinner injection in his abdomen, he should receive subsequent before-dinner injections there.

The reason for this approach is that the body absorbs insulin differently from different parts of the body. Using the same area at the same time every day ensures more consistent dosing and smoother control of diabetes. Choose from the recommended injection sites shown at top right.

Remember that each injection should be given at least 1″ (2.5 cm) away from the previous one. And the patient shouldn't reuse an injection site for at least 1 month. One way to avoid reuse is to mark the first injection site with a spot bandage and give later injections clockwise from that site, as shown at bottom right. After the fourth injection, start a new pattern whose perimeter is at least 1″ away from the first.

**Insulin injection sites**

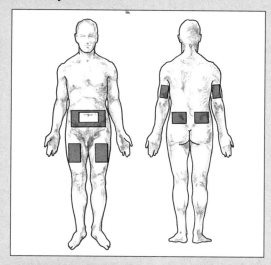

**Insulin injection pattern**

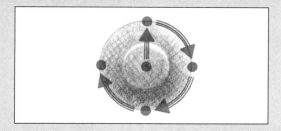

***Oral antidiabetic therapy.*** Administer an oral antidiabetic agent as prescribed.
● Before starting sulfonylurea therapy, check the patient's history for conditions that may contraindicate use of these agents, such as pregnancy, lactation, known allergies to sulfa agents, and stressful concurrent conditions or illnesses with variable but increased insulin requirements.
● If your patient is receiving phenformin, instruct him to avoid alcohol and make sure he knows how to recognize signs and symptoms of lactic acidosis.
● If your patient is receiving an alpha-glucosidase inhibitor, use antacids, bile acids, and in-

testinal absorbents with great caution because they could very well inhibit the drug's antidiabetic effect.
● Monitor the patient for adverse reactions.

***Glucose monitoring.*** Changes in blood glucose levels may cause misleading signs and symptoms — or none at all. Consequently, the diabetic patient must measure his blood glucose level several times a day.
● Encourage the patient to monitor blood glucose instead of urine glucose. Although urine testing may help monitor blood glucose control, it's rapidly being replaced by blood testing. Despite the convenience of urine tests,

# Recognizing the Somogyi phenomenon

The Somogyi phenomenon—or insulin rebound syndrome—can occur when your patient receives too much insulin. Normally, you'd expect excessive insulin administration to cause *hypoglycemia*. But when the Somogyi phenomenon takes place, the body's normal defense mechanisms overreact to hypoglycemia and cause abundant *secretion of counterregulatory hormones*—glucocorticoids, epinephrine, glucagon, and growth hormone. Because these hormones counter insulin's action, *hyperglycemia* sets in, suggesting a need for an *increase in insulin dosage*. Of course, administering more insulin only worsens the problem, causing even more severe hypoglycemia and rebound hyperglycemia (see diagram). At this point, the patient needs less insulin.

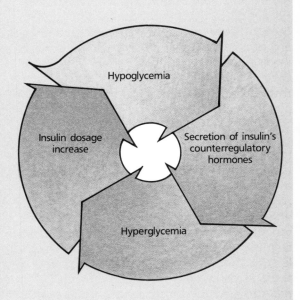

## Assessment

You can't correct this problem unless you recognize it—and recognition can be tricky. Rule out dietary deviations as the cause of poor control, and consider that patients under unusual stress (as with pregnancy or surgery) are at greater risk for the Somogyi phenomenon.

First, check for classic hypoglycemia signs and symptoms—sweating, warmth, restlessness, lightheadedness, tremors, palpitations, weakness, hunger, night sweats, pallor, drowsiness, insomnia, personality changes, and visual disturbances. But remember, these changes may be too subtle to detect—especially if hypoglycemia occurs only at night, which it commonly does. So blood glucose levels should be monitored throughout the night as well if you suspect the Somogyi phenomenon.

Your patient will probably have hypoglycemia for a day and then hyperglycemia for one or more days. However, his blood glucose level may fluctuate between hyperglycemia and hypoglycemia within a single day; if you test at only one time, your result may be misleading.

Evaluate urine or blood glucose trends for several negative results followed by several positive results. To confirm the pattern, monitor blood glucose levels every few hours. Glucose testing proves crucial in detecting this phenomenon because signs and symptoms of recurring hypoglycemia may be subtle enough to escape detection.

Characteristic temperature and blood pressure changes also suggest the Somogyi phenomenon. During a hypoglycemic episode, body temperature and diastolic pressure typically drop slightly while systolic pressure increases slightly.

## Intervention

Treatment involves cautiously decreasing the insulin dosage. If the patient has the Somogyi phenomenon, he'll show improved control with less insulin. Type I diabetic patients may need a reduction of only a few units of insulin; Type II patients on insulin may need reductions of up to 30%.

they don't always reflect blood glucose levels accurately. The renal threshold for glucose spillage into urine increases with age, making glycosuria harder to detect. Also, a time lag separates the development of hyperglycemia and the appearance of glucose in the urine, and urine tests can't reveal hypoglycemia.

Urine tests *can* detect ketone bodies, however — particularly important for the ketosis-prone diabetic patient. Encourage urine ketone testing for all Type I diabetic patients and for any diabetic patient who feels ill.
• Blood glucose self-monitoring allows the patient to determine his metabolic status quickly and as often as needed, permitting more immediate feedback about dosage adjustments or the effects of noncompliance with his diet or medication regimen. It's especially useful for patients on tight-control regimens, which aim to maintain the blood glucose level as close to normal as possible while avoiding hypoglycemia. For the same reasons, blood glucose self-monitoring has become an important bedside assessment tool for nurses caring for diabetic patients.
• Blood glucose monitoring may be done using various types of meters, which read a test strip coated with blood (usually in 1 minute or less) and provide a digital readout. Alternatively, it can be done by visual inspection. The patient (or nurse) compares a test strip coated with blood to a color chart after a brief waiting period. Because so many different types of equipment are available to perform blood glucose monitoring, be sure to follow the manufacturer's instructions precisely and use the technique prescribed for your patient.
• Monitor the patient's blood glucose level on schedule. The doctor may order blood glucose testing before meals, after meals, and at bedtime. He may order a less frequent schedule for a patient who has established a stable blood glucose level.
• Monitor the patient's hemoglobin $A_{1C}$ level as ordered to assess long-term diabetes control. The degree of glycosylation (glucose adherence to the hemoglobin protein) directly correlates with the blood glucose level. Because hemoglobin $A_{1C}$ accumulates over the 120-day life span of red blood cells, its level reflects the average blood glucose level over the preceding several months.

Ideally, hemoglobin $A_{1C}$ should measure no more than one and a half times the normal level (which ranges from 3% to 6%). A high hemoglobin $A_{1C}$ value suggests hyperglycemia over several weeks, regardless of the blood glucose level. A low value coupled with a high blood glucose level suggests recent hyperglycemia onset.

**Supportive care**
• Besides monitoring the patient's blood glucose and urine ketone body levels, be sure to keep accurate records of his vital signs, weight, fluid intake, urine output, and caloric intake.
• Monitor the patient closely for signs and symptoms of hyperglycemia and hypoglycemia. If a hypoglycemic reaction occurs, obtain a blood glucose level. Immediately give a concentrated carbohydrate, such as fruit juice, hard candy, honey or, if the patient is unconscious, glucagon or I.V. dextrose. Notify the doctor of any significant change in the patient's blood glucose level.
• To help avoid problems associated with peripheral vascular disease and neuropathy, provide meticulous skin care. Even a tiny skin break (particularly on the legs or feet) eventually can lead to devastating complications that may, ultimately, necessitate amputation. Treat all injuries, cuts, and blisters immediately and aggressively. Avoid constricting hose, slippers, or bed linens. Refer the patient to a podiatrist for foot care.
• Monitor the patient's compliance with his prescribed diabetes regimen.
• Encourage the patient to express his feelings about diabetes and its effects on his life-style and life expectancy. Offer emotional support and a realistic assessment of his condition. Stress that with proper treatment, he can have a near-normal life-style and life expectancy. Assist him in developing coping strategies. Refer him and his family to a counselor if necessary. Encourage them to join a support group.

**Patient teaching**
Before the patient is discharged, be sure to cover the following teaching points.
• Explain what diabetes is, how it occurs, and what form of diabetes the patient has.
• Review the prescribed diet and reinforce the dietitian's instructions. Teach the patient how to adjust his diet when he exercises.
• If the patient eats many meals in restaurants, teach him how to select a meal that fits his

# How exercise affects the diabetic patient

To understand the physiologic effects of exercise, think of the body as the energy supplier, the circulatory system as the energy pipeline, and the muscle as the energy user. Here—as with other bodily functions—the law of supply and demand prevails, and that means the energy in the pipeline must remain even at all times. That's where the diabetic patient runs into trouble. To understand why, first consider the physiologic effects of exercise on a nondiabetic person.

## Normal effects of exercise
A resting muscle gets by on the energy it draws from free fatty acids (FFAs). But once that muscle starts exercising, it needs an extra energy source. At first, intramuscular glycogen, adenosine triphosphate, and creatinine supply the extra energy. But soon even that's not enough and the muscle starts drawing on blood glucose.

After just 10 minutes of exercise, the muscle's glucose uptake may be 15 times higher than basal value; after 60 minutes, more than 35 times higher. At that point, FFAs provide only about 40% of the muscle's energy, with the rest coming from blood glucose and glycogen. After 3 to 4 hours of activity, the muscle reverts to FFAs as its primary energy source. Even so, it continues using more blood glucose than it did before it started exercising.

The hormonal system keeps blood glucose on an even keel by regulating glucose and FFA metabolism. The insulin level drops, so hepatic output and lipolysis improve. Catecholamine, cortisol, glucagon, and growth hormone levels increase, which also stimulates hepatic output and lipolysis. As a result, the blood glucose level doesn't climb or drop. Increased glucose use balances greater glucose production, so glucose levels in the "pipeline" stay even.

## How diabetes alters the formula
For a person with diabetes, increased glucagon, cortisol, and growth hormone levels may greatly exceed what's needed, so he produces too much glucose. His plasma catecholamine levels may rise twofold or threefold, increasing not just glucose production but pulse rate and blood pressure, too. His injected insulin may be mobilized prematurely, causing his insulin level to rise rather than drop. If his insulin level is too low or inadequate, exercise will increase the blood glucose level. That's because his body continues to release glucose from the liver but can't move it into the exercising muscle. Consequently, his blood glucose can't remain on an even keel.

You can see why a diabetic patient might easily become discouraged from exercising. But he needn't be. If he exercises when his insulin level is adequate, he might *reduce* his blood glucose level. That's because circulating insulin both suppresses glucose formation in the liver and increases the muscles' glucose uptake.

Even after he finishes exercising, his body needs a few hours to replenish hepatic and muscle glycogen, so his blood glucose level stays low. With this prolonged blood glucose de-

diet plan; if appropriate, tell him how he can obtain nutrient composition lists from fast-food restaurants.
• Encourage the patient with Type II diabetes to control his weight. Suggest a support group, such as Weight Watchers or Overeaters Anonymous, if necessary.
• Advise the patient about aerobic exercise programs, and emphasize that he must exercise at least three times a week, with each session lasting 45 to 60 minutes, for the program to be effective. Teach him the components of a safe, effective exercise program. Explain the effects of exercise on the blood glucose level, and review safety guidelines to follow. (See *How exercise affects the diabetic patient.*)
• Instruct the patient on all facets of insulin ad-

ministration, if prescribed, including the insulin type, when the insulin will peak, the proper dosage, proper technique for drawing up insulin, insulin mixing (if applicable), administration technique, site rotation, and insulin storage.
• Teach the patient about oral antidiabetic therapy, if prescribed, including the name of the drug, dosage, frequency, administration times, and adverse reactions to look for and report. Stress that the drug doesn't replace dietary measures but works in conjunction with them to improve blood glucose control. Advise the patient to take the drug only as ordered and never to alter the frequency or dosage without consulting his doctor. Stress that he must never discontinue the drug without medical advice because uncontrolled hyperglycemia might re-

crease, the need for exogenous insulin may drop dramatically and the need for sulfonylureas may be eliminated. But the patient must perform the right exercise program—and he must perform it regularly. If he stops, the benefits stop.

Use the chart below to select the exercise that's right for your diabetic patient, from mild (strolling) or moderate (bowl-ing, golf) to vigorous (skiing, tennis). The chart also tells you how many calories per hour are burned by mild, moderate, marked, and vigorous exercise and what dietary guidelines your patient should follow before or during exercise to avoid a potentially life-threatening diabetic crisis.

| EXERCISE | | | | DIET | |
|---|---|---|---|---|---|
| INTENSITY | CALORIES/ HOUR | EXAMPLES | DURATION | 15 to 30 MINUTES BEFORE EXERCISE | DURING EXERCISE |
| Mild | 50 to 199 | Standing, strolling (1 mph), light housework | Less than 30 minutes<br>More than 30 minutes | None<br>None | None<br>None |
| Moderate | 200 to 299 | Walking (2 mph), vacuuming, bowl-ing, playing golf | Less than 30 minutes<br>More than 30 minutes | None<br>None | None<br>5 g simple carbohydrate every 30 minutes |
| Marked | 300 to 399 | Jogging (3 to 4 mph), swimming, scrubbing floors | Less than 30 minutes<br><br>More than 30 minutes | 15 to 20 g complex carbohydrate, plus pro-tein<br>15 to 20 g complex carbohydrate, plus pro-tein | None<br><br>10 g simple carbohydrate every 30 minutes |
| Vigorous | Over 400 | Jogging (5 mph), skiing, playing ten-nis | Less than 30 minutes<br><br>More than 30 minutes | 30 to 40 g complex carbohydrate, plus pro-tein<br>30 to 40 g complex carbohydrate, plus pro-tein | None<br><br>10 to 20 g simple carbo-hydrate every 30 minutes |

sult. Review guidelines for alcohol use because sulfonylureas may cause alcohol intolerance and hypoglycemia.
• Discuss hypoglycemia and hyperglycemia, including their causes, signs and symptoms, and treatment.
• Demonstrate how to test urine for ketone bodies and how to use the testing product the patient will be using at home. Have him return the demonstration until he can do it correctly.
• Demonstrate blood glucose self-monitoring and proper use of the equipment the patient will be using at home. Teach him how to stick his finger to obtain test blood, how to apply a blood droplet to the test strip, and how to read the results. Have him repeat the demonstration until he can do it correctly. Remind

him that good technique and accurate timing will help ensure reliable results. Instruct him to perform the test at the times ordered by his doctor as well as any time he feels his blood glucose level needs checking to validate subjective symptoms. Also tell him what to do if he consistently obtains blood glucose results outside the range established by his doctor.
• Explain how glycosylated hemoglobin testing is done and what the values mean.
• Inform the patient that stress, as occurs with illness or surgery, causes release of certain hormones that increase the blood glucose level. (See *When the patient with diabetes mellitus has surgery*, page 174.) Illness also may alter dietary intake, causing further complications

# When the patient with diabetes mellitus has surgery

When a diabetic patient undergoes surgery, he faces a greater risk of complications. This is especially true if his diabetes is poorly controlled, because chronic hyperglycemia can cause many changes in body function.

For example, it may cause atherosclerosis of the coronary, cerebral, and peripheral arteries, which may then contribute and progress to such end-stage organ disease as cerebrovascular disease, eye disease, cardiovascular disease, neuropathy, renal disease, or peripheral vascular disease. Unstable diabetes mellitus also may increase the risk of infection.

## Physiology
Surgery initiates a stress reaction that causes release of the so-called stress hormones—epinephrine, glucagon, growth hormone, and cortisol. All of these hormones can raise the blood glucose level, altering the patient's metabolic control. Anesthesia used during surgery adds to the metabolic insult by reducing the patient's blood pressure and causing release of catecholamines, especially epinephrine.

Stress hormones cause the blood glucose level to rise by triggering a series of reactions:
• Glycogen stored in the liver is converted back to glucose (glycogenolysis).
• Conversion of amino acid to glucose (gluconeogenesis) is increased.
• Breakdown of fat tissue to free fatty acids and glycerol (a glucose substance) accelerates.
• Insulin release is inhibited.

Ultimately, these metabolic events lead to release of glucose into the bloodstream at the same time that the secretion of insulin is suppressed. For the diabetic patient, who can't secrete or utilize insulin to combat these events, complications can develop quickly.

## Risks
Besides the normal risks associated with surgery, the diabetic patient also may suffer:
• impaired wound healing
• microvascular and macrovascular complications
• decreased infection resistance
• unstable metabolic control leading to an increased risk of hypoglycemia and hyperglycemia.

## Assessment
• Before surgery, obtain a thorough history. Determine the type of surgery scheduled, the form of diabetes the patient has, his current diabetes therapy, diabetes-related complications, psychosocial conditions that might interfere with diabetes management, current or previous infections, fluid and electrolyte status, and blood glucose and hemoglobin $A_{1c}$ levels.
• Perform a complete preoperative physical examination, staying alert for abnormalities that suggest diabetes complications. For example, look for skin ulcers, poor capillary refill, and varicosities (which suggest peripheral vascular disease or ankle edema). Check for elevated blood pressure, abnormal heart sounds, and an altered heart rate or rhythm, which may signify cardiovascular disease.
• Review laboratory data and other test results (such as chest X-ray and electrocardiography) for abnormalities. For example, increases in serum creatinine, blood urea nitrogen, and urinary protein levels suggest underlying renal disease.

## Surgical care
• Make sure surgery is scheduled early in the day to minimize metabolic disruption. If your patient is insulin dependent, expect to administer glucose I.V. on the morning of surgery and to adjust the patient's insulin dosage upward. More insulin may be administered during surgery if needed. If your patient isn't insulin dependent, expect to administer glucose I.V. on the morning of surgery; insulin may be given during surgery if needed.
• After surgery, if your patient is insulin dependent, give glucose I.V. as ordered until he can take food orally. Also give regular insulin by subcutaneous injection in equally divided doses or added to I.V. fluids, as ordered. When he begins to eat again, give his usual intermediate insulin dose and supplemental doses of regular insulin as prescribed. Monitor the blood glucose level every 4 to 6 hours, as indicated.
• For the non-insulin-dependent postoperative patient, monitor the blood glucose level every 4 to 6 hours. Administer insulin as ordered. When blood glucose levels fall to the normal range and he can tolerate oral intake, expect to resume his oral antidiabetic agent, if prescribed.

HOME CARE

# Ensuring proper skin and foot care for the diabetic patient

The diabetic patient must take meticulous care of his skin and feet to avoid complications of peripheral vascular disease and neuropathy. Teach him to follow these guidelines:
• Inspect your skin daily. Look for small breaks, especially between the toes and around the toenails. Closely examine the soles of both feet and the skin under fat folds.
• Clean your skin daily with soap and warm water. Check water temperature first; otherwise, neuropathy may cause a bad burn. Bath water should range from 90° to 95° F (32.2° to 35° C).
• Always dry your skin gently. To prevent tissue damage, avoid vigorous rubbing of your legs and feet.
• After bathing, apply lotion to alleviate dry skin. But *don't* put lotion between your toes—this moist area promotes bacterial growth.
• Wear clean socks and underwear each day. Use only cotton garments, which absorb perspiration best, and make sure they fit well. Avoid tight-fitting garments (such as tight stockings), which may impair leg and foot circulation.
• Wear leather shoes, if possible. Synthetic materials

trap perspiration and may cause fungal infections and blisters. Buy new shoes late in the day, when your feet are swollen. Break in new shoes gradually to avoid blisters and subsequent infection.
• Never go barefoot.
• Always wear socks with shoes.
• Have a podiatrist remove corns and calluses. Avoid using commercial preparations because they may be too harsh for your skin. Never use a razor blade to remove calluses—this may cause injury leading to infection.
• Cut your toenails straight across and no shorter than the toe tip. If your vision is impaired, have a family member or podiatrist cut your toenails for you.
• If an injury occurs, wash the area with soap and warm water and apply a dry, sterile dressing. Don't use iodine or other harsh antiseptics, which may cause further damage. Change the dressing several times daily and inspect the area closely. If it becomes red, hot, swollen, or painful or if you see drainage on the dressing, call the doctor at once. If the injury involves a leg, don't use that leg until the injury heals. Elevate your leg as much as possible to increase circulation and help it heal.

---

for the diabetic patient receiving insulin or an oral antidiabetic.
• Emphasize that the patient must adhere to the following sick-day rules to help balance the metabolic upsets that illness can cause: Call your doctor before taking your prescribed insulin—he may adjust the dosage. Increase your fluid intake. Monitor your blood glucose level and test your urine for ketone bodies more frequently than usual. If illness reduces your dietary intake, spread your daily carbohydrate allowance over 24 hours. If you can't tolerate solid foods, eat foods with more simple sugars than normally allowed (for example, custard, gelatin, and nondiet soft drinks). Return to your normal prescribed diet as soon as possible. Call your doctor if blood glucose testing shows steadily increasing hyperglycemia, constant hyperglycemia above your normal pattern, or urine ketone bodies. Also call the

doctor if you're insulin dependent and become too sick to eat normally or remain active. Don't stay alone because your hyperglycemia may get worse and reduce your awareness and perception. Have a family member or friend contact the doctor at once if you can't do so yourself—for instance, if you have difficulty breathing or if you become sleepy and have trouble concentrating.
• Review guidelines for skin and foot care. (See *Ensuring proper skin and foot care for the diabetic patient.*)
• Stress the importance of complying with the prescribed treatment plan to prevent or minimize long-term effects of diabetes. Emphasize the need for regular follow-up doctor's visits.
• Encourage the patient and his family to contact the ADA, Juvenile Diabetes Foundation, or American Association of Diabetes Educators for further information, as appropriate.

# Potassium imbalances

Potassium, a cation that's the dominant intracellular electrolyte, is maintained in the blood within a narrow range of concentration (3.5 to 5 mEq/liter). When it exceeds or falls below this range, a potassium imbalance — hyperkalemia or hypokalemia, respectively — occurs.

## Causes

*Hyperkalemia* usually results from reduced potassium excretion by the kidneys — for example, from acute or severe chronic renal failure, oliguria caused by shock or severe dehydration, or use of potassium-sparing diuretics (such as triamterene) in patients with renal disease. Inadequate potassium excretion also may result from hypoaldosteronism or Addison's disease. Other causes of hyperkalemia include failure to excrete excessive amounts of potassium that have been infused I.V. or administered orally, and massive release of intracellular potassium — for example, from burns, crushing injuries, severe infection, or acidosis.

*Hypokalemia* rarely results from a dietary deficiency because many foods contain potassium. Instead, potassium deficiency is caused by excessive GI losses (for example, from vomiting, gastric suctioning, diarrhea, villous adenoma, or laxative abuse); chronic renal disease with tubular potassium wasting; certain drugs, especially potassium-wasting diuretics, steroids, and some sodium-containing antibiotics (such as carbenicillin); and alkalosis or insulin effect, which causes potassium to shift into cells without true depletion of total body potassium.

Hypokalemia also may occur during prolonged potassium-free I.V. therapy, or secondary to hyperglycemia (causing osmotic diuresis and glycosuria), Cushing's syndrome, primary hyperaldosteronism, excessive licorice ingestion, or severe serum magnesium deficiency.

## Pathophysiology

Potassium promotes contraction of skeletal, smooth, and cardiac muscle. It also figures prominently in nerve impulse conduction, acid-base balance, enzyme action, and cell membrane function. Because the normal serum potassium level has such a narrow range, a slight deviation in either direction can have profound effects on neuromuscular function.

A rising serum potassium level decreases the resting membrane potential of muscle cells, leading to increased excitability. Consequently, muscle cell membranes respond to even minor stimuli and may even react spontaneously. This can cause arrhythmias and neuromuscular dysfunction, such as muscle twitching and cramps, which if left untreated may lead to profound weakness (from exhaustion) followed by flaccid paralysis. The increased response of smooth muscles in the GI tract may increase motility, resulting in diarrhea.

Conversely, a falling serum potassium level heightens the resting membrane potential of muscle cells, causing decreased excitability. Muscle cell membranes then require a stronger stimulus. Neuromuscular dysfunction results, as exhibited by slow or weak muscle contraction. Impaired neuromuscular action can cause a decreased level of consciousness, generalized skeletal muscle weakness and, if left untreated, flaccid paralysis. Respiratory and cardiac muscles are especially affected by neuromuscular impairment; shallow ineffective respirations, heart block, and hypotension may occur. The decreased response of smooth muscles in the GI tract can slow motility, leading to constipation and abdominal distention.

## Complications

Complications of potassium imbalance are extensions of neuromuscular dysfunction. Profound changes in neuromuscular function can lead to confusion, coma, paralysis, life-threatening arrhythmias, cardiac or respiratory arrest (or both), and paralytic ileus.

## Assessment

The history and physical examination may reveal cardiovascular irregularities, manifested by dizziness, postural hypotension, and arrhythmias. The patient with *hyperkalemia* may complain of nausea, diarrhea, and abdominal cramps. The patient with *hypokalemia* may have nausea and vomiting, anorexia, abdominal distention, constipation, paralytic ileus, and decreased peristalsis.

# ECG changes in potassium imbalance

Hyperkalemia and hypokalemia may induce abnormal waveforms, as shown by the dotted lines (a depressed ST segment) on these electrocardiogram (ECG) strips.

## Hyperkalemia

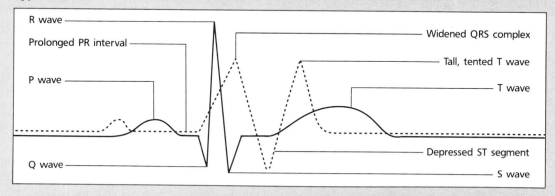

R wave

Prolonged PR interval

P wave

Q wave

Widened QRS complex

Tall, tented T wave

T wave

Depressed ST segment

S wave

## Hypokalemia

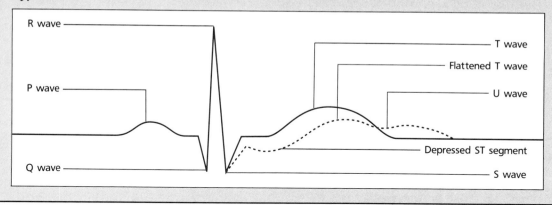

R wave

P wave

Q wave

T wave

Flattened T wave

U wave

Depressed ST segment

S wave

Note any neuromuscular complaints, such as skeletal muscle weakness, numbness, and tingling (with hyperkalemia); weakness and hyporeflexia (with hypokalemia); and flaccid paralysis or respiratory paralysis (with either imbalance).

### Diagnostic tests

Serum potassium measurement definitively diagnoses a potassium imbalance. Serum potassium will measure less than 3.5 mEq/liter in hypokalemia and more than 5 mEq/liter in hyperkalemia. Electrocardiography (ECG) may re-

veal characteristic changes. (See *ECG changes in potassium imbalance.*) Additional tests may be needed to determine the underlying cause of the imbalance.

### Treatment

For *hyperkalemia,* treatment consists of withholding potassium supplements and administering a cation exchange resin orally or by enema. Sodium polystyrene sulfonate with 70% sorbitol causes exchange of sodium ions for potassium ions in the intestine.

For severe hyperkalemia, rapid infusion of

# Administering I.V. potassium safely

You should give potassium replacement I.V. only if the patient has severe hypokalemia or can't take oral supplements. Follow these guidelines to ensure safe I.V. potassium therapy:
• Don't administer potassium by I.V. infusion in concentrations exceeding 60 mEq/liter. Don't infuse it at a rate higher than 20 mEq/hour, or approximately 200 to 250 mEq/day, unless indicated.
• Never administer potassium by I.V. push or bolus; this can cause cardiac arrest.
• During rapid potassium infusion, monitor the patient's heart rhythm to help prevent cardiac toxicity from inadvertent hyperkalemia. Report any irregularities immediately.
• Carefully monitor the patient to prevent or minimize toxic effects. Check the patient's serum potassium levels periodically and evaluate him for such signs and symptoms of potassium toxicity as muscle weakness and paralysis.
• Monitor the I.V. site for signs and symptoms of infiltration, phlebitis, and tissue necrosis.

10% calcium gluconate decreases myocardial irritability and temporarily prevents cardiac arrest, although it doesn't correct the serum potassium excess. This agent is contraindicated in patients receiving digitalis glycosides.

Sodium bicarbonate I.V., another emergency therapy, increases pH and causes potassium to move back into cells. Insulin and glucose I.V. (10% to 50% solution) also cause potassium to shift into cells. Infusions of these agents should be followed by dextrose 5% in water ($D_5W$) because a 10% to 15% solution stimulates secretion of endogenous insulin. Hemodialysis and peritoneal dialysis aid removal of excess potassium, although these techniques are slow.

For *hypokalemia,* the doctor will prescribe increased dietary potassium intake or oral supplements with potassium salts; potassium chloride is the preferred supplement. An edematous patient with diuretic-induced hypokalemia should receive a potassium-sparing diuretic such as spironolactone.

The patient with GI potassium loss or severe potassium depletion requires an I.V. potassium replacement. If he also has hypocalcemia, he'll need a calcium supplement.

## Nursing care
### Immediate care
Focus on restoring a normal serum potassium level and preventing or minimizing complications.
• Frequently monitor the patient's serum potassium and other electrolyte levels, and carefully record his intake and output.
• For the patient with *hyperkalemia,* immediately stop any infusion containing potassium and substitute a potassium-free solution, as prescribed. Also withhold any prescribed oral potassium supplement. Notify the doctor immediately.
• If hyperkalemia is severe, expect to administer regular insulin and glucose I.V. in the prescribed dosage. Remember to follow insulin and glucose therapy with an infusion of $D_5W$, as prescribed, to avoid stimulating endogenous insulin secretion. If the patient has metabolic acidosis, expect to administer sodium bicarbonate I.V.
• If hyperkalemia isn't severe, administer sodium polystyrene sulfonate orally, or rectally by retention enema, as prescribed. Instruct the patient to retain the enema for 30 to 60 minutes.
• When administering repeated insulin and glucose therapy, assess for signs and symptoms of *hypoglycemia* (muscle weakness, syncope, hunger, and diaphoresis). With prolonged use of sodium polystyrene sulfonate, watch for signs of hypokalemia. Monitor for and report arrhythmias.
• For the patient with hypokalemia, notify the doctor immediately and administer I.V. potassium slowly and cautiously, as prescribed, to prevent arrhythmias and vein irritation. Never give potassium supplements to a patient whose urine output measures less than 600 ml/day. (See *Administering I.V. potassium safely.*)

Carefully monitor the patient who's receiving digitalis glycosides because hypokalemia enhances the action of these drugs. Assess for signs and symptoms of digitalis toxicity (anorexia, nausea, vomiting, blurred vision, and arrhythmias). Monitor heart rhythm and report any irregularities immediately. Measure GI losses from suctioning or vomiting.

### Continuing care

Monitor the patient's serum potassium level daily, and assess regularly for signs and symptoms of potassium imbalance.

If your patient has *hyperkalemia*, determine the cause of the imbalance and carry out measures aimed at eliminating or managing the underlying condition. Provide enough calories to prevent tissue breakdown and potassium release into extracellular fluid. Implement safety measures if the patient exhibits muscle weakness.

Assess the patient for GI complications, such as abdominal distention, intestinal cramping, and diarrhea. Watch for signs of hyperkalemia in predisposed patients — especially those with poor urine output and those receiving I.V. or oral potassium supplements. Before giving a blood transfusion, check to see when the blood was donated; in older blood cells, hemolysis releases potassium. Infuse only *fresh* blood if the patient has an average to high serum potassium level.

If your patient has *hypokalemia*, administer a daily oral potassium supplement, as prescribed. If he's receiving a liquid oral potassium supplement, have him sip it slowly to prevent GI irritation. Give the supplement with or after meals, accompanied by a full glass of water or fruit juice. Implement safety measures if the patient has muscle weakness or postural hypotension.

Monitor the patient for abdominal distention, decreased bowel sounds, and constipation. Obtain an order for a laxative if constipation occurs.

### Patient teaching

Teach the patient how to recognize signs and symptoms of hyperkalemia and hypokalemia, including weakness and an irregular pulse. Stress the importance of reporting these changes to the doctor.

• To help prevent hyperkalemia, teach the patient who uses salt substitutes containing potassium to discontinue these if his urine output decreases.

• Inform the patient that he can help prevent hypokalemia by consuming potassium-rich foods, such as oranges, bananas, tomatoes, milk, dried fruits, apricots, peanuts, and dark-green, leafy vegetables.

• Emphasize the need to take potassium supplements as prescribed, particularly if the patient is also taking digitalis glycosides or diuretics.

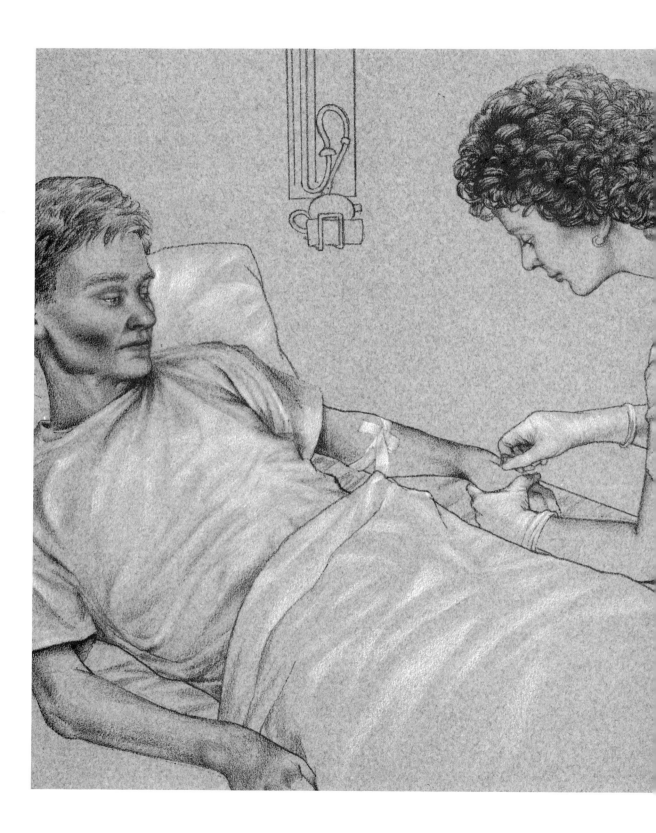

# CHAPTER 8

# Hematologic and immune disorders

Caring for acutely ill patients with hematologic and immune disorders can be both a challenging and rewarding nursing assignment, particularly if your patient has acquired immunodeficiency syndrome (AIDS). You're likely to meet a great deal of anger and despair in AIDS patients and their loved ones, which can make your assignment that much more trying. But it's just as likely to reaffirm your nursing and caring skills.

A successful vaccine or cure may eventually be developed for AIDS, but until then, it's up to you to care for these patients and their severe, long-lasting opportunistic infections, such as meningitis, Kaposi's sarcoma, and the most common infection, *Pneumocystis carinii* pneumonia. This chapter presents the latest theories on the pathophysiology of AIDS, drug therapies offering new hope for AIDS patients, such as zalcitabine in combination with zidovudine (AZT), and coping strategies—for you and your patient.

Before discussing AIDS, however, the chapter covers two of the more common hematologic disorders you'll see—anemia, caused by a red blood cell (RBC) deficiency, and leukemia, a white blood cell (WBC) disorder that's the most common form of cancer in children. You'll learn about their causes, complications, and treatments, such as bone marrow transplantation, along with nursing care, such as managing hemorrhage and transfusion reactions in anemia patients and administering chemotherapy to leukemia patients.

# Aplastic anemias

Potentially fatal, aplastic (hypoplastic) anemias are characterized by pancytopenia (anemia, leukopenia, thrombocytopenia) and bone marrow hypoplasia. Such abnormalities reflect injury to or destruction of stem cells in the bone marrow or bone marrow matrix.

Although the term *aplastic anemias* often is used interchangeably with other terms for marrow failure, it properly refers to pancytopenia caused by the decreased functional capacity of a hypoplastic, fatty marrow. These disorders usually produce fatal bleeding or infection, particularly when they're idiopathic or stem from chloramphenicol use or infectious hepatitis. Mortality for aplastic anemias with severe pancytopenia is 80% to 90%.

### Causes
Aplastic anemias usually develop when damaged or destroyed stem cells inhibit RBC production. Less commonly, they occur when the damaged bone marrow microvasculature creates an unfavorable environment for cell growth and maturation. About half of such anemias result from drugs, toxic agents, and radiation. The rest result from severe disease (especially hepatitis), preleukemic and neoplastic infiltration of the marrow, or immunologic factors (this, however, has not been confirmed).

*Drugs.* Many drugs administered to treat other disorders may cause aplastic anemia and must

be stopped to evaluate the progression of aplastic anemia if the disorder is suspected. Such drugs include:
• antibiotics, including chloramphenicol, cephalosporins, sulfonamides and, rarely, penicillins
• anti-inflammatory drugs, such as phenylbutazone, indomethacin, gold salts, and penicillamine
• anticonvulsants, especially phenytoin, ethosuximide, and carbamazepine
• antineoplastics
• diuretics
• antidiabetic, antithyroid, and antimalarial drugs
• zidovudine.

*Chemicals and toxins.* Aplastic anemias have been linked to prolonged exposure to lindane (an insecticide), benzene, heavy metals, carbon tetrachloride, and kerosene.

*Radiation.* Bone marrow aplasia is a major acute sequela of radiation exposure. Dependent on active mitosis, the marrow is particularly susceptible to radiation effects.

*Infections.* Infectious mononucleosis, hepatitis C, Epstein-Barr virus, Venezuelan equine encephalitis, cytomegalovirus (CMV), and miliary tuberculosis have been implicated in the development of aplastic anemias.

*Other conditions.* Some aplastic anemias may stem from rheumatoid or autoimmune diseases, such as rheumatoid arthritis, systemic lupus erythematosus, and graft-versus-host disease; paroxysmal nocturnal hemoglobinuria; thymoma; and pregnancy. Other anemia forms, such as Fanconi's anemia, may be congenital.

### Pathophysiology
The exact pathogenesis of aplastic anemia is unknown. Presumably, stem cells have an excessive vulnerability to toxic agents that can cause the disease. The toxins target and damage actively dividing cells, resulting in aplasia.

### Complications
Life-threatening mucous membrane hemorrhage is the most common complication of

aplastic anemias. Immunosuppression can lead to secondary opportunistic infections. Other complications of aplastic anemias are associated with the treatment regimen and include transfusion reactions and sequelae of bone marrow transplantation.

## Assessment

### Signs and symptoms

Clinical features of aplastic anemias vary with the severity of pancytopenia, although they often arise insidiously. Assess your patient for symptoms of anemia, such as progressive weakness and fatigue, shortness of breath, headache, pallor and, ultimately, tachycardia and congestive heart failure.

Inspect for the effects of thrombocytopenia — ecchymosis, easy bruising and bleeding (especially from the mucous membranes), petechiae, retinal bleeding, or bleeding into the central nervous system (CNS). Neutropenia may give rise to infection, so note any fever, sore throat, or oral or rectal ulcers. Other findings may include an altered level of consciousness (LOC), bibasilar crackles, and opportunistic infections.

### Diagnostic tests

Confirming aplastic anemia requires a series of laboratory tests, including a complete blood count (CBC) with differential, coagulation studies, and serum iron levels and iron-binding capacity. Bone marrow biopsy aids the diagnosis. (See *Laboratory findings in aplastic anemia.*)

Bone marrow biopsies from several sites may yield a dry tap or show severely hypocellular or aplastic marrow, with a varying amount of fat, fibrous tissue, or gelatinous replacement; absence of megakaryocytes and iron because the iron is deposited in the liver rather than in the marrow); and depression of erythroid cells.

Differential diagnosis must rule out paroxysmal nocturnal hemoglobinuria and other diseases in which pancytopenia is common.

## Treatment

Treatment must eliminate any identifiable cause of aplastic anemia and provide vigorous supportive measures. The doctor will prescribe

## Laboratory findings in aplastic anemia

If your patient has aplastic anemia, expect blood studies to show the following:
• red blood cell (RBC) count of 1 million/mm³ or less, usually with normochromic and normocytic cells (although macrocytosis [larger-than-normal RBCs] and anisocytosis [excessive variation in RBC size] may exist)
• very low absolute reticulocyte count
• elevated serum iron levels (unless bleeding occurs), but normal or slightly reduced total iron-binding capacity; hemosiderin is present, and tissue iron storage is visible with a microscope
• decreased platelet, neutrophil, and white blood cell counts
• abnormal coagulation results, reflecting a decreased platelet count.

plenty of rest and discontinue any medications that may further damage the bone marrow.

If the patient is neutropenic, he'll be monitored for fever and receive antibiotics, if needed (although prophylactic antibiotics aren't given). The doctor may order transfusions of blood and blood components. However, transfusions usually are avoided early in the course of treatment because they may cause sensitization to human leukocyte antigen (HLA), which can make subsequent platelet transfusion and bone marrow transplantation ineffective.

Bleeding can be controlled by pressure application or topical vasoconstriction with cold compresses. Prednisone may be given to reduce bleeding caused by vascular fragility. Platelet transfusions may be indicated if the patient has a severe bleeding disorder that can't be controlled by other methods. (See *Transfusing blood products,* page 184.)

A patient with mild aplastic anemia may have sufficient marrow reserves to avoid infection. If his blood count worsens, though, he may undergo a trial of an anabolic steroid, such as oxymetholone or nandrolone decanoate, to help stabilize his blood count.

# Transfusing blood products

| PRODUCT | APPROPRIATE USES | INAPPROPRIATE USES | EFFECT |
|---|---|---|---|
| Red blood cells (RBCs) | • For anemic patients who need increased oxygen-carrying capacity | • For volume expansion<br>• As an hematinic<br>• To accelerate wound healing | 1 unit of RBCs raises hematocrit by 3% and hemoglobin level by 1 g/dl in a hematologically stable adult. Check patient's hematocrit 24 hours after transfusion to assess effectiveness of transfusion. |
| Platelets | • For control or prevention of bleeding due to platelet deficiencies or dysfunction<br>• For prophylaxis in platelet counts less than 10,000 to 20,000/mm³<br>• For bleeding patients whose platelet counts are less than 50,000/mm³ | • For patients with immune thrombocytopenic purpura (except for life-threatening bleeding)<br>• For prophylaxis in massive blood transfusion<br>• For prophylaxis after cardiopulmonary bypass | 1 unit of platelets raises peripheral platelet count of a 70-kg adult by 5,000/mm³ if underlying cause of thrombocytopenia is resolved or controlled. Obtain platelet count within 1 hour after transfusion to verify effect. |
| Fresh frozen plasma (FFP) | • To increase clotting factors in patients with demonstrated deficiency. (However, FFP transfusion is rarely warranted if prothrombin time [PT] and partial thromboplastin time [PTT] are less than 1.5 times normal.) | • For volume expansion<br>• As a nutritional supplement<br>• For prophylaxis in massive blood transfusion<br>• For prophylaxis after cardiopulmonary bypass | Effectiveness of FFP is measured indirectly, by monitoring coagulation function with PT and PTT or with specific factor assays within 2 to 4 hours after transfusion. |

## Surgery

Some patients are candidates for bone marrow transplantation. In this procedure, 500 to 700 ml of marrow are aspirated from the pelvic bones of an HLA-compatible donor (allogeneic donor) or from the patient himself during periods of complete remission (autologous donor). The aspirated marrow is filtered, then infused into the patient in an attempt to repopulate his marrow with normal cells. Use of alternative donors, such as unrelated histocompatible volunteers or closely, but imperfectly, matched family members, remains experimental. (See *Comparing autologous and allogeneic bone marrow transplantation.*)

In patients with severe aplastic anemia who have undergone a bone marrow transplant, about half have survived in good health. It's also used for some patients with acute leukemia, certain immunodeficiency diseases, and solid-tumor cancers.

For a young patient with a sibling marrow donor who's fully histocompatible, a transplant is the best therapy and should be considered early to help avoid the need for transfusions after the procedure. Transfusions increase the risk of graft-versus-host rejection, which is already high in patients with aplastic anemia and is the major obstacle to a successful outcome. Survival of minimally transfused patients is close to that of patients who've had an identical twin as donor. The procedure produces higher survival rates in patients younger than 20 — approximately 80%.

The risk of graft-versus-host disease after marrow transplantation rises progressively with age, occurring in about 90% of adults over age 30. In older persons, transplantation also carries a significant risk of interstitial pneumonitis and opportunistic infections secondary to the preoperative conditioning regimen (usually chemotherapy alone or in combination with total-body radiation therapy). As a result, bone marrow transplantation is rarely recommended for patients over age 40.

Management of patients in the intermediate range (ages 20 to 40) depends on their transfusion history, their general clinical condition and, unfortunately, perhaps also on their medical insurance.

Before or after a bone marrow transplant, the doctor may order such drugs as methylprednisolone, cyclosporine, corticosteroids, antithymocyte globulin, cyclophosphamide, and

# Comparing autologous and allogeneic bone marrow transplantation

A patient who needs a bone marrow transplant may donate the marrow himself (autologous donor) during a period of complete remission. If his own marrow is inappropriate, another donor is sought (allogeneic donor). Human leukocyte antigen testing determines if allogeneic donor marrow is genetically compatible with the patient's marrow.

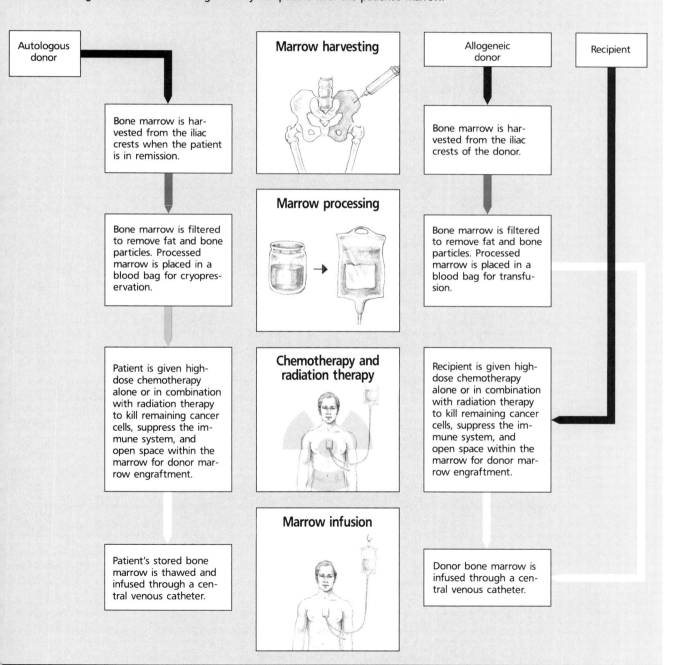

Autologous donor

Bone marrow is harvested from the iliac crests when the patient is in remission.

Bone marrow is filtered to remove fat and bone particles. Processed marrow is placed in a blood bag for cryopreservation.

Patient is given high-dose chemotherapy alone or in combination with radiation therapy to kill remaining cancer cells, suppress the immune system, and open space within the marrow for donor marrow engraftment.

Patient's stored bone marrow is thawed and infused through a central venous catheter.

**Marrow harvesting**

**Marrow processing**

**Chemotherapy and radiation therapy**

**Marrow infusion**

Allogeneic donor

Recipient

Bone marrow is harvested from the iliac crests of the donor.

Bone marrow is filtered to remove fat and bone particles. Processed marrow is placed in a blood bag for transfusion.

Recipient is given high-dose chemotherapy alone or in combination with radiation therapy to kill remaining cancer cells, suppress the immune system, and open space within the marrow for donor marrow engraftment.

Donor bone marrow is infused through a central venous catheter.

azathioprine to promote immunosuppression and help prevent graft rejection. After a transplant, hormonal factors may be given to increase marrow production. These may include granulocyte-macrophage colony-stimulating factor, stem cell factor, and erythropoietin.

## Nursing care

• If the patient's platelet count is low (less than 20,000/mm³), help prevent hemorrhage by avoiding I.M. injections, suggesting the use of an electric razor and a soft toothbrush, humidifying oxygen to prevent dry mucous membranes (which may bleed), and promoting regular bowel movements to avoid constipation (which can cause rectal mucosal bleeding). To further reduce the risk of rectal bleeding, give a stool softener and provide an appropriate diet.
• Apply pressure to venipuncture sites until bleeding stops. Detect bleeding early by checking for blood in the patient's urine and stool and assessing his skin for petechiae.
• Help prevent infection by washing your hands thoroughly before entering the patient's room, providing a diet high in vitamins and proteins to boost his resistance, and providing or encouraging meticulous mouth and perianal care.
• Make sure throat, urine, nasal, stool, and blood cultures are done regularly and correctly to monitor for infections.
• If the patient has a low hemoglobin level (which can cause fatigue), schedule frequent rest periods. Administer oxygen therapy as needed and ordered.
• To prevent aplastic anemia in the patient receiving anemia-inducing drugs, monitor blood studies carefully.

## Blood transfusions

• Be sure to follow safe administration guidelines closely and check for signs and symptoms of transfusion reactions.
• Ensure that blood isn't out of a refrigerator for more than 30 minutes before starting the transfusion. Don't store blood in the refrigerator on the nursing unit.
• Warm blood only in a monitored blood warmer.

• Make sure only 0.9% sodium chloride solution comes in contact with blood components or the administration set.
• Administer all blood components with a blood filter.
• Avoid adding medications (including those intended for I.V. use) to blood or blood components or infusing them through the same administration set as the blood component.
• Monitor for transfusion reactions by measuring the patient's temperature and checking for rash, urticaria, pruritus, back pain, restlessness, and shaking chills.

## Surgical care

• If the patient is scheduled for a bone marrow transplant, teach him and his family about chemotherapy and total-body radiation therapy if he'll undergo these therapies before a transplant, and about strategies to decrease the risk of endogenous infections. Instruct them in meticulous hand washing, routine oral and perineal care, and proper skin care. (See *Problems of bone marrow transplantation.*)
• Teach the patient and his family how to care for a central venous catheter early in the course of hospitalization.
• Administer prophylactic antibiotics postoperatively as ordered. For instance, you may give nystatin for fungal infections, co-trimoxazole (trimethoprim-sulfamethoxazole) to prevent *Pneumocystis carinii* pneumonia, acyclovir to prevent herpes, I.V. immunoglobulin and ganciclovir to prevent CMV, and oral, nonabsorbable antibiotics to decontaminate the GI tract.
• Perform routine surveillance cultures for bacteria, fungi, and viruses.
• As ordered and needed, transfuse CMV-negative blood products for CMV-negative patients who received CMV-negative marrow.
• For patients receiving high-dose cyclophosphamide, implement strategies to prevent hemorrhagic cystitis, a potential adverse effect. For instance, administer continuous bladder irrigation as ordered. If such irrigation isn't ordered, push oral fluids and schedule voiding every 2 hours. Administer mesna (a uroprotective agent), antispasmodics, and analgesics, if ordered.

COMPLICATIONS

## Problems of bone marrow transplantation

| COMPLICATION | CHARACTERISTICS | MANAGEMENT | NURSING ACTIONS |
|---|---|---|---|
| Graft-versus-host disease | • Results from engraftment of immunocompetent donor; T cells react against immunoincompetent recipient tissues (skin, GI tract, and liver)<br>• Occurs in 30% to 60% of allogeneic marrow transplant recipients<br>• Can be acute or chronic | • *Prophylactic immunosuppressants:* cyclosporine, methotrexate, monoclonal antibodies, immunotoxins<br>• *Therapeutic immunosuppressants:* cyclosporine, high-dose steroids, antithymocyte globulin, azathioprine, thalidomide, monoclonal antibodies, immunotoxins | • Irradiate all blood products.<br>• Monitor for delayed marrow reconstitution.<br>• Monitor for prolonged lymphopenia and neutropenia.<br>• Evaluate blood cyclosporine levels and notify doctor of significant abnormalities.<br>• Monitor for adverse effects of immunosuppressants. |
| Pulmonary interstitial pneumonitis | • Usually affects patients over age 30, those with a history of chest irradiation or bleomycin therapy, and patients who test positive for cytomegalovirus (CMV)<br>• Caused by CMV (in 50% of patients), *Pneumocystis carinii* pneumonia (5%), and idiopathic and other agents (45%) | • Use of CMV-negative blood products in CMV-negative patients with CMV-negative donor marrow<br>• *Antimicrobial therapy:* ganciclovir, acyclovir, co-trimoxazole, foscarnet, I.V. immunoglobulins | • Monitor for adverse effects of antimicrobial therapy.<br>• Implement turning, coughing, and deep-breathing regimen. |

• Consult with an occupational therapist to develop a plan for diversional activities during isolation, if the doctor determines the need for strict infection prevention, or while the patient is sequestered in a laminar flow room. Implement a program of range-of-motion and isometric exercises during the isolation period.

**Patient teaching**
• Teach the patient to avoid contact with potential sources of infection, such as crowds, soil, and standing water, which may harbor pathogenic microorganisms.
• If the patient doesn't require hospitalization, inform him that he can continue his normal life-style with some modifications (such as regular rest periods).
• Refer the patient to the Aplastic Anemia Foundation of America for additional information and assistance.

# Acute leukemia

Acute leukemia is a malignant proliferation of WBC precursors (blasts) in the bone marrow or lymph tissue and their accumulation in peripheral blood, marrow, and body tissues. In the United States, an estimated 11,000 persons develop acute leukemia annually. The disease is more common in males than in females, in whites (especially those of Jewish ancestry), in children between ages 2 and 5, and in those who live in urban and industrialized areas. Among children, acute leukemia is the most common cancer form. Acute leukemia ranks 20th among causes of cancer-related death in people of all ages.

Unless treated, acute leukemia is always fatal, usually because of complications stemming from leukemic cell infiltration of the marrow or vital organs. Prognosis varies with treatment.

Among the most common leukemia forms are acute lymphoblastic (lymphocytic) leukemia (ALL) and acute myeloblastic (myelogenous) leukemia (AML). ALL affects the development of lymphoid cells and involves lymphocytes that regulate the immune response; it accounts for 80% of leukemias in children ages 2 to 5. AML affects the development of myeloid cells and involves monocytes or granulocytes whose main function is controlling infection.

## Causes

The causes of acute leukemia are varied. Factors implicated in the disease include:
• genetic disorders, such as Down's syndrome, agammaglobulinemia, and Fanconi's anemia
• exposure to radiation (atomic bomb victims have an increased incidence of both ALL and AML)
• drugs, such as chemotherapeutic agents
• exposure to certain chemicals
• viruses, including human T-cell leukemia and lymphoma viruses
• immunologic factors.

## Pathophysiology

Abnormal proliferation of immature, nonfunctioning WBCs is the hallmark of leukemia. As these cells reproduce, they spill out of the tissue where they originate (lymphocytes in lymph tissue, granulocytes in marrow), and then enter the bloodstream and other tissues. (See *What happens in leukemia.*)

Eventually, these abnormal cells invade vital organs and glands, causing them to enlarge and malfunction. Leukemic cells also impair the production of normal WBCs, RBCs, and platelets in the marrow.

## Complications

Acute leukemia increases the risk of infection and eventually causes organ malfunction.

## Assessment

### Signs and symptoms

Common assessment findings in acute leukemia include fatigue, weakness, headache, pallor, lethargy, shortness of breath, decreased appetite, weight loss, and loss of body mass. Check for signs of bleeding abnormalities, such as bruising after minor trauma, nosebleeds, gingival bleeding, purpura, ecchymoses, petechiae, prolonged menses, hematuria, and melena.

Also note signs or symptoms of infection, including pain, fever, chills, skin redness, celluli-tis, cough, sore throat, sputum production, abnormal breath sounds, increased respiratory rate, frequent or painful voiding, perirectal pain, and rectal drainage.

Assess your patient for altered neurologic function as well, evidenced by headache, nausea and vomiting, blurred vision, slurred speech, facial neuropathies, drooling, changes in LOC, papilledema, and meningeal irritation.

Suspect organ infiltration if you detect abdominal fullness, anorexia, enlarged lymph nodes, bone or joint pain, painless and nontender skin nodules, hepatosplenomegaly, or abdominal tenderness.

### Diagnostic tests

Laboratory tests that help diagnose acute leukemia include CBC with differential and clotting studies (prothrombin time, partial thromboplastin time, and fibrin split products). Radiographic studies help rule out other causes of the patient's symptoms. (See *Diagnostic findings in acute leukemia,* page 190.)

## Treatment

### Chemotherapy

Chemotherapy, which aims to eradicate leukemic cells and induce remission, should begin at once. Specific chemotherapeutic agents depend on the leukemia form. Agents used to treat ALL include daunorubicin, mercaptopurine, methotrexate, prednisone, and vincristine. Drugs used to treat AML include cytarabine, daunorubicin, doxorubicin, cyclophosphamide, mitoxantrone, etoposide, prednisone, and vincristine. To help avert renal dysfunction, allopurinol therapy is initiated before chemotherapy starts.

### Other measures

Additional treatment measures are supportive and depend largely on the patient's symptoms. To treat fatigue, weakness, and headaches, the doctor typically orders rest, oxygen therapy, and analgesics and monitors the patient through serial laboratory tests, electrocardiography, and pulse oximetry.

If the patient has lost significant weight, improve his nutritional status by increasing his calorie and protein intake and ensuring ade-

PATHOPHYSIOLOGY

# What happens in leukemia

This illustration shows how white blood cells (agranulocytes and granulocytes) proliferate in the bloodstream in leukemia, overwhelming red blood cells (RBCs) and platelets.

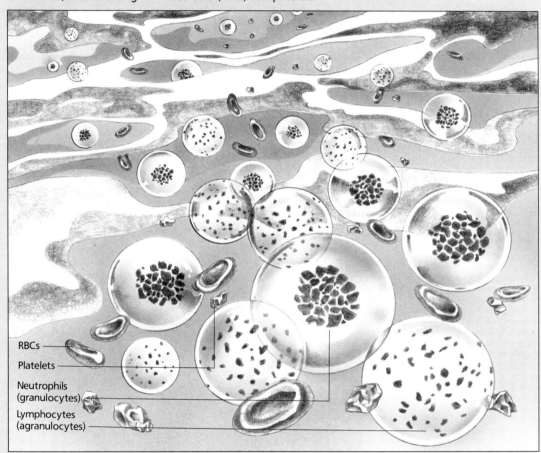

RBCs

Platelets

Neutrophils (granulocytes)

Lymphocytes (agranulocytes)

quate hydration. To treat bleeding abnormali-ties, the patient usually receives blood and blood components as needed. Use a blood warmer to avoid hypothermia and a WBC filter to avoid antibody reactions.

To manage infection, the doctor may order antibiotics, adequate nutrition and hydration, topical antibiotic therapy for skin infections, and cultures of appropriate sources.

If the patient has organ infiltration, he'll re-ceive analgesics, as needed, and undergo labo-

ratory studies, biopsy (as indicated), and radiologic bone studies to assess disease pro-gression.

**Surgery**
The patient may undergo a bone marrow transplant so that he can receive high-dose chemotherapy or radiation therapy while avoid-ing lethal marrow toxicity. Many leukemias ex-hibit a dose-related response to chemotherapy: the greater the dose, the more leukemic cells

# Diagnostic findings in acute leukemia

| FINDINGS | CAUSES |
|---|---|
| Anemia, hypocalcemia, hypomagnesemia | • Marrow failure, release of cellular ions and metabolites<br>• Reduced food intake, hepatosplenomegaly, increased catabolism |
| Thrombocytopenia, hypofibrinogenemia, reduced coagulation factors V or VIII, increased fibrin split products | • Marrow failure, disseminated intravascular coagulation (DIC) |
| Granulocytopenia; radiographic evidence of pneumonia and sinusitis | • Marrow failure, immunodeficiency |
| Pleocytosis, reduced cerebrospinal fluid (CSF) sugar, increased CSF protein | • Meningeal or nerve infiltration or compression |
| Periosteal elevation, bone destruction on X-rays, abnormal marrow, pressure fibrosis | • Local leukemic infiltration |
| Hyperfibrinogenemia, elevated serum aspartate aminotransferase (formerly SGOT) or serum alanine aminotransferase (formerly SGPT), and elevated alkaline phosphatase | • Infiltration of abdominal viscera |
| Abnormal results on liver or spleen biopsy or on bone scan | • Local tumor growth or infiltration |
| Concentrated urine, elevated blood urea nitrogen and uric acid levels | • Dehydration, uric acid nephropathy, DIC |

destroyed. However, toxic effects of chemotherapy often limit the dose. Bone marrow transplantation can "rescue" the marrow from these effects.

## Nursing care

### Immediate care

• Administer blood and blood components, as ordered.
• Protect the patient from potential sources of infection: Bar infected persons from entering the patient's room.
• Monitor laboratory studies and body functions, intake and output, and hematest excretions for occult blood.
• Note that surgical care procedures for bone marrow transplantation in leukemia patients will be the same as for patients with aplastic anemia.

### Continuing care

• Give blood transfusions, if ordered, to help maintain adequate blood counts. Monitor the patient closely for transfusion reactions. Measure his temperature at least every 4 hours and check his WBC count.

*Diet and nutrition.* A high-protein diet is important for the patient with acute leukemia.
• If your patient has lost much weight, promote good nutrition by encouraging him to consume high-calorie, high-protein foods and beverages. However, chemotherapy and adjunctive prednisone may cause weight gain, so dietary counseling and teaching are helpful.
• Determine your patient's food likes and dislikes. Provide small, frequent meals at nonstressful times, especially if he feels ill or nauseated.
• Make sure the patient's diet contains an adequate amount of essential vitamins.
• Ensure adequate hydration.

*Medication.* Administer chemotherapy, as ordered. Stay alert for adverse drug effects.
• After giving an antifungal agent, withhold food and drink for 20 minutes to allow time for the medication to coat the mouth.
• Start antibiotics, as ordered, if the patient has any signs of infection (such as fever or chills)—no matter how slight.

### Supportive care

Focus supportive measures on comfort, minimizing adverse effects of chemotherapy, helping preserve veins, managing complications, and providing psychological support.
• For the patient with fatigue, weakness, and headache, restrict activity, provide undisturbed periods, elevate the head of the bed, and take precautions against falls.
• Good mouth care is essential for a leukemia patient. Before chemotherapy begins, identify preexisting oral problems. Obtain your patient' dental history. Assess him for gingivitis, bleeding gums, loose teeth, and mouth pain. If he wears dentures, check their fit. Check for den-

tal debris, amount and viscosity of saliva, and ability to swallow. Provide frequent mouth care and saline rinses. If you find small, isolated ulcerations or red or white patches in the patient's mouth, instruct him to use a soft toothbrush after meals and at bedtime.
• Check for signs and symptoms of stomatitis and oral infection, and report these to the doctor. Inspect for white, cheesylike patches on the tongue and mucous membranes that scrape off easily, leaving ulcerated areas. Also assess for a red, dry, swollen tongue.
• To manage bleeding abnormalities, monitor vital signs, CBC with differential, prothrombin time, and partial thromboplastin time. To relieve epistaxis, apply ice to the bridge of the nose. Administer transfusions, as ordered. For prolonged menses, maintain an obstetrical pad count. Avoid medications in suppository form.
• To combat infection, administer antibiotics as ordered and monitor vital signs and laboratory studies. For a neutropenic patient, restrict fresh flowers, fruits, and vegetables. Teach the patient proper hand-washing technique.
• To manage a patient with altered neurologic function, conduct ongoing neurologic assessment, decrease environmental stimuli, and administer medications, as ordered.
• Take steps to prevent hyperuricemia, a possible reaction to rapid, chemotherapy-induced leukemic cell lysis. Provide the patient with about 2 liters of fluid daily, and give acetazolamide, sodium bicarbonate tablets, and allopurinol, as ordered. Check the patient's urine pH often; it should be above 7.5. Watch for a rash, nausea, vomiting, drowsiness, and other signs of sensitivity to allopurinol.
• If the patient fails to respond to treatment and enters the terminal disease phase, take steps to manage pain, fever, and bleeding. Make sure he's comfortable. Provide emotional support. If he wishes, arrange for religious counseling. Discuss the option of home or hospice care.

## Patient teaching

• Before treatment begins, help establish an appropriate rehabilitation program for the patient to follow during remission.
• Inform the patient that drug therapy is tailored to his leukemia form. Explain that he'll probably need a combination of drugs; teach him about the ones he'll receive. Make sure he understands adverse drug reactions and the measures he can take to prevent or alleviate them.
• If the patient will receive cranial radiation therapy, explain what this treatment is and how it will help him. Be sure to discuss potential adverse reactions, and review the steps he can take to minimize these.
• Instruct the patient to consume high-calorie, high-protein foods and beverages if chemotherapy causes weight loss and anorexia. If he loses his appetite, advise him to eat small, frequent meals. If chemotherapy and adjunctive prednisone instead cause weight gain, he'll need dietary counseling.
• Teach the patient and his family how to recognize signs and symptoms of infection (fever, chills, cough, and sore throat). Tell them to report these to the doctor at once.
• Inform the patient that his blood may lack adequate platelets for proper clotting. Teach him how to identify signs of abnormal bleeding (such as bruising and petechiae). Instruct him to apply pressure and ice to the area to stop bleeding. Urge him to report excessive or abnormal bleeding.
• Instruct the patient to use a soft toothbrush and to avoid hot or spicy foods and commercial mouthwashes, which can irritate mouth ulcers caused by chemotherapy.
• Teach him to gargle with a solution of 2 teaspoons of salt in 1 quart of warm water after brushing his teeth. Instruct him to avoid mouthwashes containing alcohol, which dry the mucous membranes. Advise him to remove dentures and other orthodontic appliances for at least 8 hours daily (overnight is acceptable). Tell him to use a dental spray three times a day to clean his mouth.
• Advise the patient to limit his activities and to plan rest periods during the day.
• Teach the patient that he can help avoid infection by practicing good skin, mouth, and perirectal care and by avoiding crowds and persons with known infections.
• Refer the patient to the social services department, a home health care agency, and ed-

ucational and support groups such as the American Cancer Society.

# Acquired immunodeficiency syndrome

A problem of epidemic proportions, AIDS is one of the most serious health challenges of our time. The World Health Organization reported over 600,000 AIDS cases worldwide in 1993 and estimates nearly 1.5 million cases by the year 2000. According to the Centers for Disease Control and Prevention (CDC), there have been 194,344 deaths from AIDS in the United States. Approximately one million Americans currently test positive for the human immunodeficiency virus (HIV).

Since first describing the syndrome in 1982, the CDC has declared a case surveillance definition for AIDS and modified it several times. Most patients are diagnosed by these criteria.

The CDC defines AIDS as an illness characterized by laboratory evidence of HIV infection coexisting with one or more "indicator" conditions. According to the CDC, a patient has AIDS if he has HIV infection, a CD4$^+$ T-cell count of less than 200 cells/$\mu$l, and one or more of the conditions A, B, or C from the CDC's clinical HIV classification categories. (See *Classifying HIV infection*.)

AIDS is known by progressive destruction of cell-mediated (T cell) immunity. Humoral immunity and even autoimmunity are affected because of the central role of the CD4$^+$ T (T4 helper or inducer) lymphocyte in immune reactions. The resulting immunodeficiency makes the patient vulnerable to opportunistic infections, unusual cancers, and other abnormalities.

AIDS starts with infection by the HIV retrovirus and ends with the severely immunocompromised, terminal stage of this disease. Depending on individual variations and the presence of cofactors that influence disease progression, the time elapsed from acute HIV infection to the appearance of symptoms to a diagnosis of AIDS and eventually to death varies greatly. Current antiretroviral treatment and prophylaxis of common opportunistic infections can delay the natural progression of HIV disease and prolong survival.

The pathology of HIV infection falls into three types:
• immunodeficiency (opportunistic infections and unusual cancers)
• autoimmunity (lymphoid interstitial pneumonitis, hypergammaglobulinemia, and production of autoimmune antibodies)
• neurologic dysfunction (AIDS dementia complex or HIV encephalopathy, and peripheral neuropathies).

## Causes
AIDS is caused by infection with HIV, a retrovirus belonging to the lentivirus family. This virus is transmitted by direct inoculation during intimate sexual contact, transfusion of contaminated blood or blood products (a risk diminished by routine testing of all blood products), sharing of or accidental injection with contaminated needles, or transplacental or postpartum transmission from an infected mother to a fetus or an infant. No evidence suggests HIV is transmitted by insect bite, saliva, casual contact, or sharing eating or drinking utensils.

## Pathophysiology
HIV infection leads to profound pathology, either through direct destruction of CD4$^+$ T cells or other immune cells and neuroglial cells, or indirectly, through the secondary effects of CD4$^+$ T-cell dysfunction and resulting immunosuppression. HIV selectively invades cells bearing the CD4$^+$ antigen, which acts as a receptor for the virus and allows it to enter the cell. Once inside the cell, HIV replicates, leading to cell death; in some cases, it lies latent within the cell.

Although the patient may lack clinical signs of advancing viremia, HIV continues to invade CD4$^+$ T cells and to replicate. CD4$^+$ T cells act as the body's army to fight off infection; thus, as the CD4$^+$ T cell level falls, the risk of devel-

# Classifying HIV infection

The classification system used by the Centers for Disease Control and Prevention (CDC) groups human immunodeficiency virus (HIV) infection into three categories reflecting clinical disease and three categories reflecting CD4$^+$ T-cell counts. These groups form a matrix of nine mutually exclusive categories for defining HIV in adolescents and adults, but not in children.

## Clinical categories
• A: The patient has asymptomatic, acute HIV or persistent generalized lymphadenopathy (PGL).
• B: The patient doesn't have conditions in category A or C but does have symptoms such as bacillary angiomatosis, oropharyngeal or persistent vulvovaginal candidiasis, fever or diarrhea lasting over 1 month, idiopathic thrombocytopenic purpura, pelvic inflammatory disease, and peripheral neuropathy.
• C: The patient has what the CDC defines as acquired immunodeficiency syndrome (AIDS)-indicator conditions: candidiasis of the bronchi, trachea, lungs, or esophagus; cervical cancer; coccidioidomycosis (disseminated or extrapulmonary); cryptococcosis (extrapulmonary); cryptosporidiosis (chronic, intestinal); cytomegalovirus (CMV) disease affecting organs other than the liver, spleen, or lymph nodes; CMV retinitis with vision loss; encephalopathy related to HIV; herpes simplex involving chronic ulcers or herpetic bronchitis, pneumonitis, or esophagitis; histoplasmosis (disseminated or extrapulmonary); isosporiasis (chronic, intestinal); Kaposi's sarcoma; lymphoma (Burkitt's, or its equivalent); lymphoma (immunoblastic, or its equivalent); lymphoma of the brain (primary); *Mycobacterium avium-intracellulare* or *M. kansasii*, (disseminated or extrapulmonary); *M. tuberculosis* at any site (pulmonary or extrapulmonary); and any other species of *Mycobacterium* (disseminated or extrapulmonary); *Pneumocystis carinii* pneumonia (recurrent); progressive multifocal leukoencephalopathy; *Salmonella* septicemia (recurrent); toxoplasmosis of the brain; and HIV wasting syndrome.

## T-cell categories
The CD4$^+$ T-cell ranges listed below are positive markers for HIV infection (along with various test results identifying HIV or the HIV antibody). The categories are:
• 1: More than 500 CD4$^+$ T cells/$\mu$l
• 2: 200 to 499 CD4$^+$ T cells/$\mu$l
• 3: Less than 200 CD4$^+$ T cells/$\mu$l

| | CLINICAL CONDITIONS | | |
| --- | --- | --- | --- |
| T-CELL CATEGORIES | ASYMPTOMATIC ACUTE (PRIMARY) HIV or PGL | SYMPTOMATIC (NOT A OR C) CONDITIONS | AIDS-INDICATOR CONDITIONS |
| More than 500/$\mu$l | A1 | B1 | C1 |
| 200 to 499/$\mu$l | A2 | B2 | C2 |
| Less than 200/$\mu$l | A3 | B3 | C3 |

oping opportunistic infections increases sharply. (See *What happens in HIV infection*, page 194.)

**New theories.** Research into HIV and how it relates to AIDS is ongoing. Some recent studies suggest that macrophages may play a larger role in AIDS than previously thought. In fact, some researchers think AIDS may be more of a macrophage disease than a T-cell disease. This may help explain why AIDS has such a long latency period and why the virus seems to escape immune detection.

Infected macrophages appear to act as reservoirs for HIV, perhaps transporting the virus to and from various parts of the body. HIV-infected macrophages also may prevent T-cell activation. Diagnostic tests that detect the virus in macrophages (such as the Cetus test) are being developed for commercial use.

## Complications
HIV can infect many human cell types. Besides macrophages, the virus attacks GI, lung, and kidney cells. It also can attack brain cells, causing AIDS dementia complex, a subcortical dementia characterized by changes in cognition,

PATHOPHYSIOLOGY

# What happens in HIV infection

In acquired immunodeficiency syndrome (AIDS), the number of CD4$^+$ T (lymphocyte) cells declines, mainly because the human immunodeficiency virus (HIV) selectively binds with and destroys these cells. The primary glycoprotein in HIV's lipid envelope, a substance called gp 120, binds HIV to CD4$^+$ T receptor sites.

## Entrance of HIV into cell

After binding to a target cell, HIV enters the cell and sheds its envelope. Just how the virus enters the cell isn't known, but its mechanism may be similar to receptor-mediated endocytosis. Or the HIV envelope might fuse directly with the cell membrane, mediating entry into the membrane.

Once HIV enters the cell, the enzyme reverse transcriptase transcribes the genomic ribonucleic acid (RNA) into deoxyribonucleic acid (DNA). Afterward, during cell division, DNA is integrated into the host genome by a virus-encoded enzyme. At this point, HIV's replication cycle may be suspended until the infected CD4$^+$ T cell becomes activated.

## Activation of CD4$^+$ T cells

CD4$^+$ T cells can be activated by such pathogens as cytomegalovirus, Epstein-Barr virus, hepatitis A and B virus, and herpes simplex virus (especially type 2). They can also be stimulated allogeneically by exposure to such body fluids as semen or blood. Activation is followed by transcription, protein synthesis with posttranslational processing (protein cleavage and glycosylation), and assembling of viral proteins and genomic RNA at the cell surface, where mature viral particles (virions) bud and break free of the cell. HIV reproduction kills CD4$^+$ T cells, although no one knows exactly how.

Because CD4$^+$ T cells are critically important in the immune response, destruction of even part of their population can cause immunodeficiencies, leaving the patient vulnerable to potentially fatal opportunistic infections and cancers.

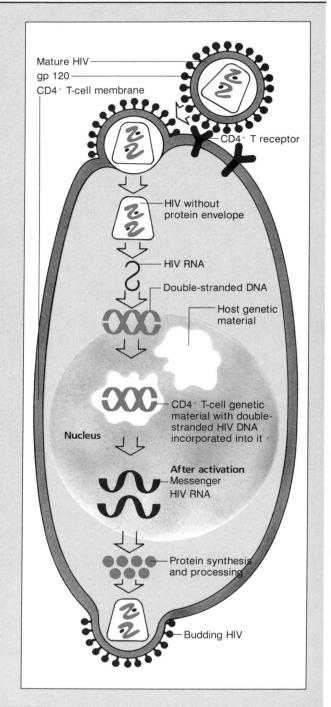

behavior, and motor function (such as confusion, apathy, and paranoia), along with coordination loss. Some patients suffer a wasting syndrome defined as loss of 10% or more of body weight with persistent diarrhea, weakness, and fever.

*Cancers.* Some AIDS patients develop severe malignancies, such as Kaposi's sarcoma, non-Hodgkin's lymphoma, and other lymphomas. Kaposi's sarcoma, the most common form of cancer in AIDS patients, affects endothelial tissue, compromising all blood vessels. In its original form, the disease affects the cutaneous tissues, usually of the legs; it can exist for a decade or longer without harming internal organs. However, the AIDS-associated form, a far more aggressive disease, invades the deeper organs and tissues, especially of the GI tract. In advanced states, the disease obstructs the lymphatic system, causing leg, head, and neck edema.

*Opportunistic infections.* Various opportunistic infections may develop in AIDS patients. Like any infection in an immunocompromised host, they tend to be severe, longer lasting, recurrent, and disseminated. Common infections include cryptococcal meningitis and other brain infections, oropharyngeal and esophageal infections (such as candidiasis and herpes simplex), CMV, *Mycobacterium avium-intracellulare,* and *Pneumocystis carinii* pneumonia. (See *Opportunistic infections associated with AIDS,* page 196.)

# Assessment
## Signs and symptoms
HIV infection manifests itself in many different ways. After inoculation with the virus, an infected person may experience a mononucleosis-like syndrome (which may be attributed to a flu or other virus) and then may remain asymptomatic for years. In this latent stage, the only sign of HIV infection is laboratory evidence of seroconversion. Some patients are asymptomatic until the abrupt onset of complications.

When symptoms appear, they may take many forms: persistent generalized adenopathy, nonspecific symptoms (weight loss, fatigue,

night sweats, fevers), neurologic symptoms resulting from HIV encephalopathy, opportunistic infection, or malignancy.

## History
Obtaining a thorough history is important for the patient who is known to have HIV infection. If he has advanced disease, he may provide a history that includes periods of illness followed by periods of well-being.

For the patient with suspected HIV infection, explore the history for blood transfusions, high-risk sexual behavior, and past infections. However, be sure to maintain a nonjudgmental approach.

Obtain a medication history, noting any immunosuppressant agents. Ask the patient if he currently smokes or previously did, and find out if he's ever received radiation therapy. Smoking and radiation therapy may contribute to immunosuppression.

In AIDS, even vague symptoms may require prompt intervention. Thus, when obtaining the history, stay alert for any of the following findings, which may indicate a serious infection:
• fever above 103° F (39.4° C) at any time
• fever above 101° F (38.3° C) for 3 or more days
• shortness of breath
• persistent diarrhea
• unusual bleeding
• persistent headache
• localized weakness
• paralysis
• change in balance or sensation
• seizures or loss of consciousness, visual changes, or a change in mental status.

## Physical examination
To detect all possible indications of AIDS, which may vary widely, use a thorough, body-system approach. Keep in mind that any unusual finding may signal the need for further diagnostic testing.

To assess the patient's respiratory status, auscultate all lung fields and note cough, dyspnea, sputum production, or hemoptysis. These findings may signal respiratory disease caused by bacteria, viruses, or fungi. Opportunistic respiratory infections may include *Pneumocystis*

# Opportunistic infections associated with AIDS

Acquired immunodeficiency syndrome (AIDS) leaves its victims vulnerable to a host of serious infections. For instance, *cytomegalovirus* (CMV) may cause pneumonia, diarrhea, colitis, retinal hemorrhages and exudates, visual changes leading to blindness, and encephalitis. Treatment may include foscarnet or ganciclovir.

## Viruses
The *herpes simplex* virus may cause lesions on the perineal, perianal, and scrotal areas, the face, and the esophagus. In the colon, mucocutaneous herpetic ulcers may last longer than 1 month. Drugs used to treat herpes simplex include acyclovir, vidarabine, and the investigational drug fiacitabine. *Disseminated herpes zoster* causes a weeping, raised, coalesced pruritic rash, usually on the buttocks, back, and legs. To treat the infection, the doctor may prescribe acyclovir, vidarabine, or foscarnet.

## Fungi
*Candida albicans* causes an infection that may result in difficult, painful swallowing, a white coating or plaque in the oral or rectal mucosa, and skin lesions in the axilla and groin. Some patients may have systemic candidiasis. Drug therapy may include miconazole, nystatin, clotrimazole, ketoconazole, I.V. amphotericin B, fluconazole, or flucytosine. *Cryptococcus neoformans,* also a fungal infection, causes meningitis and fungemia. It's treated with amphotericin B, fluconazole, or miconazole.

## Protozoa
Disseminated *Pneumocystis carinii* pneumonia initially causes diarrhea, night sweats, fever, weight loss, and unexplained lymphadenopathy. Later, the patient may experience dyspnea, dry cough, tachypnea, cyanosis, diffuse crackles, and severe hypoxemia. Retinal manifestations include cotton-wool exudates. Treatment involves co-trimoxazole, pentamidine, or trimetrexate with leucovorin. Investigational therapy includes dapsone with trimethoprim; pyrimethamine with sulfadoxine, eflornithine hydrochloride, or combined therapy with investigational drugs such as piritrexim isethionate.

The protozoan *Toxoplasma gondii* causes brain abscess, diffuse encephalopathy, and meningoencephalitis. Drugs used to combat this infection include sulfadiazine and pyrimethamine with leucovorin. *Cryptosporidium,* another protozoan, causes GI symptoms ranging from soft stools to severe diarrhea. Treatment may include paromomycin, quinine, and clindamycin. The patient may receive supportive therapy, such as octreotide acetate, somatostatin, opiate-based antidiarrheal drugs, total parenteral nutrition, and fluid replacement.

## Bacteria
*Mycobacterium avium-intracellulare* and *M. tuberculosis* cause chronic cough, hemoptysis, fatigue, weakness, weight loss, and fever. Usually, the patient receives two or more of the following drugs: rifampin, isoniazid, ethambutol, ethionamide, streptomycin, clarithromycin, azithromycin, capreomycin, cycloserine, or pyrazinamide. Investigational drug therapy includes ansamycin and clofazimine.

*carinii* pneumonia (the most common), CMV, *Mycobacterium avium-intracellulare,* and tuberculosis.

GI findings may include signs of infection, such as candidiasis, thrush, or herpes simplex virus; gingivitis; hairy leukoplakia; and aphthous ulcers. The patient may complain of pain on swallowing, diarrhea, nausea, vomiting, and weight loss. Assess his nutritional status (often compromised in AIDS).

Neurologic findings may include a persistent headache, seizures of new onset, visual alterations, and changes in LOC. Such findings typically reflect opportunistic infections and neoplasms that directly invade the CNS. Stay alert for psychiatric symptoms, such as depression, psychosis, and anxiety over health changes and poor prognosis.

Inspect your patient's skin for cutaneous Kaposi's sarcoma. Look for small, multicentric, cherry-red, purple, or blue patches; plaques; or nodular skin lesions. These lesions may appear

# Pediatric AIDS

Children make up a small proportion (less than 2%) of the total population infected with human immunodeficiency virus (HIV). However, the number more than doubles yearly and will climb even higher as more HIV-infected women bear children. Twenty percent of acquired immunodeficiency syndrome (AIDS) patients are between ages 20 and 29. This means hundreds of infants will be born to women who carry the virus but who may not show signs of illness for months or years.

## How children acquire HIV infection

Although the exact transmission route isn't always clear, HIV travels from mother to fetus or infant in one of three ways:
• across the placenta before birth
• from the mother's body fluids during birth
• from infected breast milk after birth.
   In children, HIV infection may result from:
• maternal HIV infection
• transfusion of HIV-contaminated blood
• sexual abuse.

## Classifying HIV infection

In children under age 13, HIV infection may be classified as P-0, P-1, or P-2. Class P-0 indicates indeterminate HIV infection. Class P-1 indicates asymptomatic infection and can be divided into:
• normal immune function (subclass A)
• abnormal immune infection (B)
• unknown immune function (C).
   Class P-2 indicates symptomatic infection and can be divided into six subclasses:
• nonspecific findings (subclass A)

• progressive neurologic disease (B)
• lymphoid interstitial pneumonitis (C)
• secondary infectious disease (D)
• secondary neoplastic disease (E)
• other disease possibly resulting from HIV infection (F).

## Comparing pediatric AIDS to adult AIDS

AIDS in children may present a strikingly different clinical picture than in adults. For instance, pediatric patients rarely develop Kaposi's sarcoma. They do fail to thrive, as their growth lags and neurologic complications reverse previously attained developmental milestones. As they live longer with AIDS, they succumb to the common opportunistic infections that strike adult AIDS patients, including recurrent candidiasis, *Pneumocystis carinii* pneumonia (PCP), and *Mycobacterium avium* complex.

## Providing treatment

Therapy, especially with zidovudine or didanosine, improves and prolongs life. Prophylaxis for PCP, the most common and frequently fatal AIDS-related infection, should be given to:
• HIV-exposed infants with CD4$^+$ counts of less than 1500 cells/$\mu$l.
• HIV-positive infants and children who've had PCP.
• HIV-positive infants and children with a CD4$^+$ percentage of less than 20% or a CD4$^+$ count of less than 1500 cells/$\mu$l in ages 1 to 12 months, less than 750 cells/$\mu$l in ages 1 to 2, less than 500 cells/$\mu$l in ages 2 to 6, and less than 200 cells/$\mu$l in children over age 6.

over the entire body or they may be isolated or follow a linear pattern. Although they seldom drain, they may cause irritation, swelling, and pain in the areas they affect. Kaposi's lesions also may appear on the oral mucosa and in the lymph nodes, GI tract, lungs, and visceral organs.

   Other physical findings in AIDS patients may include signs of cardiac disorders, such as cardiomyopathy from opportunistic infections, and signs of renal disorders related to infec-

tions and the toxic effects of treatment. Children with AIDS may present strikingly different effects. (See *Pediatric AIDS.*)

## Diagnostic tests

Laboratory evidence of seroconversion typically occurs 8 to 12 weeks after infection by HIV. Antibody tests, the most commonly performed studies, indirectly indicate infection by revealing HIV antibodies. The recommended protocol calls for initial screening with an enzyme-linked

## Using the CD4⁺ T-cell count to guide AIDS therapy

Some doctors may use the CD4⁺ T-cell count of an acquired immunodeficiency syndrome (AIDS) patient as a therapeutic benchmark, as described below.

• CD4⁺ T-cell count above 600/µl: No intervention is needed. The CD4⁺ T-cell test should be repeated in 6 months, however.

• CD4⁺ T-cell count between 500 and 600/µl: Zidovudine (AZT) may be indicated in the near future. The patient needs closer surveillance, with repeat testing every 3 months.

• CD4⁺ T-cell count between 300 and 500/µl, and CD4⁺ T-cell percentage above 22: Zidovudine may be prescribed, as indicated. The patient should repeat the test every 6 months.

• CD4⁺ T-cell count between 200 and 300/µl, or CD4⁺ T-cell percentage of 20 to 22: The patient may receive zidovudine and may soon need *Pneumocystis carinii* pneumonia prophylaxis. He requires closer surveillance and repeat testing every 3 months.

• CD4⁺ T-cell count below 200/µl, or CD4⁺ T-cell percentage less than 20: *Pneumocystis carinii* pneumonia prophylaxis is indicated. Repeat testing is optional.

immunosorbent assay (ELISA) test. If results are positive, the ELISA test should be repeated. If still positive, the findings should be confirmed by an alternative method, usually the Western blot or an immunofluorescence assay.

However, antibody testing isn't always reliable because the duration needed to produce a detectable HIV antibody level varies from one patient to another. An infected patient can test negative anywhere from a few weeks to (in one documented case) 35 months. Transferred maternal antibodies, lasting for up to 10 months, make neonatal antibody tests unreliable.

Direct testing, although more involved, overcomes these problems by detecting HIV itself. Such testing includes antigen tests, HIV cultures, nucleic acid probes of peripheral blood lymphocytes, and the polymerase chain reaction.

Further blood tests support the diagnosis

and help evaluate the severity of immunosuppression: CD4⁺ T-cell and CD8⁺ T-cell lymphocyte subset counts, erythrocyte sedimentation rate, CBC, serum beta₂-microglobulin count, p24 antigen level, neopterin levels, and anergy testing. The CD4⁺ T-cell count may help determine treatment. (See *Using the CD4⁺ T-cell count to guide AIDS therapy.*)

*Other tests.* Because many infections in AIDS patients are reactivations of previous infections, patients commonly are tested for syphilis, hepatitis B, tuberculosis, toxoplasmosis and, in some areas, histoplasmosis.

Chest X-rays and sputum analysis may be needed to determine the cause of respiratory symptoms. AIDS dementia requires a three-step diagnosis:

• Western blot confirmation of HIV infection
• identification of signs of dementia
• exclusion of other conditions that may cause dementia, such as hypoxia, hypoglycemia, CNS tumors, and brain atrophy.

### Treatment

No known cure for AIDS exists. To help the patient through a crisis, the health care team must support each affected organ or system. However, whether to alleviate symptoms completely or treat them palliatively is an ethical issue of growing importance. The health care team must consider the patient's prognosis and other factors, including whether the risks of treatment outweigh the benefits and whether such treatment will significantly reduce his remaining quality of life.

#### Drug therapy

Drugs used to treat HIV and AIDS fall into several categories:

• those that slow replication of the virus
• those that prevent or stop recurrence of opportunistic infections
• those that boost the immune system.

Drugs currently available to treat HIV include zidovudine, didanosine (ddI), and zalcitabine. These nucleoside analogs inhibit HIV replication through inhibition of reverse transcriptase. They've been shown to increase survival and decrease the incidence of

# Drugs used in patients with AIDS

This chart describes drugs used to fight conditions related to human immunodeficiency virus (HIV) infection and acquired immunodeficiency syndrome (AIDS), such as pneumonia.

| DRUG | INDICATIONS | DOSAGE | ADVERSE EFFECTS |
|---|---|---|---|
| Co-trimoxazole | • Prevention or treatment of *Pneumocystis carinii* pneumonia | • 15 to 20 mg/kg (based on trimethoprim component) I.V. every 6 hours daily for 14 to 21 days | • Nephrotoxicity<br>• Hypotension<br>• Blood dyscrasias<br>• Anaphylaxis |
| Didanosine (ddI) | • Treatment of HIV patients intolerant or unresponsive to zidovudine | • Adults weighing 60 kg or more: 200 mg P.O. every 12 hours | • Headache<br>• Nausea<br>• Peripheral neuropathy |
| Interferon alfa-2a | • Treatment of Kaposi's sarcoma | • 36 million units S.C. or I.M. daily for 10 to 12 weeks<br>• Thereafter, 36 million units S.C. or I.M. 3 times a week | • Flulike syndrome<br>• Myalgia<br>• Bronchospasm<br>• Rash<br>• Acute hypersensitivity reaction |
| I.V. immune globulin | • Prevention of infection in children | • 400 mg/kg every 28 days | • Rigors<br>• Chills<br>• Fever |
| Pentamidine | • Prevention of *Pneumocystis carinii* pneumonia | • 300 mg every 4 weeks (may be given by nebulizer) | • Leukopenia<br>• Hypotension<br>• Hypoglycemia |
| Zalcitabine | • Treatment of advanced HIV infection in patients with significant immunologic deterioration | • Adults weighing 30 kg or more: 0.75 mg P.O. every 8 hours<br>• Must be taken with zidovudine 200 mg P.O. every 8 hours | • Headache<br>• Nausea<br>• Pancreatitis<br>• Peripheral neuropathy |
| Zidovudine (AZT) | • Treatment of HIV infection | • 200 mg P.O. every 4 hours around the clock (1200 mg/day) for 1 month<br>• Thereafter, 100 mg P.O. every 4 hours (600 mg/day) | • Nausea<br>• Headache<br>• Anemia<br>• Granulocytopenia |

opportunistic infections.

Zidovudine is recommended for initiating antiretroviral therapy. However, long-term therapy may cause drug resistance in HIV as well as the emergence of resistant strains of HIV. The drug didanosine has been approved for use after failure of zidovudine; zalcitabine has been approved for use in combination with zidovudine. (See *Drugs used in patients with AIDS.*)

Studies of zidovudine and zalcitabine in different dosages and combinations show that two drugs are indeed better than one. Concomitant use of two or more agents that target different points in the HIV life cycle can attack the virus more aggressively. This approach restricts viral replication, minimizes the toxicity of each drug, and decreases the emergence of resistant strains. Alternating the drugs at 1-week intervals seems to be a successful protocol.

## Fighting Kaposi's sarcoma

Therapy for Kaposi's sarcoma depends on the patient's clinical status. If he doesn't have a history of fever, infections, night sweats, or weight loss, the doctor may prescribe experimental immunomodulators, antiviral drugs, or both. Alternatively, the patient may receive vinblastine alternating with vincristine or other single-agent chemotherapy. The latter therapy also is indicated for the patient who does have a history of infections, fever, night sweats, or weight loss — although this patient may receive experimental drugs instead.

Advanced cutaneous, rapidly progressing, or pulmonary Kaposi's sarcoma may warrant etoposide, low-dose doxorubicin, other single-agent chemotherapy, or experimental drugs. Kaposi's sarcoma with neutropenia or thrombocytopenia calls for vincristine or bleomycin. Radiation therapy may be used to treat painful, bulky Kaposi's sarcoma or lymphedema.

Antiretroviral drugs, antimicrobials, cancer chemotherapy, radiation therapy, and immunotherapy may all be used for the AIDS patient during the course of the disease. Some AIDS patients undergo chemotherapy or radiation therapy for malignant tumors while receiving antiviral drugs. This puts them at high risk for increased immunosuppression and other adverse effects, which must be treated symptomatically.

### Managing *Pneumocystis carinii* pneumonia
The most common life-threatening opportunistic infection in AIDS patients, *Pneumocystis carinii* pneumonia is usually managed with pentamidine or co-trimoxazole. If either drug is ineffective or not tolerated by the patient, the doctor may order an alternative agent, such as dapsone, clindamycin, primaquine, trimetrexate, or atovaquone.

Adjunctive therapy includes treatment of hypoxemia with oxygen therapy and possibly mechanical ventilation.

Steroids recently have proved somewhat effective in patients who have *Pneumocystis carinii* pneumonia with acute respiratory failure. The response rate is 60% to 80%. Although signs and symptoms of *Pneumocystis carinii* pneumonia may worsen for the first few days of treatment, most patients respond within 5 to 7 days. Prophylactic therapy for pneumonia includes dapsone, co-trimoxazole, and pentamidine.

### Managing Kaposi's sarcoma
Treatment for this cancer depends on whether the disease is restricted to the skin or involves deeper tissues. Cutaneous lesions are treated for cosmetic reasons with electron-beam therapy. (See *Fighting Kaposi's sarcoma.*)

For deeper lesions, chemotherapy is the treatment of choice, although these lesions also may be irradiated. Kaposi's sarcoma carries a better prognosis than *Pneumocystis carinii* pneumonia and other opportunistic infections associated with AIDS.

### Ongoing research
Clinical research is actively looking at all areas of treatment, and each year several new approaches to treatment are approved. Trichsanthin (GLQ223) destroys HIV-infected macrophages; however, it has caused significant neurologic toxicities during phase I trials. BI-RG-587 has an action similar to zidovudine but may be less toxic. Three vaccines — rGP120, rGP160 (both recombinant), and GP160 — have successfully protected chimpanzees from HIV. HIV immunogen, a postinfection vaccine under development by Jonas Salk, may stimulate production of protective antibodies.

In another avenue of research, some AIDS patients are receiving thymic tissue transplants in an attempt to restore the immune system. Preliminary results show that patients exhibit prompt, partial, selective, and transient repopulation of the circulating T-cell pool, along with clinical improvement. However, researchers doubt that transplanting thymic tissue alone will regenerate the immune system. Combined

# Preventing HIV transmission

Human immunodeficiency virus (HIV) can be transmitted by unprotected sex; by sharing contaminated needles; and by other means, such as transplacental or postpartum transmission from an infected mother to a fetus or an infant, blood transfusion, artificial insemination, organ transplant, needle stick, or exposure to an open wound. This chart describes ways to reduce the risk of HIV transmission.

| RISK FACTOR | TRANSMISSION MODE | PREVENTIVE MEASURES |
|---|---|---|
| Sex | • Rectal intercourse | • Tell the patient to use a latex condom prelubricated with nonoxynol-9 and a lubricant containing nonoxynol-9 for every occurrence. |
| | • Vaginal intercourse | • Same as above. |
| | • Cunnilingus (rare) | • Tell the patient to use a barrier, such as a dental rubber dam or plastic wrap (may reduce transmission risk to near zero). |
| | • Fellatio (rare) | • Tell the patient to use a barrier, such as a condom (may reduce transmission risk to near zero). |
| I.V. drug use | • Sharing HIV-contaminated hypodermic equipment | • Tell the patient not to use drugs or, if he does, to stop now and get treatment. Further, tell him to avoid sharing needles and "shooting galleries" and to clean needles after each use with soap, running water, and bleach. |
| Other exposure to blood, tissue, and semen | • Transmission from mother to infant | • Tell the patient to obtain prepregnancy and prenatal screening and risk assessment, and to avoid breast-feeding. |
| | • Blood transfusion, organ donation, artificial insemination | • Ensure that screening questionnaires are filled out properly and reviewed, and that the patient is fully informed about autologous blood transfusions. |
| | • Needle-stick or sharp instrument exposure | • Never recap a needle.<br>• Handle sharp instruments and specimen tubes with the greatest of care.<br>• Use only puncture-proof containers for waste.<br>• Follow Centers for Disease Control and Prevention (CDC) guidelines for universal precautions. |
| | • Exposure to an open wound | • Follow CDC guidelines for universal precautions. |

with drug treatment, though, the technique may improve the patient's prognosis.

Prevention still remains the most potent weapon against HIV infection. (See *Preventing HIV transmission*.)

## Nursing care
### Immediate care
• If your patient is acutely ill, focus your interventions on stabilizing him, providing appropriate organ support, controlling pain, relieving anxiety, and discussing treatment options (if his physical and psychological condition warrant it).
• As the patient's condition worsens, monitor for signs of major organ system failure. Provide support as appropriate.

### Continuing care
• Throughout your care, monitor the patient for fever, noting its pattern. Assess for tender and swollen lymph nodes, and check laboratory studies frequently.

• Be especially alert for signs of infection, such as skin breakdown, cough, sore throat, and diarrhea.

• If your patient has an oral infection, advise him to rinse his mouth daily with 0.9% sodium chloride or bicarbonate solution to relieve discomfort. A solution of diphenhydramine hydrochloride mixed with kaolin and pectin mixtures also may be effective. Teach him to avoid glycerin swabs because these may dry the mucous membranes.

• Record the patient's caloric intake. If needed and ordered, administer total parenteral nutrition (TPN) to maintain adequate caloric intake. However, keep in mind that TPN is a potential source of infection, and meticulous aseptic management of the tubes and infusion site is vital to prevent sepsis.

• If your patient has cutaneous Kaposi's sarcoma, monitor the progression of lesions. Provide meticulous skin care, especially if he's debilitated.

• Always follow universal precautions to prevent exposure to contaminated blood, body fluids, and secretions. Diligently practicing universal precautions can prevent inadvertent transmission of AIDS and other infectious diseases transmitted by similar routes.

• Recognize that the diagnosis of AIDS is emotionally charged because of the disease's social impact and poor prognosis. The patient may face the loss of his job, financial security, and the support of his family and friends. Coping with an altered body image and the emotional burden of untimely death may overwhelm him. Be supportive to him, his family, and significant others. Encourage him to discuss his feelings. If needed, refer him to outside sources.

### Patient teaching

• If the patient must remain in isolation, explain the rationale for this measure. Describe how AIDS affects the immune response and makes him susceptible to opportunistic infections. Discuss ways to prevent infections, such as avoiding crowds and people with known infections, washing all fresh fruits and vegetables thoroughly, and cooking meat until it's well done.

• Caution the patient to avoid using alcohol and recreational drugs such as opiates and marijuana, because these substances can make him more vulnerable to opportunistic infections. Explain the danger of using inhaled nitrates; although these agents don't cause AIDS, they may increase the risk of Kaposi's sarcoma.

• Be sure to teach all of your patients, not just AIDS patients, about all possible HIV transmission modes. Discuss measures to help prevent the spread of AIDS, such as wearing a condom during vaginal or anal intercourse; not sharing needles or syringes; and with HIV-positive patients, not donating blood, body organs or tissue, or sperm. With HIV-positive women, discuss contraception. Explain that mother-to-infant transmission of AIDS can occur during pregnancy or breast-feeding.

# Suggested readings

Baird, S.M., and Grant, M. *Cancer Nursing: A Comprehensive Textbook.* Philadelphia: W.B. Saunders Co., 1991.

Blevins, S., and Hicks, D. "Laparoscopic Cholecystectomy," *Canadian Nurse* 88(4):42-43, April 1992.

Chmielewski, C. "Renal Anatomy and Overview of Nephron Function, Pt. 1," *ANNA Journal* 19(1):34-40, February 1992.

Coe, F.L., et al. "The Pathogenesis and Treatment of Kidney Stones," *New England Journal of Medicine* 327(16):.141-51, October 15, 1992.

Cohen, J.R. *Vascular Surgery for the House Officer,* 2nd ed. Baltimore: Williams & Wilkins Co., 1991.

Currie, P.J. "Valvular Heart Disease: A Correctable Cause of Congestive Heart Disease," *Postgraduate Medicine* 89(6):123-36, May 1, 1991.

Emma, L.A. "Chronic Arterial Occlusive Disease," *Journal of Cardiovascular Nursing* 7(1):14-24, October 1992.

Epstein, C.D. "Changing Interpretations of Angina Pectoris Associated with Transient Myocardial Ischemia," *Journal of Cardiovascular Nursing* 7(1):1-13, October 1992.

Failla, S., and Radoslovich, N. "Ask the OR," *AJN* 93(1):76, January 1993.

Fuller, C., and Hartley, B. "Systemic Lupus Erythematosus in Adolescents," *Journal of Pediatric Nursing* 6(4):251-57, August 1991.

Guthrie, D.W., and Guthrie, R.A. *Nursing Management of Diabetes Mellitus,* 3rd ed. New York: Springer Publishing Co., 1991.

Haire-Joshu, D., ed. *Management of Diabetes Mellitus: Perspectives Across the Life Span.* St. Louis: Mosby–Year Book, Inc., 1992.

Hickey, J. *Clinical Practice of Neurological and Neurosurgical Nursing.* Philadelphia: J.B. Lippincott Co., 1992.

Holechek, M.J. "Glomerular Filtration and Renal Hemodynamics," *ANNA Journal* 19(3):237-45, June 1992.

Ignatavicius, D.D., and Bayne, M.V. "Interventions for Clients with Acute and Chronic Renal Failure," in *Medical-Surgical Nursing: A Nursing Process Approach.* Edited by Ignatavicius, D.D, and Bayne, M.V. Philadelphia: W.B. Saunders Co., 1991.

Ignatavicius, D.D., and Bayne, M.V. "Interventions for Clients with Urologic Disorders," in *Medical-Surgical Nursing: A Nursing Process Approach.* Edited by Ignatavicius, D.D., and Bayne, M.V. Philadelphia: W.B. Saunders Co., 1991.

Jackson, D.C., et al. "Endoscopic Laser Cholecystectomy," *AORN Journal* 51(6):1546-52, June 1990.

Lawler, M. "Managing Other Complications Beyond the Respiratory System," *Nursing91* 21(11):40-46, November 1991.

Leondike, M., and Shattuck, M. "Intravenous Cyclophosphamide in Lupus Nephritis," *Journal of Intravenous Nursing* 16(1):23-27, January-February 1993.

Letterer, R., et al. "Learning to Live with Congestive Heart Failure," *Nursing92* 22(5):34-42, May 1992.

Lewis, S., and Collier, I., eds. *Medical-Surgical Nursing: Assessment and Management of Clinical Problems,* 3rd ed. St. Louis: Mosby–Year Book, Inc., 1992.

Litwack, K. "Managing Postanesthetic Emergencies," *Nursing91* 21(9):49-51, September 1991.

Matrisciano, L. "Unstable Angina: An Overview," *Critical Care Nurse* 12(8):30-40, December 1992.

McKenna, M. "Management of the Patient Undergoing Myocardial Revascularization: Percutaneous Transluminal Coronary Angioplasty," *Nursing Clinics of North America* 27(1):231-42, March 1992.

Meyrier, A., and Guibert, J. "Diagnosis and Drug Treatment of Acute Pyelonephritis," *Drugs* 44(3):356-67, September 1992.

Moran, E. "Surgery Adds to Arsenal Against Gallstones," *Hospitals* 64(7):53-54, April 5, 1990.

Oncology Nursing Society. *Core Curriculum For Oncology Nursing,* 2nd ed. Philadelphia: W.B. Saunders Co., 1992.

O'Sullivan, C.K. "Mitral Regurgitation as a Complication of MI: Pathophysiology and Nursing Implications," *Journal of Cardiovascular Nursing* 6(4):26-37, July 1992.

Pak, C.Y. "Etiology and Treatment of Urolithiasis," *American Journal of Kidney Diseases* 18(6):624-37, December 1991.

Pierce, C.D. "Acute Post-MI Pericarditis," *Journal of Cardiovascular Nursing* 6(4):46-56, May 1992.

Price, C. "Continuous Renal Replacement Therapy: The Treatment of Choice for Acute Renal Failure," *ANNA Journal* 18(3):239-44, June 1991.

Rogers, M.L. "Pericarditis: A Different Kind of Heart Disease," *Nursing90* 20(2):52-58, February 1990.

Rosen, R.L. "Acute Respiratory Distress in Persons with COPD: Diagnosis and Treatment," *Choices in Respiratory Management* 21(5):99-101, September-October 1991.

Smeltzer, S.C., and Bare, B.G. "Management of Patients with Urinary and Renal Dysfunction," in *Brunner and Suddarth's Textbook of Medical-Surgical Nursing,* 7th ed. Edited by Smeltzer, S.C., and Bare, B.G. Philadelphia: J.B. Lippincott Co., 1992.

Spera, M., et al. "Acute Care for the Elderly: A New Approach," *Nursing Management* 22(2):36-38, February 1991.

Spilman, P., and Whelton, A. "Nonsteroidal Anti-inflammatory Drugs: Effects on Kidney Function and Implications for Nursing Care," *ANNA Journal* 19(1):19-28, February 1992.

Stewart, J., et al. "Cardiomyoplasty: Treatment of the Failing Heart Using the Skeletal Muscle Wrap," *Journal of Cardiovascular Nursing* 7(2):23-31, January 1993.

Surratt, S., et al. "Troubleshooting a Sump Tube," *AJN* 93(1):42-47, January 1993.

Toto, K.H. "Acute Renal Failure: A Question of Location," *AJN* 92(11):44-53, November 1992.

Wen, S.F., et al. "Acute Renal Failure Following Binge Drinking and Nonsteroidal Anti-inflammatory Drugs," *American Journal of Kidney Diseases* 20(3):281-85, September 1992.

# Advanced skilltest

*This self-test presents case histories with related multiple-choice questions as well as general multiple-choice questions on caring for the acutely ill patient. The questions begin on this page and continue to page 209. You'll find the answers along with rationales on pages 210 and 211.*

## Case history questions

*Marc Johnson, age 48, suffered an acute hemolytic transfusion reaction several days ago. He's admitted to your unit in acute renal failure. Mr. Johnson's vital signs are as follows: blood pressure, 170/100 mm Hg; heart rate, 110 beats/minute; respiratory rate, 28 breaths/minute; and temperature, 100° F (37.8° C). His urine output is 100 ml over the past 8 hours, and his serum electrolyte values are: sodium, 120 mEq/liter; potassium, 7 mEq/liter; and chloride, 90 mEq/liter. His blood urea nitrogen (BUN) level is 60 mg/dl, and his partial pressure of arterial carbon dioxide (PaCO$_2$) is 30 mm Hg.*

**1.** The most significant sign of acute renal failure is:

    a.  decreased BUN levels.

    b.  a rise in body temperature.

    c.  hypertension.

    d.  oliguria.

**2.** Acute renal failure usually results from:

    a.  spasms of the renal arteries.

    b.  acute tubular necrosis.

    c.  sodium intoxication.

    d.  water intoxication.

**3.** Which of these assessment findings is the most worrisome?

    a.  Serum sodium level

    b.  Serum potassium level

    c.  Heart rate

    d.  PaCO$_2$ value

**4.** Based on Mr. Johnson's vital signs, you should monitor him for:

    a.  cardiac standstill.

    b.  constipation.

    c.  tetany and leg cramps.

    d.  all of the above.

*Two hours after eating lunch, Amy Kirkland, age 29, experiences sudden diaphoresis, anxiety, nervousness, hunger, and weakness. She feels better after eating several peanut butter crackers and drinking some milk. But several weeks later, she has a second episode and sees her doctor. Based on a comprehensive history and physical examination, the doctor diagnoses reactive hypoglycemia.*

**5.** Which of the following conditions can cause reactive hypoglycemia?

    a.  Hepatic disease

    b.  Insulinoma

    c.  Excessive alcohol ingestion

    d.  Dumping syndrome

**6.** Which foods should Ms. Kirkland avoid?

    a.  Those high in fats

    b.  Simple carbohydrates

    c.  Spicy foods

    d.  Red meat

*Joey Mason, age 7, develops polyuria, polydipsia, polyphagia, weight loss, and fatigue over the course of a week. His parents bring him to the emergency department, where you find that he's semicomatose. A blood glucose test measures 459 mg/dl. Joey is admitted with a diagnosis of diabetes mellitus.*

**7.** Based on Joey's clinical presentation, you would monitor him for which complication of unstable diabetes mellitus?

    a. Hypoglycemia
    b. Diabetic ketoacidosis (DKA)
    c. Hyperosmolar nonketotic syndrome (HNKS)
    d. Autonomic neuropathy

**8.** Joey is started on insulin therapy. However, he's reluctant to learn how to self-administer the injections and he gets upset about having daily injections. Which insulin delivery system would be best for Joey?

    a. NovoPen
    b. An insulin pump
    c. A jet-injection device
    d. Micronized glyburide

**9.** When discussing sick-day rules for diabetic patients, Joey's mother asks you when she should withhold his insulin. Which instruction should you give her?

    a. Withhold insulin only if he is vomiting.
    b. Withhold insulin if he is vomiting and has diarrhea.
    c. Give the same insulin dose regardless of his symptoms.
    d. Give an adjusted insulin dose after conferring with the doctor.

*George Richter, age 34, has been in a head-on motor vehicle collision and suffered extensive contusions and abrasions. X-rays reveal open fractures of the right tibia and fibula and a closed fracture of the right femur at midshaft. Two hours after he's admitted, he undergoes surgery for open reduction and internal fixation of his femur and has an external fixator device applied to his right tibia and fibula. Later, in the recovery room, his heart rate measures 134 beats/minute. After assessing him and reviewing the operating room record, you determine that Mr. Richter has a fluid volume deficit.*

**10.** The most likely source of blood loss in Mr. Richter is:

    a. an undiagnosed head injury.
    b. his tibia and fibula fractures.
    c. his multiple abrasions.
    d. his right femur fracture.

**11.** Mr. Richter receives a transfusion of two units of packed red blood cells (RBCs) and a liter of lactated Ringer's solution over 3 hours. His heart rate then drops to 88 beats/minute.

  The next day, his heart rate increases again. You note that he appears tachypneic, dyspneic, and slightly agitated and doesn't remember you. Based on the history and your assessment findings, you would suspect:

    a. fat embolism syndrome.
    b. osteomyelitis.
    c. hemorrhage.
    d. compartment syndrome.

**12.** Which dermal finding is characteristic of fat embolism syndrome?

    a. Palmar erythema
    b. Generalized flushing
    c. Petechial rash of the chest
    d. Pale, cool, clammy skin

**13.** You're concerned about Mr. Richter's tachypnea, tachycardia, and dyspnea. The most appropriate intervention would be to:

    a.  obtain a 12-lead electrocardiogram.

    b.  check his oxygen saturation with a pulse oximeter and administer oxygen as needed and as ordered.

    c.  medicate him for pain as ordered.

    d.  administer a bolus of I.V. fluids.

## General questions

**14.** When preparing your patient for surgery, you assess his preoperative baseline breath sounds and breathing patterns. If the patient has a preexisting respiratory condition (such as chronic obstructive pulmonary disease), which preoperative intervention would *not* be appropriate?

    a.  Administering bronchodilators

    b.  Administering antibiotics if the patient has purulent sputum

    c.  Administering morphine sulfate

    d.  Performing chest physiotherapy

**15.** Preoperative drugs are given for all of the following reasons *except* to:

    a.  impede blood coagulation.

    b.  reduce anxiety.

    c.  decrease discomfort.

    d.  protect the airway during surgery.

**16.** Factors that influence the nature of a patient's pain include its duration, severity, and source. Which of the following is *not* a potential source of pain?

    a.  Cutaneous tissue

    b.  Subcutaneous tissue

    c.  Visceral organ tissue

    d.  Deep somatic (nerve, bone, muscle, and supportive) tissue

**17.** Which of the following agents is a nonsteroidal anti-inflammatory drug (NSAID)?

    a.  Aspirin

    b.  Ibuprofen

    c.  Naproxen

    d.  All of the above

**18.** What's the most important supportive nursing measure when caring for a dying patient?

    a.  Being honest and realistic when talking to the patient and his family

    b.  Being silent to avoid saying the wrong thing

    c.  Listening to the patient

    d.  Not crying in front of the patient and his family

**19.** Which combination drug therapy is most helpful in treating unstable angina?

    a.  Anticoagulant and antiplatelet therapy

    b.  Calcium channel blocker and beta blocker therapy

    c.  Thrombolytic and nitrate therapy

    d.  Calcium channel blocker, nitrate, and beta blocker therapy

**20.** Congestive heart failure may result from which of the following conditions?

    a.  Pulmonary embolism

    b.  Anemia

    c.  Pregnancy

    d.  All of the above

**21.** The usual cause of mitral stenosis is:

    a.  infection.

    b.  coronary insufficiency.

    c.  rheumatic fever.

    d.  pulmonary emboli.

**22.** Which of the following is *not* a risk factor for arterial occlusive disease?

    a.  Myocardial infarction

    b.  Cigarette smoking

    c.  Hyperlipidemia

    d.  Infection

**23.** Assessment findings for the patient with cor pulmonale may include all of the following *except:*

    a.  bradycardia.

    b.  dependent edema.

    c.  distended neck veins.

    d.  weak pulse.

**24.** Which condition is characterized by a resting pulmonary artery systolic pressure (PASP) above 30 mm Hg and a mean pulmonary artery pressure (PAP) above 18 mm Hg, with no obvious cause?

    a.  Vascular obstruction

    b.  Alveolar hypoventilation

    c.  Secondary pulmonary hypertension

    d.  Primary or idiopathic pulmonary hypertension

**25.** The chief treatment goals for a patient with acute asthma are to achieve or maintain adequate oxygen saturation and to rapidly reverse airflow obstruction. To reverse airflow obstruction quickly, drug therapy centers on inhaled beta agonists. Which beta agonist has the most potent bronchodilating activity with the fewest adverse effects?

    a.  Albuterol

    b.  Cromolyn sodium

    c.  Isoetharine

    d.  Metaproterenol

**26.** Which factor increases a patient's risk of developing pneumonia?

    a.  Human immunodeficiency virus (HIV) or acquired immunodeficiency syndrome (AIDS)

    b.  Chronic illness

    c.  Smoking

    d.  All of the above

**27.** Cerebrovascular accident (CVA) is defined as the sudden, nonconvulsant onset of neurologic deficits related to an altered cerebral blood supply. The most common cause of CVA is:

    a.  a thrombus.

    b.  an embolism.

    c.  a tumor.

    d.  a hemorrhage.

**28.** To evaluate and diagnose a CVA, all of the following studies are done *except:*

    a.  a magnetic resonance imaging (MRI) scan.

    b.  a perfusion scan.

    c.  a computed tomography (CT) scan.

    d.  a cerebral arteriogram.

**29.** The most important means of diagnosing Alzheimer's disease is:

    a.  a neurologic examination.

    b.  psychological testing.

    c.  a CT scan.

    d.  a cerebral angiogram.

**30.** Which of the following statements best describes pancreatitis?

    a. It is an autoimmune disease associated with alcoholism.

    b. It is a genetic or familial disease characterized by autodigestion of the pancreas.

    c. It is an inflammatory disease leading to pancreatic edema and obstruction of the pancreatic ducts.

    d. It is an infectious process associated with the hepatitis B virus.

**31.** Which elevated serum substance is the best indicator for diagnosing pancreatitis?

    a. Creatinine

    b. Glucose

    c. Lipids

    d. Amylase

**32.** Eight days ago, your patient underwent a permanent ileostomy with formation of a continent ileostomy to treat ulcerative colitis. When teaching him about home care, you should include which of the following points?

    a. Perform frequent perianal skin care.

    b. Irrigate the pouch daily with 500 ml of 0.9% sodium chloride solution.

    c. Insert a drainage catheter into the ileal stoma.

    d. Include high-fiber foods in the diet.

**33.** Intestinal obstruction results from mechanical or nonmechanical (neurogenic) blockage of the intestinal lumen. Causes of nonmechanical obstruction include spinal cord lesions, paralytic ileus, and peritoneal irritation. Causes of mechanical obstruction include all of the following *except:*

    a. hernia.

    b. adhesions.

    c. peritonitis.

    d. neoplasms.

**34.** The hallmark of leukemia is an abnormal proliferation of white blood cell (WBC) precursors. Granulocytes, a type of WBC, initially form in the:

    a. bloodstream.

    b. bone marrow.

    c. organs.

    d. RBCs.

**35.** A leukemia patient may receive a bone marrow transplant to spare his marrow from the toxic effects of radiation or chemotherapy. The basis for determining whether donor marrow is compatible with the patient's marrow is:

    a. blood typing.

    b. genetic compatibility testing.

    c. human leukocyte antigen (HLA) testing.

    d. sex.

**36.** Aplastic anemia results from injury to or destruction of stem cells in the bone marrow, causing pancytopenia. Which category of drugs has *not* been implicated in causing aplastic anemia?

    a. Antibiotics

    b. Antineoplastics

    c. Anticonvulsants

    d. Antiarrhythmics

**37.** Which of the following is *not* a direct complication of HIV infection?

    a. AIDS dementia complex

    b. Hemorrhage

    c. Opportunistic infections

    d. Wasting syndrome

# Answers and rationales

**1. d.** Oliguria (urine output below 500 ml/day) is a classic sign of acute renal failure. BUN levels increase in acute renal failure because of retention of waste products. Acute renal failure is characterized by hypotension, not hypertension, and doesn't cause a rise in temperature.

**2. b.** Acute tubular necrosis is the most common cause of acute renal failure. Renal artery spasms don't play a role in acute renal failure. Sodium and water intoxication don't occur in acute renal failure because the patient can't conserve sodium or water.

**3. b.** The serum potassium level of 7 mEq/liter is the most serious finding because hyperkalemia is the most life-threatening sign of acute renal failure.

**4. a.** Cardiac standstill could be caused by the patient's markedly elevated serum potassium level. Acute renal failure doesn't cause constipation or tetany.

**5. d.** Reactive hypoglycemia can result from alimentary hyperinsulinism caused by dumping syndrome. Patients who've had gastric surgery may develop this form of hypoglycemia because the rapid gastric emptying that accompanies these disorders causes rapid glucose absorption and excessive insulin release. Hepatic disease, insulinoma, and excessive alcohol ingestion are not causes of reactive hypoglycemia.

**6. b.** The patient with reactive hypoglycemia must modify her diet to delay glucose absorption and gastric emptying. This means avoiding simple carbohydrates and eating small, frequent meals that are high in protein and fiber.

**7. b.** DKA most often occurs in patients with Type I diabetes, which typically presents with rapidly developing symptoms, as in Joey's case. HNKS occurs in patients with Type II diabetes, in which symptoms are mild and develop gradually.

**8. c.** A jet-injection device delivers insulin to subcutaneous tissue without using a needle. Other devices require needles.

**9. d.** When an insulin-dependent diabetic patient becomes sick, he must still take insulin but must notify the doctor first in case his dosage should be adjusted.

**10. d.** Although the patient should be assessed for potential thoracic, abdominal, and pelvic bleeding, the femur fracture the probable source of blood loss. Up to 3 liters can be lost into the thigh around a fracture site and, despite this patient early repair, fluid replacement may not have been adequate.

**11. a.** In a patient with a recent history of a long-bone fracture (especially of the femur), these findings should lead you to suspect fat embolism syndrome.

**12. c.** A petechial rash of the chest, axillae, and conjunctivae occurs in about 50% of patients with fat embolism syndrom It usually disappears within a few hours of onset.

**13. b.** Checking oxygen saturation values and providing supplemental oxygen as needed are the most appropriate emergency measures to combat fat embolism syndrome. In fat embolism syndrome, the embolized fat globules are filtered and trapped in the lungs, where they set off a chain of chemcal reactions that can cause severe respiratory compromise (including adult respiratory distress syndrome).

**14. c.** Before surgery, morphine sulfate wouldn't be given to a patient with a respiratory condition because it can cause respiratory depression. Bronchodilators, antibiotics, and chest physiotherapy might be ordered for this patient.

**15. a.** Anticoagulants, such as heparin and warfarin, aren't given preoperatively because they prevent blood from clotting and could cause hemorrhage in the surgical patient. Drugs may be given to reduce anxiety, decrease discomfort, and pro tect the airway during surgery.

**16. b.** Pain doesn't arise from subcutaneous tissue. Sources pain include cutaneous tissue, visceral organ tissue, and deep somatic tissue.

**17. d.** Aspirin, ibuprofen, and naproxen are all NSAIDs.

**18. a.** You should be honest and sincere with a dying patien If you're silent, fearing you'll say the wrong thing, the patien may sense your discomfort and become alienated. Although listening is important, it's not enough. You should ask questions that will encourage the patient to share his thoughts and feelings about being seriously ill. Crying with him in a controlled manner is acceptable in appropriate situations, bu avoid sobbing in front of him or his family.

**19. d.** Some studies show that the triple regimen of a calci channel blocker, a nitrate, and a beta blocker is the most be eficial treatment for unstable angina. Thrombolytics, antiplatelets, and anticoagulants are crucial in managing unstable angina, but they must be used in conjunction with a calcium channel blocker, a nitrate, and a beta blocker.

**20. d.** Congestive heart failure may be caused by pulmonary embolism, infections, anemia, thyrotoxicosis, pregnancy, arrhythmias, myocarditis, infective endocarditis, systemic hypertension, and physical and emotional distress.

**21. c.** Mitral stenosis is usually caused by rheumatic fever. The latency period from the time of rheumatic fever to the onset of clinical symptoms of mitral stenosis can range from 10 to 40 years.

**22. d.** Infection doesn't predispose a patient to arterial occlusive disease. Besides those mentioned, risk factors include hypertension, aging, diabetes, a family history of vascular disorders, and CVA.

**23. a.** Cor pulmonale causes tachycardia, not bradycardia. All the other findings may be present.

**24. d.** Primary or idiopathic pulmonary hypertension is characterized by a resting PASP above 30 mm Hg, a mean PAP above 18 mm Hg, and increased pulmonary vascular resistance, without obvious causes. Secondary pulmonary hypertension results from existing cardiac or pulmonary disease or both.

**25. a.** Along with terbutaline, albuterol is the most potent bronchodilator and causes the fewest adverse reactions.

**26. d.** All of these factors may increase a patient's risk of developing pneumonia. Other predisposing factors include cancer, abdominal and thoracic surgery, atelectasis, common cold, chronic respiratory disease, influenza, malnutrition, alcoholism, sickle cell disease, tracheostomy, exposure to noxious gases, aspiration, and immunosuppressive therapy.

**27. a.** A thrombus, which results from atherosclerosis, is the most common cause of CVA. Embolism and hemorrhage are less common causes, and tumors rarely cause a CVA.

**28. b.** A perfusion scan is the only study that's usually not done to diagnose a CVA. MRI scans, CT scans, and cerebral arteriography can confirm the diagnosis and reveal important information about how the CVA might affect the patient.

**29. c.** A CT scan is the most useful tool in diagnosing Alzheimer's disease because it shows the frontal lobe atrophy characteristic of the disease.

**30. c.** Pancreatitis is an inflammatory disease leading to pancreatic edema and obstruction of the pancreatic ducts. It's not an autoimmune or genetic disease, and it's not related to the hepatitis B virus.

**31. d.** A dramatically elevated serum amylase level confirms pancreatitis and rules out perforated ulcer, acute cholecystitis, appendicitis, and bowel infarction. Serum glucose levels usually also rise in pancreatitis, but this finding isn't as characteristic. Elevated serum lipid and creatinine levels aren't diagnostic indicators of pancreatitis.

**32. c.** The continent ileostomy pouch normally is drained with a catheter. It doesn't require daily irrigations. Instructions on frequent perianal skin care aren't needed because the stoma is on the abdomen. The stoma is irrigated with 30 ml, not 500 ml, of 0.9% sodium chloride solution — and only if the drainage tube becomes clogged. This patient shouldn't eat high-fiber foods because they might aggravate his condition.

**33. c.** Peritonitis may be a nonmechanical cause of intestinal obstruction. Hernia, adhesions, neoplasms, stenosis, intussusception, volvulus, and foreign bodies are forms of mechanical obstruction.

**34. b.** Granulocytes initially form in the bone marrow. WBCs are released into, not produced in, the bloodstream. RBCs and WBCs form separately.

**35. c.** HLA testing is the main method of determining bone marrow compatibility. Genetic compatibility testing is done but isn't the major focus. Sex and blood typing aren't the main concerns regarding compatibility.

**36. d.** Antiarrhythmics don't cause acquired aplastic anemia. Drugs implicated in this disease include antibiotics, antineoplastics, anticonvulsants, anti-inflammatory drugs, antidiabetic drugs, antithyroid agents, antimalarial drugs, and zidovudine.

**37. b.** Hemorrhage isn't a direct complication of HIV infection. Direct complications include AIDS dementia complex, opportunistic infections, wasting syndrome, subcortical dementia, and secondary cancers (such as Kaposi's sarcoma, non-Hodgkin's lymphoma, and other lymphomas).

# Index

i refers to illustration; t refers to a table